WORKING WITH OLDER PEOPLE

Denise Tanner and John Harris

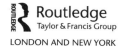
Routledge
Taylor & Francis Group

LONDON AND NEW YORK

communitycare

9007777703

First published 2008 by Routledge
2 Park Square, Milton Park, Abingdon, Oxon OX14 4RN

Simultaneously published in the USA and Canada
by Routledge
270 Madison Ave, New York, NY 10016

Routledge is an imprint of the Taylor & Francis Group, an informa business

© 2008 Denise Tanner and John Harris

Typeset in Sabon
by Keystroke, 28 High Street, Tettenhall, Wolverhampton
Printed and bound in Great Britain
by TJ International Ltd, Padstow, Cornwall

British Library Cataloguing in Publication Data
A catalogue record for this book is available from the British Library

Library of Congress Cataloging in Publication Data
Tanner, Denise, 1960–
Working with older people / Denise Tanner and John Harris.
p. cm. — (Social work skills series)
Includes bibliographical references and index.
ISBN 0–415–35421–8 (pbk.) — ISBN 0–415–35420–X (hardback)
1. Social work with older people.
2. Older people. I. Harris, John, 1952– II. Title.
HV1451.T36 2007
362.6—dc22
2007004046

ISBN10: 0–415–35420–X (hbk)
ISBN10: 0–415–35421–8 (pbk)
ISBN10: 0–203–00090–0 (ebk)

ISBN13: 978–0–415–35420–2 (hbk)
ISBN13: 978–0–415–35421–9 (pbk)
ISBN13: 978–0–203–00090–8 (ebk)

WORKING WITH OLDER PEOPLE

...ant part of social work
...adult services, human
...tions, this book will be

...vledge, skills and values
...alifying award in Social

...e

...his key text facilitates
...s for each chapter, case
...ctivities throughout the
book and the final chapter contains pointers to consider for all of the activities. It will
be essential reading for social work students and qualified social workers.

Denise Tanner is an Associate Professor in Social Work in the School of Health and
Social Studies, University of Warwick, UK.

John Harris is a Professor in the School of Health and Social Studies, University of
Warwick, UK.

the social work skills series

published in association with *Community Care*

series editor: Terry Philpot

the social work skills series

- builds practice skills step by step
- places practice in its policy context
- relates practice to relevant research
- provides a secure base for professional development

This new, skills-based series has been developed by Routledge and *Community Care* working together in partnership to meet the changing needs of today's students and practitioners in the broad field of social care. Written by experienced practitioners and teachers with a commitment to passing on their knowledge to the next generation, each text in the series features: *learning objectives; case examples; activities to test knowledge and understanding; summaries of key learning points; key references; suggestions for further reading.*

Also available in the series:

Commissioning and Purchasing
Terry Bamford
Former Chair of the British Association of Social Workers and Executive Director of Housing and Social Services, Royal Borough of Kensington and Chelsea.

Managing Aggression
Ray Braithwaite
Consultant and trainer in managing aggression at work. Lead trainer and speaker in the 'No Fear' campaign.

Tackling Social Exclusion
John Pierson
Senior Lecturer at the Institute of Social Work and Applied Social Studies at the University of Staffordshire.

Safeguarding Children and Young People
Corinne May-Chahal and Stella Coleman
Professor of Applied Social Science at Lancaster University.
Senior Lecturer in Social Work at the University of Central Lancashire.

The Task-Centred Book
Mark Doel and Peter Marsh
Research Professor of Social Work at Sheffield Hallam University.
Professor of Child and Family Welfare, University of Sheffield.

Using Groupwork
Mark Doel
Research Professor of Social Work at Sheffield Hallam University.

Practising Welfare Rights
Neil Bateman
Author, trainer and consultant specialising in welfare rights and social policy issues.

CONTENTS

FIGURES AND TABLES

FIGURES

TABLES

BOXES

ACTIVITIES

ACKNOWLEDGEMENTS

The authors would like to thank the following for permission to reproduce copyright material:

Jessica Kingsley Publishers for Littlechild, R. and Blakeney, J. (1996) 'Risk and older people', in H. Kemshall and J. Pritchard (eds) *Good Practice in Risk Assessment and Risk Management*; and Craig, C. (2004) 'Reaching out with the arts: meeting with the person with dementia', in A. Innes, C. Archibald and C. Murphy (eds) *Dementia and Social Inclusion: Marginalised Groups and Marginalised Areas of Dementia Research, Care and Practice*.

Community Care for Simey, M. (2002) 'I want something to do', *Community Care* 24–30 October: 20.

INTRODUCTION

Social work with older people is sometimes seen as epitomising what is wrong with current social work more generally, namely responses to needs that evoke Lipsky's telling reference to 'people processing' (1980: xvi). We meet social workers and social work students who feel that working with older people has turned them into just such people-processors. They are frustrated by the bureaucratic and instrumental nature of much of the work they undertake with older people, or rather, as it so often seems, on behalf of older people, as a common complaint is the amount of time they have to spend sitting at a computer keyboard, tapping in information required by care management software, in order to ensure that older people receive 'care packages' on the basis of their assessments. In contrast to Lipsky's description of people at the front line of public services as 'street-level bureaucrats' with considerable day-to-day discretion, these social workers feel that they have become 'screen-level bureaucrats' (Bovens and Zouridis 2002), working within the narrow constraints imposed by eligibility criteria and anchored to their workstations for many hours at a time. Working with older people can, then, appear to be at the cutting edge of the 'McDonaldization' (Ritzer 2000) of social work, shaped by its principles of efficiency, predictability, calculability and control by non-human technology. In this vein, Lloyd provides a roll call of the strands in contemporary social work with older people that can have a negative impact on access to services and may result in organisational perspectives dominating assessments of and responses to needs:

- the inadequacy of resources and restrictions on their use;
- contradictions in the policy framework within which practice is located;
- insecurity associated with the privatisation and marketisation of services;
- the development of care management;
- the standardisation of practice and the imposition of procedural rules.

(Lloyd, L. 2006a: 1172)

However, this is only part, albeit a major part, of the story. Consider this account of someone's experience of social work, as relayed to us:

My 87-year-old father collapsed in the street and was admitted to hospital. After a few weeks, he was offered an operation to replace his aortic valve. The consultant explained to my father and the family the risks involved and the possible outcomes. My father decided to take up the offer. The operation was successful although, as he was warned, 'it made him very poorly'. After the operation, the doctors, nurses and therapists sought to aid my father's recovery through their different fields of specialist expertise and they recorded their activity and opinions in the patient's notes. To the family it seemed that their inputs to my father's care were quite fragmented, with the specialists sometimes making little reference to one another's opinions and conclusions. It was different with the hospital social worker; she sought to treat my father as a whole person. She spent time talking and listening; coaxing his feelings from him during the recovery process and helping him to express his hopes, fears and wishes for the future. The social worker then liaised with the other professionals and coordinated the timing of his discharge, bringing together a recovery plan and a workable care package. The social worker was my father's advocate and always treated him with respect. She was available to the family when we had concerns and questions. It was very reassuring, both for my father and the family, to have the social worker as an essential and dependable point of reference during what was a distressing, stressful and emotional time.

(Jones, J. 2006)

John Jones' experience of being on the receiving end of social work was a positive one, suggesting that the social worker had salvaged the possibility of good practice, despite being in the midst of the difficult conditions described by Lloyd. This reflects the spirit in which this book has been written. Our stance is to confront head-on the issues, tensions, dilemmas and contradictions that social workers and social work students experience every day, as they go about their work with older people, located within what often seems like a whirlwind of policy change and a plethora of restrictions. However, as we face these problems, we do not give up on the possibility of achieving worthwhile outcomes in the current context by seeking to achieve good practice in working with older people.

For us, the starting point for good practice is taking seriously the experiences, perceptions and perspectives of older people themselves and this is where Chapter 1 begins, before moving on to the ways in which 'old age' is constructed socially, culturally and economically. The impact of ageism on policy, practices, attitudes and behaviours is explored, together with ageism's interaction with other forms of difference, diversity and inequality. This exploration suggests that the social category of 'older people' is highly diverse, even more so because whilst there may be certain shared themes between some older people, influenced by wider structural factors and age-cohort experiences, each situation is also unique, affected by individual personalities, life course experiences and individual subjectivities. In order to respond effectively to this diversity of experiences, social workers need to draw critically on a wide range of theories, building their understanding in each situation and incorporating the 'theories' of older people themselves.

The historical context has shaped current practice with older people and Chapter 2 shows that policy concerning social services for older people was not a central consideration in the post-war Welfare State. In contrast, the community care reforms of the early 1990s are seen as having been of lasting significance for social work with older people through their introduction of an enduring system of assessment and care management. More recent policy initiatives[1] within that system, under New Labour, are reviewed in the light of their central political concern with resources and in terms of whether and, if so, how they might contribute to improving the well-being of older people.

Chapter 3 focuses on assessing the needs of older people and examines the use of the law in doing so. It quickly becomes apparent that there is no coherent legal framework underpinning social work with older people but a complex myriad of different pieces of legislation, dating back to 1948. It is important for social workers to grapple with the practice issues raised by the complexities of the legal framework for assessment and to be aware of the impact of relevant policy, in particular, the *Single Assessment Process* and *Fair Access to Care Services*. Two points of tension emerge: needs-led versus service-led assessment and the nature and extent of unmet need. Within these tensions, good practice indicates that assessment should focus on promoting individuals' well-being. This seems to be reflected in recent policy relating to older people, notwithstanding conflicts within policy and contradictions at the level of practice.

The stages in care management that follow assessment are planning, implementing and reviewing services, which are the subject of Chapter 4. The legal and policy framework relevant to the provision of community care services, both non-residential and residential, is provided, together with the arrangements for regulating care provision. In the current context, the changing nature of the 'care market' is seen as having important implications for older people. A key trend that runs through planning, implementing and reviewing services is that, despite the emphasis in policy on promoting well-being, in practice services remain targeted on those with high levels of need.

The relationship between social work skills and particular methods and approaches, including care management, are considered in Chapter 5 and the potential of the exchange model is set out. Whilst acknowledging the obstacles an exchange approach encounters in practice, social workers are encouraged to work within and around the constraints raised by such barriers. In doing so, social work with older people is seen as requiring a range of skills within a 'person-centred' and 'holistic' framework, which requires social workers to recognise and respond to the 'whole' person within the context of her/his 'whole' social system, rooted in an appreciation of older people's biographies. The ways in which information is recorded and shared with older people, often regarded as simply a 'technical' aspect of practice, is seen as influencing the way in which older people are regarded within the social work process.

A current buzzword, 'partnership', is the focus of Chapter 6, which unpicks the nature of effective partnership working in planning and delivering services for older people. Key issues are identified in the relationship between social work and health services and the often-neglected area of housing support for older people is highlighted. The increasingly significant role of the voluntary sector in providing services for older people is noted and the legal framework for working with carers is outlined, with the stress placed on how the legal provisions can be used to meet the needs of carers, including older carers. A central theme is that partnership is an increasingly significant aspect of policy. It faces a number of barriers to its implementation but there are principles that can form the basis for effective partnership, given the right conditions.

In Chapter 7, we assert the centrality of values in social work with older people but emphasise that realising values-based practice is often complex and contradictory as social workers encounter a range of value conflicts, for example, those raised by dilemmas in dealing with risk versus protection or when faced with the differing needs and perspectives of service users and carers. The importance of working with different and conflicting perspectives is stressed, with social workers being encouraged to think critically about the nature and level at which they involve older people and seeking to maximise their involvement wherever possible.

Activities are provided in each of the chapters. These are designed for use either by individual readers or as the basis for exercises in group learning. In Chapter 8 we have provided pointers to the issues raised by these activities. We wish to stress that these pointers are not 'answers'. They are simply our suggestions for you to think about. Your thinking may well raise issues that we have not considered.

Finally, we hope that you will engage with this book in the spirit in which it is offered in three senses. First, that you will be committed to seeking to understand the contexts and circumstances in which social work with older people is located. Second, notwithstanding the constraints and problems you encounter, that you will look for the possibilities for good practice. Third, that you will join in the debate about social work with older people. We have used the writing of the book to try and think of ways through some of the tensions, dilemmas and contradictions of current social work with older people but none of what we say is an attempt to come up with the definitive last word on any issue or topic; we wish to provoke debate, not to curtail it. We hope that you will be committed to taking that debate further and that, by so doing, you will make your own contribution to advancing good practice in social work with older people.

CHAPTER 1

UNDERSTANDING LATER LIFE

OBJECTIVES

By the end of this chapter you should have an understanding of:

- older people's experiences and perceptions of later life;

- ageism and anti-ageist practice;

- issues of difference, diversity and inequality;

- the critical use of theory to inform practice;

- the importance of drawing on a range of theoretical perspectives.

This chapter's consideration of the nature and experiences of later life is intended to help you prepare for working with older people. It begins by exploring later life from the perspective of the experiences of older people and moves on to stressing the need for anti-ageist perspectives to permeate practice, highlighting issues of difference and diversity in older age. The chapter argues that whilst it is vital to anchor our practice in the ways that older people understand their situations, we also need to be familiar with wider theoretical perspectives. The diversity of service users' needs and values and the complexity of social situations that social workers encounter require us to be able to draw on a range of theories. The chapter aims to help us to adopt a critical approach towards theories and to use them creatively in making sense of situations.

SERVICE USER INVOLVEMENT

We want to begin with the experiences and perspectives of older people themselves. The rationale for doing this can be found within the wider movement for service user involvement. Service user involvement is a central theme in the planning and delivery of health and social care services and in the provision of social work education. Strong mandates for service user involvement emanate from social policy and legislation, the professional value base of social work and service user movements (Braye 2000). The key thrust of the service user involvement agenda is that service users are experts by virtue of their experience and that, for too long, this expertise has been ignored, marginalised or colonised by others (Beresford and Croft 2001; Beresford 2003). As far as older people are concerned, despite the prevalence in policy and practice of concepts such as empowerment and participation, and some engagement with the voices of older people themselves (see, for example, Barnes and Bennett 1998; Harris, John 2001), ageism remains widespread in institutions, professional practice and the experiences of older people (Nolan 2000). In research, too, there has been a tendency to pathologise and marginalise older people. Their perspectives and voices have frequently been missing within academic and policy literature (Hey 1999), although there have been attempts at redressing their absence (see, for example, older people acting as research advisers in Tozer and Thornton 1995). The importance of narrowing the gap between knowledge and experience has been increasingly recognised because 'the greater the distance between direct experience and its interpretation, then the more likely the resulting knowledge is to be inaccurate, unreliable and distorted' (Beresford 2003: 22). Beresford puts forward a number of principles aimed at taking forward service user involvement, based on improving our understanding of other people's experience:

- listening to what people say;
- seeking to develop empathy with the perspectives and situations of others;
- working to be open-minded and non-judgemental and challenging discrimination in ourselves and other people;
- recognising what we do and don't 'know';
- valuing people's direct experience;
- accepting the possibility that there are knowledges different from our own;
- being prepared to accept something we may not fully understand instead of rejecting it without consideration;
- being willing to move out to people, meet people on their own territory and see how things are for them;
- acting upon knowledge that is based on direct experience – not just saying that we accept that this is how it is for someone else, but also being prepared to work with them to change it (active knowledge);
- involving people with direct experience (for example, service users) in the development and provision of professional education and training;
- valuing the direct experience of service users in health and social care and encouraging the recruitment of service users as workers;
- increasing access to research training for people with direct experience and supporting their involvement in research so that they can influence the process of knowledge production.

(Beresford 2003: 55–6)

These principles reflect widespread recognition of the different kinds of knowledge and understanding that service users can contribute and that must be incorporated, alongside other sources and types of knowledge, at all levels in social work and social care services (Pawson *et al.* 2003). In planning the reform of social work education, the General Social Care Council set up a series of service user focus groups. The first theme identified by the groups was the need for social workers to understand the experiences and perspectives of service users. The second was the importance of social workers having effective skills in communicating and helping (Department of Health 2002a). We now turn to that first key theme in seeking to understand the experiences and perspectives of older people. (The second key theme – the skills required for working effectively with older people – will be considered in Chapter 5.)

OLDER PEOPLE'S EXPERIENCES AND PERCEPTIONS OF LATER LIFE

ACTIVITY 1.1: WHAT IS IT LIKE TO BE 'AN OLDER PERSON'?

Drawing on a range of perceptions and experiences of older people themselves, try to build up a picture of what it is like to be 'an older person' by carrying out one or more of the following:

- Read first hand accounts written by older people, for example autobiographical material, magazine articles, poetry. (One example can be found in Box 1.1, page 8.)
- Read qualitative research accounts that include quotations from older people about their perceptions and experiences.
- Listen to television or radio interviews or documentaries that feature older people giving accounts of their lives.
- Browse older people's websites (for example, www.hellsgeriatrics.co.uk).
- Have informal talks with older friends, relatives or neighbours.
- Talk to older people at a local residential or day centre or at a social club for older people. (You will need to explain the purpose and ensure that they are happy to talk to you.)

(*Remember*: people you are defining as 'older people' may not see themselves in this way.)

Make notes on some of the following:

- How do older people define 'being old'? Do they perceive themselves as old? Why/why not?
- What is it like to be 'old'? What are some of the difficulties encountered? What strategies are used to deal with these difficulties?
- What do older people enjoy about being older? What gives life meaning and value?

- How do they view their situations now compared with the past? In what ways are their lives the same/different?
- Have their relationships with their families, friends and communities changed over time? If so, in what ways? How do they feel about these changes?
- What services do older people value? What outcomes and processes do they want to see?
- If they need assistance, now or in the future, who would they prefer to provide this and what things are important to them about how this is provided?
- How does their experience of later life compare with what they thought it would be like?
- What hopes or concerns do older people have about their future?
- If they had a magic wand, what changes would they make to improve their lives?

BOX 1.1   I WANT SOMETHING TO DO

MARGARET SIMEY

I grew up in the tradition that working life ended for women at 60 and for men at 65. Then followed a few years when older people were entitled to rest after their labours until terminal decrepitude finally released them from this weary world. It is on this assumption that the provision of care for older people is apparently still based.

There is no recognition of the fact that instead of dying off before we reach our mid-70s, it is much more likely that many of us will live until we are 90 or even 100. The implications of this for housing, pensions, welfare and family life are simply ignored. There is a gap, a black hole, in our concept of community care.

At first, retirement is for many a happy release from regular employment – an opportunity to travel, take up voluntary work or go fishing. But inevitably, for all of us decrepitude relentlessly overtakes us. In my own case it came with an abruptness that was shocking. I had led a happy life as a voluntary worker and councillor until my 90s. I tripped on a paving stone and my subsequent state of dependency brought home to me the startling realisation that I had fallen into the gap.

Unable to bathe myself, I applied to the ever-helpful social services for assistance only to be told that there was a two-year waiting list for domiciliary care because the funds for that service had been spent. I had outlived the available resources. What an experience this life in the gap is proving to be. Social services has organised transport to take me to a day centre for a weekly bath.

A plethora of caring services are offered to me, for which I am deeply grateful. Yet I remain dissatisfied, hungry for something, I know not what. Despairing sociologists beg me and my kind to tell them what we need or want. Struggling to articulate what it is that I hanker after, I have come to realise that my trouble is that all this concern focuses on my physical needs. The well-being of me, Margaret, is nobody's business.

What, then, do I want? It is assumed that I must be lonely and that being lonely means a lack of company. In fact I am fortunate in having so many visitors that my son proposes to stick a notice on my door saying: 'Do not disturb. Keep out'.

Peel away the assumptions and what is left is, in fact, a deep sense of exclusion. I don't belong. I am not one of 'them'. I have no role, no place in our community. 'They' come to do 'good' to me. My relationship with 'them' is all get and no give, a sad and demeaning experience.

The clue to the problem of the exclusion of older people lies in the relationship between those who run the services and those who are supposed to benefit from them. Older people must be emancipated from their present state of helpless dependency. They must be allowed their fair share of responsibility for their own well-being and that of the community to which they belong. Here is the last cause I mean to fight.

(A 'This Life' feature, published in *Community Care*, 24–30 October 2002: 20. Margaret Simey, a notable Liverpool politician, died in July 2004, aged 98.)

One area worthy of reflection is how you defined whom you would regard as 'an older person' for the purposes of Activity 1.1. It may be that you used chronological age or perhaps you referred to signs of physical ageing or took account of someone's health, abilities and/or behaviour. You may also have considered subjective perceptions; whether or not people see themselves as old. If chronological age is used to define someone as 'an older person', it is important to remember that a wide age range can be encompassed. For example, defining the threshold of old age at 65 means that the category of 'older people' may span three or four decades. To deal with this, some studies distinguish the 'older old', for example, those aged over 75 or 80, suggesting that particular social and psychological processes may characterise this phase of later life (Johnson, C. and Barer 1997) but even amongst the 'older old', chronological age may indicate very little beyond being a process of general social categorisation. In response to the problems of defining an 'older person' simply in relation to the numbers of years lived, it is tempting to regard biological ageing as an alternative starting point for defining old age and to see this as more 'objective' and 'scientific'. However, the rate of biological ageing is influenced by social and economic conditions. For example, a study of minority ethnic older people across Europe noted premature ageing and poorer health amongst certain minority ethnic groups despite their, in some cases, younger chronological age (Policy Research Institute on Ageing and Ethnicity 2004). This finding illustrates how dimensions of inequality encountered at earlier stages in the life course can impact on biological processes and the lived experience of later life. Notwithstanding the limitations involved, research studies involving older people usually adopt a chronological definition of old age (for example, selecting samples of people who are over the age of 60 or 65).

Research that has sought to uncover older people's views and experiences has identified important themes common to many older people but has also highlighted key aspects of diversity within the category of those defined as 'older people'. In relation to common themes, Thompson *et al.* (1990) explored the life stories of people aged 60 to 80 who were grandparents. This study found that regardless of chronological age, physical signs of ageing or health status, participants did not perceive themselves as 'old'. Nor did their lives fit stereotypical views of old age. Rather, the authors noted, 'their lives are characterised by variety, vitality, diversity, activity, energy, interest; by "youthfulness" in attitude, outlook and activity (including paid employment), regardless of their age' (Thompson *et al.* 1990: 121).

It was crucial to these older people's sense of well-being that life had a meaningful purpose. Lack of material resources and hostile public attitudes were experienced as barriers to their being able to pursue opportunities to make life meaningful. (As the sample for this research was people who were grandparents, it is likely that the more isolated older people without family support networks were excluded.) Similar themes were identified in a study by Langan *et al.* (1996), which was based on interviews with 39 older people. Activities and social relationships outside of the home and maintaining the structure of everyday routines were highly valued by older people, with home seen as an important place of privacy, independence and autonomy. A much larger scale study, using a national survey and semi-structured follow-up interviews with 999 older people, found that older people defined quality of life in terms of: positive relationships with their family, friends and neighbours; having a good home and neighbourhood; having a positive outlook on life; having activities and hobbies; being in good health; having meaningful roles and activities; enjoying an adequate income; and feeling independent and in control of their lives (Gabriel and Bowling 2004). The themes of autonomy and being in control also emerged strongly in a study based on in-depth interviews, focus groups and participant observation with older people. Here, it was not so much independence, but interdependence that was central to older people's sense of well-being:

> Success in managing the changes that accompanied ageing . . . was in large part determined by the extent to which people were able to maintain inter-dependent lives: being able to view themselves as both givers and receivers of emotional, social and practical support.
>
> (Godfrey *et al.* 2004: 213)

This section has focused on some *common themes* in older people's experiences and perspectives. Dimensions of difference and diversity will be considered later in the chapter.

ACTIVITY 1.2: COMPARING EXPERIENCES

Compare your findings from Activity 1.1 with the research findings outlined in the paragraphs above. From what you have learned about older people's experiences and perceptions of later life (in your work for Activity 1.1 and through the research findings above), identify five key messages for social work policy and/or practice.

It has become apparent that older people's experiences of later life and younger people's perceptions of older people are shaped by a range of processes and influences. These are interwoven with ageism, which acts as a decisive constraining factor, impacting on how later life is perceived and experienced.

AGEISM

Butler defined ageism as 'a process of systematic stereotyping of, and discrimination against, people because they are old, just as racism and sexism accomplish this for skin colour and gender' (1987: 22).[1] Bytheway argues that ageism is not simply located within individual attitudes and behaviour but is an ideology that legitimates inequalities based on age, leading to the exclusion and 'othering' of older people. He sets out a working definition of ageism:

1   Ageism is a set of beliefs originating in the biological variation between people and relating to the ageing process.
2   It is in the actions of corporate bodies, what is said and done by their representatives, and the resulting views that are held by ordinary ageing people, that ageism is made manifest.

In consequence of this it follows that:

(a) Ageism generates and reinforces a fear and denigration of the ageing process, and stereotyping presumptions regarding competence and the need for protection.
(b) In particular, ageism legitimates the use of chronological age to mark out classes of people who are systematically denied resources and opportunities that others enjoy, and who suffer the consequences of such denigration ranging from well-meaning patronage to unambiguous vilification.

(Bytheway 1995: 14)

Bytheway argues that we need to understand people within the context of the whole of the life course, rather than using older age as a defining category and marking it out as somehow different and distinct. However, in service delivery the latter approach is often used with services organised according to age-based categorisations, such as 'Older People's Teams'. At the same time, services are rarely provided on the basis of older age alone but in circumstances where it is accompanied by, for example, disability, ill health or mental distress. These difficulties may be related to ageing or they may be a continuation of problems from earlier in the life course. It is often the case that people with longstanding physical impairments or learning disabilities are transferred from specialist disability teams to 'Older People's Teams' when they reach the age of 65. The implication is that age becomes the dominant defining identity, subsuming other more specific needs, difficulties and requirements. As a consequence, particular needs, such as those associated with learning disabilities (discussed further later in the chapter), may be overlooked.

These specific examples of ageism occur in a wider context. Hughes (1995 – see Figure 1.1) shows how ageism stems from the social construction of ageing through the combination of a range of factors and highlights its manifestations in the areas of policy, personal values and the experiences of older people.

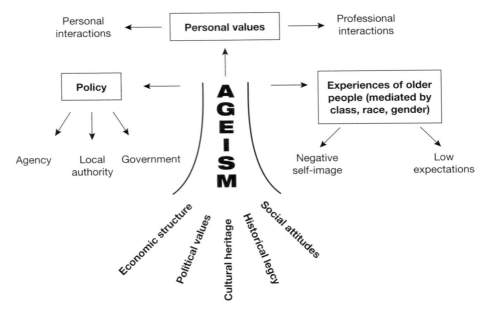

FIGURE 1.1 Ageism
Source: Adapted from Hughes 1995: 43

ACTIVITY 1.3: THE SOCIAL CONSTRUCTION OF AGEISM

Write down one example of how ageism is constructed by each of the following systems/processes:

- economic structures;
- political values;
- cultural heritage;
- historical legacy;
- social attitudes.

A report by Age Concern (2006a) found that ageism is pervasive and is the most prevalent form of discrimination. Given the endemic nature of ageism in western societies, it is all too easy to assume that ageism is a universal phenomenon, but this is not the case. In some cultures, old age does not imply a devalued status. It may give enhanced status or may not be a significant source of status at all. Wilson (2000) refers to the importance in some cultures of life stages, rather than age, in determining status. For example, for adult men in many African societies, seniority may be defined in relation to the accumulation of wealth and power, not by chronological age. In Hinduism, seniority is related to a phase of social withdrawal and religious contemplation; this life stage is reached when a son is able to assume responsibility for the family and there is only a tenuous connection between achievement of this life stage and chronological age. In such cultures, seniority may be seen as a desirable state, rather than one to be feared and resisted. Cross-cultural and historical perspectives are helpful in reinforcing our understanding of the ageist social construction of old age as the dominant discourse in western societies. Unfortunately, in that discourse, old age is socially constructed as a 'problem'. This social construction of old age confers a loss of status and a devalued identity on older people. It has consequences in terms of older people's self-perception, how they are perceived by others, their exclusion from some social activities and relationships and the approaches taken to policy and practice in health and social care services. Even when there is an awareness of ageism, this can fail to permeate actual practice. For example, Roberts *et al.* (2002) found that although managers in health and social care services understood ageism in abstract terms, they did not understand how it could be combated in day-to-day practice.

One facet of the ageist social construction of old age is the way in which age serves as a social division; it is the basis of unequal treatment in terms of policies and practices. For example, there is evidence that older people are treated less favourably on the basis of their age in access to health care (Roberts 2000) and in employment (see Box 1.2).

BOX 1.2   AGE DISCRIMINATION

It was not until October 2006 that age discrimination in employment became unlawful under *The Employment Equality (Age) Regulations* (2006) in England, Wales and Scotland (with similar regulations introduced in Northern Ireland at the same time). This legislation:

- makes it unlawful to discriminate against someone on the basis of her/his age in employment, education and training;
- more specifically, makes it unlawful to refuse to employ someone on the basis of age if s/he is under 65. Exceptions are where there is a genuine occupational requirement concerning age. People over 65 or within six months of their 65th birthday are not protected by this provision;
- creates a 'default' retirement age of 65 for both men and women. Retirement cannot be enforced before this age unless there is specific justification;
- gives people over 65 the right to pursue claims for unfair dismissal if this is believed to be on grounds related to their age;
- gives people a right to request to continue in employment after the age of 65. However, the employer does not have to comply with this request;
- gives people over 65 who are in employment entitlement to statutory redundancy pay;
- gives people over 65 who are in employment entitlement to statutory sick pay.

Evidence from the United States, which has had age discrimination legislation in place for around 30 years, suggests that this does result in increased employment rates of older workers but mainly due to them remaining longer in employment, rather than because more older workers

continued

are hired. However, whilst legislation in the United States reduced direct discrimination in employment practices, it had little impact in the short term on the attitudes of society or employers (Hornstein *et al.* 2001).

The UK Government's campaign, *Age Positive*, aims to promote the benefits to employers and individuals of a workforce that is diverse in terms of age, encouraging employers to adhere to standards contained in the *Code of Practice on Age Diversity in Employment*. However, age discrimination legislation only applies to discrimination in employment and training. While it is argued that ageism in the workplace is the most significant and damaging aspect of age discrimination (Age Positive 2005), changing demographic trends and the needs of the employment market are likely driving forces behind the focus on discrimination in employment. An ageing population has led to the need to consider mechanisms both to retain older workers in the labour market and reduce spending in terms of pensions (Phillipson 1998).

A number of factors contribute to such ageist aspects of the construction of later life. First, there are *economic* determinants. Older people are seen as unproductive and are accorded low status and value in capitalist societies (Corrigan and Leonard 1978; Phillipson 1982). As people relinquish employment roles, many lack alternative sources of power and status (Bytheway 1995). With increased participation by women in the labour force, this increasingly applies to older women, as well as men (Orme 2001). (However, some older people are able to draw on alternative sources of social status, for example social class, gender or religious or community roles.) As a consequence of compulsory retirement policies, low pensions and lack of financial power, older people have been ignored in societies dominated by consumerism (Bauman 2004). This is changing for some older people as their proportion in the population grows and widening income differentials carried over into retirement result in a larger segment of affluent older consumers. Second, there are *cultural* facets. In the dominant culture of western societies, youth is highly valued; in contrast, older age is associated with decline and decrepitude. To maintain a positive identity in a social climate hostile to older age, older people may have to distance themselves from ageist stereotypes by presenting a 'youthful' social façade (Hockey and James 1993; Biggs 1999). However, in the main older people's association with decline results in their being presented as a major problem for society. They are constructed culturally as constituting a 'demographic time-bomb' of dependent people for whom social and economic provision has to be made by the rest of society. This then serves to justify restricted pensions provision (Walker 1993). They are also presented as placing a 'burden of care' on families. This ignores the many ways in which older people are resources for, rather than consumers of, welfare (Phillipson *et al.* 2001; Godfrey *et al.* 2004). It increases attention to the support needs of carers but at the expense of the citizenship rights of older people themselves (Harris, John 2002). Third, there is an *interpersonal* dimension; we may put older people at a distance from ourselves and treat them as 'other' in order to protect ourselves from fears about our own ageing (Froggett 2002; Nelson 2005).

The ageing body

These economic, cultural and interpersonal dimensions of ageism are present in responses to physiological ageing. The changes in the body that ensue in older age are endowed with particular meanings, depending on the wider context in which they take place. In the dominant construction of ageing in western societies, physical changes are closely linked with a loss, or threatened loss, of independence and autonomy, which are highly valued. However, rather than the ageing body being connected directly with increasing dependency, Hockey and James (1993) highlight how dependency is created by particular social, economic, cultural, political and interpersonal processes. They compare the way in which dependency is created in children living in their family homes and in older people living in residential settings. They argue that older people are rendered dependent by being located within infantilisation as a powerful social discourse and that this process deprives them of full personhood by removing them from being regarded as adults: 'adults have a power and decision-making responsibility which is denied to children and elderly people' (ibid.: 37). We therefore have to think critically about how the experience of later life generally and the changes associated with physiological ageing specifically are constructed by particular societal contexts. In later work, Hockey and James (2003) argue that there is a triangular relationship between the ageing body, how the self is experienced and the society in which it is located: 'embodiment across the life course has to be understood in terms of an active self, inhabiting a body within particular social structures, producing and reproducing those structures as a set of particular cultural understandings of the ageing process' (ibid.: 214).

For social workers working with older people, this means understanding the meaning an older person gives to their experience of inhabiting an ageing body, what this represents in terms of their sense of self and how this is influenced by particular social and cultural values.

ACTIVITY 1.4: THE RELATIONSHIP BETWEEN BODY, SELF AND SOCIETY

Return to the article written by Margaret Simey (Box 1.1). How do the three components of the experience of an ageing body, a sense of self and social and cultural values interact in Margaret's description of her experience? If you were the social worker working with Margaret, how would this understanding of body, self and society inform your response to her?

Responses to ageism

We have noted the impact of ageism on the self-perception of older people, indicating that older people may internalise ageist attitudes, resulting in negative self-images and low expectations in terms of their role in society and what they can expect from services (Wilson 1995). However, research indicates that older people do not just absorb ageist attitudes passively but also find ways to challenge and manipulate meanings to reduce their disempowering effects. For example, one study explored the meanings, experiences and consequences of ageism for older people (Minichiello *et al.* 2000). Qualitative interviews were carried out with 18 older Australians and interviews were repeated with seven of them. Their perception of what 'being old' meant included loss, loneliness, being unimportant and irrelevant and having no role. They feared becoming a burden on their families as this was seen as indicating a loss of autonomy and independence. They felt that other people were 'keeping watch', monitoring their coping abilities for signs of 'oldness'. Two main strategies were used by the older people to manage ageism: accommodating ageism, for example accepting their situation and prevailing expectations ('not making waves'), and negotiating new images of ageing, adopting behaviours that prevented other people perceiving and treating them as old. Both strategies compound ageism: the first by accepting it and confirming ageist stereotypes; the second by indicating that a positive older age identity can only be achieved by distancing oneself from certain facets of becoming older (for example, an aged appearance). The researchers concluded that 'ageism is a complex phenomenon that is socially reproduced as a result of people internalising a denial of their own ageing because of ageist assumptions and associations in our language and culture which are played out in everyday situations' (Minichiello *et al.* 2000: 275). Nevertheless, seeking to negotiate new images of ageing can be seen as a form of resistance to ageism (Wilson 2001) and is not only the responsibility of older people themselves.

ACTIVITY 1.5: CHALLENGING AGEISM

It is part of a social worker's responsibility to challenge discriminatory behaviour (General Social Care Council 2002). How would you challenge the ageist attitudes reflected in the following comments?

- Old people don't make any contribution to society.
- Old people are a huge drain on taxpayers' money but are always moaning about how hard-up they are.
- 'As a GP, I'm very busy. There's no point me going to see Mrs S. just because she's a bit confused and forgetful. She's just getting old and there's no treatment for that.'
- Old people are a burden on their families.
- People change when they get old – their personalities change, they aren't interested in things and they just sit around all day. They're just waiting to die.
- 'Even though I'm 85 and struggling to manage, I'm not going to ask for help. I know there's not enough money to go round and I think it should go to helping children. I've had my life.'

Hughes (1995) outlines some values that she sees as fundamental to an anti-ageist perspective. From these values, she derives principles for anti-ageist practice. The values are:

- *personhood*: recognising the equal value and status of every individual;
- *citizenship*: recognising that every individual is an equally important member of society with rights and responsibilities;
- *celebration*: according value to old age as a life phase and celebrating diversity among older people.

The principles for anti-ageist practice that are taken from these values are:

- *empowerment*: enabling older people to control their own lives;
- *participation*: facilitating the meaningful involvement of older people;
- *choice*: facilitating older people's ability to make choices and decisions;
- *integration*: working to integrate older people into mainstream activities, rather than segregating them;
- *normalisation*: making available whatever is needed to enable older people to continue living their life as they want to.

(Hughes 1995: 45–7)

ACTIVITY 1.6: REFLECTING ON VALUES AND VALUE CONSTRAINTS

Think about the values and principles put forward by Hughes (1995). What difficulties or constraints might there be in implementing these values and principles in practice?

At the core of ageism is the 'essentialising' of older people; the assumption that everyone within the category of 'old age' is the same. If you used a range of sources in Activity 1.1, you will have probably noticed examples of difference and diversity within the experiences of those people whose perspectives you explored, an aspect of older age that we now consider in more detail.

DIFFERENCE, DIVERSITY AND INEQUALITY IN LATER LIFE

As we have seen, the category of 'older people' can easily lead to the ageist assumption that all older people are the same. However, in some cases those within the category of 'older people' will have a stronger sense of sharing key aspects of identity with people outside the category as much as, or more than, with those within it. For example, a Black or disabled identity may be more salient for a person's sense of self than being 'an older person'. As well as assuming sameness, social categories also tend to separate certain groups from others. This 'othering' process becomes problematic when certain categories of people are seen as different and a negative social evaluation is attached to them: 'The devaluing of difference is central to power relations of inequality and underpins the dynamics of oppression and the derogatory treatment of excluded persons' (Dominelli 2002: 41).

The more obvious differences are those arising from location within other social divisions such as disability, ethnicity, gender, sexuality and social class. Research with older people has begun to focus on some of these dimensions of diversity (see, for example, the collections edited by Arber and Ginn [1995] and Arber et al. [2003a] on gender and ageing). In relation to ethnicity, Nazroo et al. (2004) used quantitative and qualitative methods to explore the quality of life of older people from four ethnic groups (Jamaican Caribbean, Gujerati Indian Hindu, Punjabi Pakistani and white English). Minority ethnic older people were found to experience worse health and be at much greater risk of poverty than the white English group. Ethnic inequalities in both health and income increased considerably with advancing age and these in turn impaired people's ability to perform desired roles and activities. The disadvantages faced by the minority ethnic older people arose from their post-migration experiences of poor employment opportunities. On some dimensions – community, social and family networks – minority ethnic older people appeared to be in more favourable situations than the white group. This was also attributed to post-migration experiences through the building of ties in minority ethnic communities as a form of resistance to hostility and exclusion by the majority population.

Bigby (2004) focuses on the experiences of people ageing with lifelong disabilities, in particular learning disabilities. While the proportion of older people with learning disabilities is increasing, their overall number remains a small proportion of the total number of older people, creating a danger that their specific needs will be neglected. Older people with learning disabilities may have increased health needs, for example, people with Down's syndrome sometimes experience premature ageing and have a higher risk of Alzheimer's disease. However, Bigby argues that people with learning disabilities face reduced access to specialist disability services as they age. They are also likely to have restricted support networks and to experience high levels of disadvantage and discrimination. She points out that the voices of older people with learning disabilities remain largely silent in research. She argues that policies and programmes to promote successful ageing for older people with lifelong disabilities must be founded on the overarching principles of equal rights, citizenship, inclusion, participation, choice and self-determination.

Another dimension of difference and inequality is addressed by Langley (2001), who explores the concerns associated with ageing of 11 lesbian women and eight gay men between the ages of 51 and 68. The study notes the participants' concern with discrimination and the obstacles that historical oppression and social disapproval of same-sex relationships present in terms of older people feeling able to declare their sexuality. As a consequence, there is a danger of isolation for 'closeted' lesbian women and gay men as they age and experience the loss of partners, friends and/or mobility. Services that are insensitive to lesbian women and gay men may compound isolation rather than alleviate it. Interview respondents particularly feared residential care and the point is made that even if staff members are anti-oppressive in their practice, many residents may be homophobic. The study suggests that more specialist support services, including day and residential provision, are needed, as well as individual workers and agencies ensuring that they are sensitive to lesbian and gay cultures and lifestyles. One aspect of this sensitivity is highlighted by Connidis (2003). Unlike some other social divisions such as 'race', being gay or lesbian is not typically shared with other family members. This has two consequences: it often creates a unique standing in her/his family for the person who is lesbian or gay, and it affects relationships amongst other family members. Both of these dimensions need to be considered in relation to their impact on older people (ibid.: 83 and 91).

The studies we have considered briefly provide selected illustrative examples of areas of difference. There are many other aspects of diversity that interrelate with age that are likely to be significant for social workers working with older people. For example, social workers may work with: older people in prison; older people who are homeless; older people who have problems related to misuse of alcohol or drugs; older asylum seekers. For these older people, there will be areas of commonality with younger age groups in terms of how difficulties have arisen, are experienced and managed but there will also be differences associated with particular factors related to ageing. A further point about the potential for obscuring differences through using the label 'older people' is that identities are not static, as such fixed social categories imply, but fluid, being negotiated and renegotiated between people over time (Dominelli 2002). For example, in Margaret Simey's account (Box 1.1), it seems that what triggered a change in her self-perception, and the perception of her by others, was the disability that resulted from her fall. Despite a chronological age of 90, she did not feel or see herself as 'old' until this point.

We have already referred to 'differences' that reflect power relations of domination and oppression as 'divisions' (Williams 1996) and considered age as a social division that is cross-cut by other social divisions. As far as later life is concerned, the inequalities rooted in social divisions intersect in such a way that those who have been disadvantaged earlier in the life course are likely to experience a continuation or exacerbation of inequality in later life:

> The chances of having insufficient income in old age to ensure a healthy and socially integrated life are greatly affected by socio-demographic characteristics. The accumulated disadvantages over the life-course associated with socio-demographic variables such as gender, class, marital status and age leave certain sectors of the population much more vulnerable to income poverty in old age.
>
> (Price 2006: 261)

For example, the lower lifetime earnings of women compared with men contribute to their high rates of poverty in later life (Gough 2001), resulting in the income of women who have recently retired being only about half of that received by men in the same situation (Price 2006). It has been estimated that one in four single women pensioners lives in poverty and that in retirement twice as many women as men rely on means-tested benefits (Age Concern 2003). Women are less likely to belong to an occupational pension scheme, and when they do this is often worth on average less than a third of that received by men (Phillipson 1998). The 'oldest old' (the majority of whom are women) are especially vulnerable to poverty as improvements to pension entitlements are not made retrospectively and older cohorts do not benefit (Price and Ginn 2003; Price 2006). For example, a White Paper on pension reform (Department for Work and Pensions 2006) outlines benefits for future generations of pensioners, including women, but does not fully address the poverty of existing pensioners:

> Pensioners may not fall technically below the government's chosen (arbitrary) poverty line, but they cluster around it. This makes pensioner poverty very sensitive to the precise measures chosen. If income is taken before housing costs are deducted, pensioner poverty has barely changed since the Labour Government came to power, and if even slightly more generous 'poverty lines' are measured, then millions more pensioners are classified as 'poor'. Pensioners are also far more likely than others in the population to be in persistent poverty.
>
> (Price 2006: 256)

More radical proposals for pension reform are put forward by Age Concern England in their own 'White Paper' (Age Concern 2006b).

The impact of inequalities over the life course related to 'race' and ethnicity is also significant (Blakemore and Boneham 1994). As we saw earlier, research suggests that these inequalities are greatest in later life because of post-migration experiences. The disadvantage in employment that we have already noted also results in limited pension rights (Nazroo *et al.* 2004). Within this broad pattern of disadvantage in older age there are differences between minority ethnic groups. For example, there is evidence that Chinese and Vietnamese older people fare worse than either African Caribbean or South Asian older people in terms of income in later life (Policy Research Institute on Ageing and Ethnicity 2005).

In understanding experiences of ageing, we have argued that account must be taken of the impact of social divisions arising from gender, ethnicity, culture, religion, sexuality, health, disability, social class, income differentials and so on. However, whilst our understanding of older people's experiences and situations should be informed by knowledge of the implications of structural factors stemming from these social divisions, no assumptions can be made about the precise way in which different aspects of inequality interact in particular situations or about how they are experienced by the individuals concerned. The impact of social divisions is mediated by more personal influences such as life course experiences, personality, attitudes and values.

Recognising and valuing such diversity amongst older people is an important component of anti-oppressive practice, as shown in the values highlighted by Hughes (1995 – see above). However, concentrating solely on individual differences can obscure shared interests, weakening the potential for older people to acquire strength through uniting against common sources of injustice and exclusion (Wilson 2001). In this respect, the social construction of alternative identity categories, such as the Grey Panthers in the United States or Hell's Geriatrics in the UK, challenge dominant discourses of ageing in potentially empowering ways. Obviously there is a danger that 'by naming the difference' in this way they 'also create the possibility of discrimination' (Fook 2002: 82) but Fook suggests that one way forward is to reconceptualise 'unity' and 'diversity' so that they are not seen as opposites. We can then talk about 'unity in diversity' or 'diversity in unity' (ibid.: 160), with people from diverse backgrounds seen as unified on the basis of their shared experience of marginalisation and devalued identities. For example, in research that examined implementing equality in meeting diverse needs, it was found that minority and majority ethnic older people experienced limited choice in relation to community care services in their own homes (Bowes 2006). Similarly, Priestley and Rabiee (2002) considered the potential for closer alliances between older people's organisations and those representing disabled people. They cite figures that show that 66 per cent of people over 80 have 'moderate' or 'serious' physical impairments. Despite this, older people are underrepresented in the disability movement, with disability organisations primarily concerned with the interests of younger disabled people.

Added impetus can be given to this search for unity in diversity through the concept of citizenship (Harris, John 1999). Citizenship 'constitute(s) individuals as fully-fledged members of a socio-political community' (Turner, B. 1994: 1). As well as according this status to people, a commitment to citizenship needs to be embedded in forms of practice that promote their social rights (Twine 1994), exploring the roles social workers might play in supporting individuals, groups and movements to achieve greater autonomy and control over their lives in the face of social divisions and oppression. However, if the goal of such practice is the notion of equality as 'treating everyone the same', existing patterns of oppression will simply be perpetuated (Kymlicka and Norman 1995: 286):

> In a society where some groups are privileged while others are oppressed, insisting that persons should leave behind their particular affiliations and experiences to adopt a general point of view serves only to reinforce privilege; for the perspective and interests of the privileged will tend to dominate . . . marginalising or silencing those of other groups.
>
> (Young 1995: 185)

Using citizenship as the basis of unity in diversity, without homogenising people's needs and demands or perpetuating existing power relationships, thus involves recognising and appreciating differences. Social workers, whether they are aware of it or not, are enmeshed in reproducing day-to-day experiences of citizenship (Evans and Harris 2004a), as they engage in mediating between the state and older people (see Chapter 2).

Compounding or countering the problem?

On the one hand, we have seen some of the dangers and limitations of using 'old age' as a social category, in particular, the potential to create and reaffirm ageist assumptions and practices and to ignore the multiple and cross-cutting differences of those so categorised. On the other hand, there are also dangers of lapsing into 'agelessness', denying the changes that accompany ageing and all that the years already lived signify: 'Ironically, this denial of difference, the erasure of the years lived, further entrenches the barrier between us and them, as it strips the old *(sic)* of their history and leaves them with nothing to offer but mimicry of their youth' (Andrews 1999: 316).

One question that arises in writing a book on *Working with Older People* is whether such a project is in itself ageist. Should we be placing the spotlight on a category of people simply on the basis of age (however this is defined)? There are a number of arguments supporting this endeavour. Arber *et al.* (2003b) point out three ways in which age is significant. First, there are physiological processes associated with ageing.

The body does age, with inevitable physical changes occurring, albeit in different ways and at varying rates for different individuals. Engaging with older people's experiences of ageing means acknowledging the significance of these changes. Second, there are specific social and economic processes that shape the experience of later life, for example, retirement and pension policies and social services provision. Third, chronological age is related to membership of generational cohorts and this is linked with particular life experiences, attitudes and values. We need to reach an understanding of an older person's current situation within the context of their life course as a whole and the meanings this has for them.

Biggs *et al.* (2006) suggest, however, that the significance of older age is being denied. They analyse shifts in ideologies of ageing evident in policy trends between 2000 and 2005, particularly in terms of how people were encouraged to think about the adult life course. They conclude that there has been a policy shift that values the activities traditionally associated with work-based and mid-life identities and denies the priorities of other identities, instead advocating 'generational sameness'. They see this as being ageist:

> If the dominant ideology wishes us to see older adults as no different to any others, then rather than seeing difference as a source of ageism, it is important to interrogate this assumption of similarity and ask what we are missing and how this inhibits recognition of the special qualities of a different generational experience. Most notable here would be experiences based on special existential needs in later life and topics that run against new social norms that legitimate only limited paths of ageing . . .
>
> Rather than freeing older adults from age discrimination, this new life-plan may reproduce a new form, in which the imposition of the goals, aims, priorities and agendas of one age group are extended onto and into the lives of other age groups with little consideration being given to differences in aspiration associated with particular age-cohorts or parts of the adult life course and to an avoidance of the physical realities of later life.
>
> (Biggs *et al.* 2006: 246)

Their analysis augments Bytheway's working definition (see above), in which ageism involves making assumptions and decisions about people primarily on the basis of their chronological or biological age, by suggesting that ageism can involve denying the significance of someone's age. Steering a course between these two ageist pitfalls involves acknowledging the potential significance of age and the ageing process, but not letting this prejudice our assessment or intervention, and it requires a much more complex and nuanced understanding. It means anchoring our understanding of older people's situations in knowledge and awareness of physiological changes, social and economic processes and generational influences but at the same time moving beyond this level of understanding to exploring the meaning and significance of these factors for the individuals concerned. This second tier of understanding involves engaging with individual biographies, attitudes, values, beliefs, understandings and practices. In this way, we are able to recognise that each situation is unique, diverse, complex and constantly changing yet, at the same time, is influenced by physiological, social and structural factors. Ageing is both personal and located in an economic, social and political context.

So far we have considered a number of perspectives that can assist us in under-standing that ageing is both personal and takes place in a wider context. We now turn to social work theories that are concerned with the nature of needs, problems or situations and how to effect change. The next section will consider the need for familiarity with such theories in order to assist us in furthering our understanding of older people's experiences and situations.

THE NATURE OF THEORY

A theory is an 'organised statement of ideas about the world' (Payne 2005: 5). 'Theory' has traditionally been seen as the product of scientific knowledge, with connotations of objectivity, rationality, neutrality and detachment. Kuhn (1970), amongst others, has shown that the processes by which certain ideas come to be seen as legitimate theory are located within particular historical and social contexts and these processes are embedded in networks of interests and relations of power. Of course, it is not simply a question of ideas being imposed as theories. All sorts of ideas are put forward by a wide range of people who would like to see their ideas used to make sense of the world around them but those on the receiving end of theories can resist them, reformulate them or come up with theories of their own. In contrast to traditional depictions of theory, this alternative more critical view suggests that theory is the 'dynamic development of ideas linked to power structures in society and the interaction of dominant and countervailing ideological forces' (Thompson 1995: 34).

Social work students and qualified practitioners often struggle with the notion of 'applying theory to practice'. This may be partly due to the notion that theory can be taken in its 'raw' state from the textbook and applied to practice in a straightforward way. Then, when the theory does not 'fit' practice, it is tempting to conclude that either theory is irrelevant to practice or that it has been understood inadequately. In moving beyond the notion of straightforwardly applying theory to practice, a key point is that there is no 'magic' theory or even collection of theories that will provide all of the answers that enable a situation to be readily understood:

> Theory cannot provide simple answers which tell us 'how to do' practice. Theory can only guide and inform. Theory, practice and the relationship between them are all far too complex for there to be a clear, simple and unambiguous path for practitioners to follow. Theory provides us with the cloth from which to tailor our garment, it does not provide 'off the peg' solutions to practice problems.
>
> (Thompson 1995: 69)

A second important point about the relationship between theory and practice is that it is not a one-way relationship in which theory informs practice. Practice can generate, challenge, develop and transform theory. Thus, 'rather than "applying theory to practice", it is more accurate to see theory and practice as having an influence on each other' (Payne 2005: 26). Using theory in practice is therefore a creative process as different sources of knowledge and understanding are 'crafted' in relation to a particular situation and as the ideas generated from theory are in turn adapted and develope through their use in practice (Healy 2005).

A third point to assist in using theory in practice is clarification about what constitutes 'theory'. Postmodernism highlights the relationship between knowledge and power and questions the existence of 'universal truths' contained in modernist theories. The role of language is seen as very significant in *creating* meaning, not simply reflecting it. Power relations influence what is defined through language as knowledge and 'truth' and therefore the particular frameworks that are used for understanding and explaining situations. While there are many 'knowledges' and interpretations available, some discourses, through their connections with relationships of power, become dominant; they are heard more often and carry more 'weight' than others (Parton and Marshall 1998). Dominant discourses may be accepted by those with less power or they may be challenged or resisted. This understanding of knowledge has implications for the sources of knowledge that are seen as relevant to understanding practice and for how this knowledge is used. 'Knowledge' is not just about the 'theory' contained in academic textbooks, which, of course, reflect particular relations of power in society, for example, gender, ethnicity and social class. Postmodernist approaches emphasise that there are 'multiple truths' in any situation and stress the validity of the many different types and sources of knowledge. (This leads Fook to talk of 'ways of knowing', rather than theories [2002: 68].) In particular, practitioners are encouraged to value 'ways of knowing' from their own practice and to uncover and value the marginalised discourses of service users. To an extent, this approach is recognised in work on the types of knowledge relevant in social care, where the following categories of knowledge have been identified: organisational; policy; practitioner; research; and service user and carer (Pawson *et al.* 2003). For social workers, this indicates the need for an inclusive approach to what is regarded as valid knowledge for understanding the situations they encounter.

However, postmodernist approaches have been criticised. They have been seen as overemphasising subjectivity to the point where the individual's relationship with the social structure is ignored. This, it is argued, seriously restricts the emancipatory potential of social work in terms of challenging inequality and oppression, understood in structural terms. An alternative position, 'critical realism', seeks to reconcile agency and social structure. It builds on the insights gained from postmodernist approaches about the significance of subjectivity and individual agency but combines this with analysis of the impact of social structure on people's lives (Houston 2001), thereby accepting a 'reality' outside that of individual subjectivity. However, society is seen as complex, with numerous influences in any situation, such that simple explanations in terms of cause and effect relationships are spurious. Social structure is also not seen as determining individual experience, since individuals have the capacity to think, act, change and resist. Rather, social structure creates *tendencies*. Part of the social worker's role is to understand and explain these tendencies. Once these tendencies are understood, they can be challenged. For example, a critical realist approach would take account of evidence about the impact of poverty earlier in the life course on health inequalities in later life but would consider how this tendency related to the particular situation and to the individual older person:

> The task for social work is to (re)discover the causal mechanisms within the person, their social networks and wider society which give rise to suffering and oppression. Inevitably, this is a complex task because of the range and combined effects of these mechanisms. Some will be operating at the individual, personality level, whilst others are at the societal level.

Furthermore, we must not forget that people have the capacity to transform their situations. In other words, the effects of these mechanisms will be mediated through people's day-to-day actions. It is precisely for this reason that we must abandon any ideas that social work (or any social profession) can predict events. Our formulations will necessarily be tentative, probabilistic, cautious and refined over time.

(Houston 2001: 853)

Being critical and reflexive

As well as helping to determine *what* knowledge is relevant to practice, postmodernism has also influenced *how* it is used. The complex and changing nature of the social world and multiple sources of understanding require us to be critical and reflexive about our use of theory, continually questioning what and how we 'know' and remaining open to alternative ways of understanding. Our theories can be seen as

sets of eyeglasses through which we look at the world. Just as with our physical eyeglasses, our implicit theories may bring into focus, sharpen and angle for us our understanding of what might otherwise be a blurred stream of perception . . . these same theoretical lenses can also sometimes hamper us, can cut off angles of vision, peripheral or otherwise. We can select sets of lenses that will help us to see up close or at a distance, different sets for different purposes.

(Ely *et al.* 1997: 228)

What this suggests is that we need to start inductively from a specific situation, rather than from our favourite theories, and then work creatively with theories as 'intellectual tools, rather than as rule books' (Fook 2002: 69). In dealing with situations of diversity and complexity, we need to adopt 'a position of uncertainty' (Parton and Marshall 1998: 246), being aware of the multiple ways such situations can be understood and remaining tentative about our own evolving hypotheses. As theories are often contradictory and embody conflicting values and views about society, it is not a case of 'anything goes' in terms of how we incorporate different theoretical insights; rather, this must be a conscious and critical process (Thompson 1995). Furthermore, the use of theory in practice involves acknowledging the impact of our own involvement. It demands reflexivity on the part of the social worker; a process of 'putting ourselves in the picture' (Payne *et al.* 2002: 3), thinking about the influence we have on the social work process and the impact that it in turn has on us:

Practitioners . . . cannot occupy some detached space from which vantage point they make 'correct' decisions about their clients. They are in there too, struggling to make sense of things, to communicate, and buffeted in the same way by winds of change, by personal and cultural influences, as are service users and others. Practitioners face conflicting principles and a context that is complex and requires reflection, rather than the straightforward application of knowledge and skill.

(Brechin 2000: 29)

One issue about 'making sense of things' that makes theorising about later life (and working with older people) different from some other areas of social work is that we know that we are likely to become 'older people' ourselves. This gives added significance to being critically reflexive practitioners and 'putting ourselves in the picture', considering the impact of our attitudes, values and assumptions on our practice.

ACTIVITY 1.7: PUTTING YOURSELF IN THE PICTURE

- What are your feelings, hopes and concerns about your own ageing?
- What factors will be important in enabling you to maintain a good quality of life in old age?
- What changes do you think are needed in health and social care policy for this to happen?
- How may your feelings about your own ageing influence your social work practice with older people?

Having introduced our general stance on the nature of 'theory', we now consider the role more specific theories might play in informing social work practice with older people.

THEORETICAL 'MAPS' FOR UNDERSTANDING

Milner and O'Byrne (2002) argue that, despite the complexity of the theory–practice relationship, the perspectives we use in practice need to be made explicit. They outline five theoretical 'maps' to guide social workers. The maps are not mutually exclusive and different maps can complement each other and add further layers of understanding. They are to be used *with* service users as we generate and check out a number of possible hypotheses about 'what is going on' in a given situation. The goal is to find a 'story' that is helpful to all those involved (Milner and O'Byrne 2002: 4). The five theoretical maps summarised by Milner and O'Byrne are:

- *'a map of the ocean'*: **psychodynamic** approaches – involving 'getting below the surface of the person and their feelings';
- *'an ordnance survey map'*: **behavioural** approaches – focused on observable conduct and the 'ups and downs of action';
- *'the handy tourist map'*: **task-centred** approaches – popular brief ways of working that are easily accessible and have wide application;
- *'the navigator's map'*: **solution-focused** approaches – geared to achieving a particular destination or goal;
- *'the forecast map'*: **narrative** approaches – concerned with oppressive climates and focused on the future. (Further discussion of the use of narrative approaches with older people can be found in Chapter 5.)

In the space we have available we are unable to describe each of these approaches but a clear summary of the approaches, including evaluation of their advantages, disadvantages and outcomes, can be found in Milner and O'Byrne (2002). The key point to note here is that the 'maps' are to be used flexibly and creatively, as tools to assist with practice, as we have already stressed, not as rulebooks to be followed unthinkingly. As Milner and O'Byrne emphasise throughout, social workers should be reflexive, open-minded, consider the consequences of using particular maps and, in particular, value service users' own 'theories' about their situation. They suggest that one guide in selecting a map is to ask, 'Where is the problem/need/solution mainly located: outside the service user, within the service user, or between the user and others?' (ibid.: 73). This provides an indication (not a definitive answer) of an appropriate level of intervention.

In practice, of course, as Milner and O'Byrne acknowledge, problems may include intrapersonal, interpersonal and extrapersonal dimensions, indicating that more than one approach may be required. As well as providing a useful point of reference when considering which maps to use, the distinction between intrapersonal, interpersonal and extrapersonal dimensions is also helpful when evaluating practice. The practitioner can ask, 'On which of these levels has the intervention mainly focused?' 'At which level has change been achieved/not achieved?' This will prompt attention to issues that may have been overlooked, where further intervention may be needed.

TABLE 1.1 Guide to map selection

Nature of need/problem:	Appropriate 'map'
Intrapersonal (inside the service user)	Psychodynamic Behaviourism
Interpersonal (between service user and others)	Task-centred Family therapy
Extrapersonal (outside the service user)	Systems approach Advocacy

Source: Milner and O'Byrne 2002

Evaluating theoretical perspectives

Thinking critically about theories means taking account of the context in which they were formulated and the particular values and views about society that they reflect. There are a number of dimensions that may be useful when evaluating different theoretical perspectives on later life.

Consensual versus conflictual view of society

To what extent does a particular theoretical perspective assume a consensual view of society, accepting the status quo and assuming that society works in ways that are positive for its members as a whole? Or is a particular perspective based on the view that society contains conflicting interests and mechanisms through which some people gain and others lose?

Deficit versus heroic models of ageing

To what extent does a perspective portray later life as problematic and a time of illness, decline, passivity and dependency? Or, does it present a 'heroic model' of ageing, representing older people only in terms of activity, independence and retained 'youthfulness'?

Social determinism versus individual agency/resistance

To what extent does a perspective see older people's situations as determined by social, economic and political processes and to what extent does it allow for the capacity of older people to act within and in opposition to such processes?

Homogeneity versus diversity

To what extent does a perspective allow for differences between people or does it assume sameness, for example, making assumptions based on particular expectations about age, culture, gender, sexuality and so on?

Stasis versus change/fluidity

To what extent does a perspective assume that society and individuals are static and fixed or does it allow for change, development and fluidity?

These dimensions begin to suggest some of the ways in which theory might be linked to practice. Having acknowledged key points about using theory to inform practice, and bearing in mind these dimensions for evaluating theoretical perspectives, we turn to some of the main theoretical perspectives for understanding later life and their implications for social work practice.

THEORETICAL PERSPECTIVES ON LATER LIFE

Biological theories

Biological theories seek to understand the process of ageing in terms of biological and physiological changes that occur as people grow older. Biological theories include those that view ageing as a result of harmful environmental influences or internal defects and those that view it as an inevitable pre-programmed developmental deterioration (Bengtson *et al.* 2005). Biological theories adopt a predominantly negative view of ageing as a time of loss of function and decline and offer 'macro' level explanations that fail to take account of individual differences and social, cultural and environmental influences. As Wilson argues

> The ageing body has characteristics that can be identified in any part of the world. This does not mean that all ageing bodies are alike or that they manifest the same changes at similar chronological ages, or that physiological 'old age' will be the same in different cultures.
>
> (Wilson 2000: 18)

Because of their status as 'scientific', biological theories have been very influential in shaping attitudes and beliefs about ageing. In particular, biological theories of ageing have contributed to negative cultural attitudes towards older people through the association of ageing with frailty and incapacity. As mentioned earlier, these negative constructions also impact on the attitudes and self-perception of older people themselves. Signs of physical ageing become something to be feared or disguised, or are accepted as part of an 'aged' identity but with negative implications for selfhood (Biggs 1997). Another facet of biological understandings is that passive acceptance of the 'problems' of ageing is legitimated. Thus, professionals, carers and older people themselves may 'explain' problems such as memory loss, incontinence or declining mobility in terms of 'it's just his/her/my age', thereby excluding the possibility of interventions that may treat or alleviate the difficulties. Furthermore, biological theories of ageing do not in themselves take account of how individuals experience the process of ageing or find ways to adapt to physical changes.

Erikson's life cycle

Erikson's psychological theory sees personality as developing across the lifespan and distinguishes eight stages within the life cycle (Erikson 1977). Each stage is seen as characterised by a particular psychological conflict that has to be negotiated. Depending on how the conflict is resolved, a particular quality of ego functioning is developed in each stage. The stages are interrelated in that how conflicts are resolved at each developmental stage has implications for the subsequent stages (see Table 1.2 below).

The conflict to be negotiated in later life is between integrity and despair. To achieve ego integrity, an individual reaches an acceptance of the life lived, a sense of 'keeping things together' and a feeling that the life lived has coherence. There is an acceptance of past losses and failures and a feeling that there are no 'loose ends' (Stuart-Hamilton 2000). In contrast, a state of despair results from regret about unresolved

TABLE 1.2 Erikson's life cycle theory

Life stage	Conflict	Ego functioning
Infancy	Basic trust/mistrust	Hope
Childhood (1)	Autonomy/doubt	Will
Childhood (2)	Initiative/doubt	Purpose
Childhood (3)	Industry/inferiority	Competence
Adolescence	Ego identity/role confusion	Fidelity
Young adulthood	Intimacy/role confusion	Love
Adulthood	Generativity/stagnation	Care
Old age	Integrity/despair	Wisdom

issues, feelings of discontinuity and a fear of death. Satisfactory resolution of the conflict between integrity and despair results in the ego quality of wisdom that may be passed on to other generations.

Erikson's developmental theory connects later life with the rest of the life course and, unlike many previous psychological theories, acknowledged that learning and development are not confined to childhood but also feature in later life. However, a number of criticisms have been made of his life cycle model. First, it is seen as Eurocentric, accepting uncritically the cultural norms of society at the time (the USA in the 1950s). It takes as 'normal' and generalises from conventional expectations about life stage progression. Departure from these expectations is not seen as reflecting diversity in terms of behaviours that are different but of equal value, but rather as representing unresolved conflicts that have negative consequences for later development. Second, whilst Erikson's model is based on traditional expectations about progression through particular life stages, there is now enormous diversity in terms of the stages in the life course at which various life events or experiences occur. For example, people may have children, develop new relationships or return to education in later life. Erikson's model fixes aspects of development in particular stages rather than allowing for multiple developmental pathways, with various conflicts and challenges arising or resurfacing at different stages. Identity issues, for example, are not only encountered in adolescence but also may recur in later life through experiences such as unemployment and divorce. Erikson's theorising also remains essentially child-centred, with interest in the final two life stages being more concerned with the conditions for successfully raising children, namely passing on care and wisdom, than with understanding the subjective experiences of adulthood and later life (Biggs 1999).

Disengagement theory

This is another theory that was developed in the USA in the late 1950s and published in the early 1960s (Cumming and Henry 1961). As in Erikson's model, old age is understood in the context of an 'end of life' stage; whilst for Erikson this is about tying up loose ends, for Cumming and Henry it is about social withdrawal. Disengagement theory links the needs of ageing individuals with the needs of the social system, seeing the two as compatible. Older people are seen as disengaging from social roles and relationships in a process that is 'natural' and beneficial for them, releasing them from social expectations, and this process is regarded as of equal value for society, freeing up opportunities for younger people:

> Ageing is an inevitable mutual withdrawal or disengagement resulting in decreased interaction between the ageing person and others in the social system he (*sic*) belongs to. The process may be initiated by the individual or by others in the situation . . . When the ageing process is complete the equilibrium which existed in middle life between the individual and his (*sic*) society has given way to a new equilibrium characterised by a greater distance and an altered type of relationship.
>
> (Cumming and Henry 1961: 14)

Thus disengagement is presented as an inevitable, central and universal aspect of the ageing process, with references to 'mutual withdrawal' and 'equilibrium' conveying a consensual rather than conflictual view of society. This theory has been subject to substantial criticism on a number of counts.

First, it conveys an uncritically negative view of old age as a time of stagnation and withdrawal. Second, the theory is contradicted by research findings that reveal high levels of activity and engagement amongst many older people. While there may be some loss of social roles and activities, new roles and activities can take their place. There can be a process of reorientation or accommodation, instead of disengagement (Brandstädter and Greve 1994; Roberts and Chapman 2001). Rather than disengagement being inevitable, cross-cultural studies show that in many developing countries older people retain a very active role in their communities (Wilson 2000). Third, it is assumed that disengagement is a positive choice for older people and this is contradicted by the evidence. Gabriel and Bowling's (2004) research, referred to earlier, shows that being able to engage in hobbies and activities is an important dimension of quality of life, as defined by older people. Rather than disengagement being a positive choice, social, economic and political processes mean that in many cases older people have no option but to disengage (Walker 1981). There is evidence to suggest that those who do choose to disengage in later life are those inclined by personality to more socially isolated lifestyles (Maddox 1970). Fourth, disengagement theory suggests that in later life the needs and wishes of older people take a different turn and are distinct from their expectations and requirements earlier in the life course. Again, this is not supported by research evidence (Coleman, P. *et al.* 1998). Finally, the theory can be criticised for its negative implications for policy and practice. Through portraying disengagement as a beneficial and inevitable process, the marginalisation of older people, for example through retirement policies, segregated accommodation and 'closed off' forms of residential care, are justified. However, on a more positive note, it has been argued that while there has been little support for disengagement theory itself, it has been of value in stimulating debate and theorising that offer alternative perspectives (Estes *et al.* 2003).

Activity theory

Although activity theory predated disengagement theory, it was developed further in efforts to repudiate disengagement theory (Katz 2000). Activity theory is based on the notion that continued involvement in social roles, relationships and activities can enhance well-being in later life (Havighurst and Albrecht 1953). The dimensions important for quality of later life are seen as the same as those for earlier in the life course, in contrast to disengagement theory, where later life is seen as a distinct phase, with different requirements. Both theories are, however, based on a consensual view of society. In activity theory, it is assumed that society's need for active and hard-working citizens is matched by the needs and wishes of older people to remain active. Whereas there is limited empirical support for disengagement theory, activity theory is consistent with research evidence that suggests that older people do strive to maintain personal interests, activities and relationships (Langan *et al.* 1996; Bowling *et al.* 1997). Not only is this what many older people want, there is also evidence that social activity plays an important role in sustaining their well-being (Kendig *et al.* 2000; Fernandez-Ballesteros *et al.* 2001). For example, a research study conducted as part of the Economic and Social Research Council's *Growing Older* programme identifies keeping busy as an important means of coping for older people who are widowed (Bennett *et al.* 2004).

Whereas disengagement theory legitimates not responding or responding negatively to difficulties in retaining activities, roles and relationships, activity theory can promote positive intervention, including with older people traditionally seen as incapable of participating in social activity. In work with people with dementia, for example, occupation and play are seen as important dimensions for retaining personhood (Kitwood 1997). A review of research on rehabilitation and dementia notes that activities can improve communication, mental and emotional well-being, if activities are selected and adapted to accommodate someone's level of cognitive impairment (Mountain 2005). However, activity theory does have potential pitfalls: 'The image of hordes of social workers forcing older people to mix with others "for their own good", with compulsory whist drives and so forth, is not a pleasant one' (Stuart-Hamilton 2000: 160). In other words, older people want and benefit from continued engagement not in any activity, but in social activities that are personally meaningful and rewarding to them. The whole notion of 'activity' is more complex than its presentation in activity theory. We need to allow for the diversity of meanings that activity may have for older people; for example, older people may interpret it to include activities such as taking naps, watching television, gambling and daydreaming (Katz 2000).

Both disengagement and activity theories are prescriptive in that they are putting forward a view about how older people *should* behave (Victor 2005). Establishing a direct causal relationship between activity (or disengagement) and older people's well-being is also problematic. Indeed, one study suggests it is the social relationships as an intrinsic part of most activities that are the significant factor in promoting well-being, rather than activity itself (Litwin and Shiovitz-Ezra 2006). However, both disengagement and activity theory, though seemingly diametrically opposed, may have some relevance for understanding the situations and views of older people:

> There are discourses that see old age as a time of well-earned rest (these are usually men's discourses) and there are discourses on the importance of keeping mind and body active. In the same way older people in many cultures

think that a dignified disengagement from mid-life activities is appropriate in advanced old age, even though they also think that they should keep in touch with the rest of society as far as they possibly can. Theories may conflict logically but they often make sense to individual elders as representations of different aspects of their lives.

(Wilson 2000: 11)

ACTIVITY 1.8: USING THEORIES TO MAKE SENSE OF OLDER PEOPLE'S EXPERIENCES

Look back at your notes from Activity 1.1, the extract in Box 1.1 and the research findings on older people's experiences and perspectives presented earlier in the chapter. What evidence is there that supports either disengagement or activity theories of ageing?

Continuity theory

Continuity theory asserts that older people manage changes and choices by seeking to preserve both internal continuity, that is, continuity of ideas, preferences, skills, etc., and external continuity, that is, continuity of their physical and social environment (Atchley 1989). Whilst continuity theory has been criticised by those who argue that later life is characterised by constant change and fluidity, Atchley argues that continuity does not necessarily mean that things remain exactly the same but rather that change is negotiated within an overall framework of continuity that connects the individual with her/his past life. This is supported by Coleman, P. et al.'s (1998) longitudinal research, which found continuity in the life themes of people over the age of 80, with family relationships being the themes' main sources. Research has also demonstrated the importance to older people of maintaining habits and routines (Johnson, C. and Barer 1997; Sidenvall et al. 2001) and the significance of continuity of the physical environment of home and locality (Phillipson et al. 2001). However, while there is empirical support for some aspects of continuity theory, it tends to attribute problems encountered to individual deficits rather than social factors. For example, if people cannot meet their own needs because they are disabled or poor, Atchley sees this as 'pathological ageing'. Similarly, he sees continuity as maladaptive when someone lacks the physical or mental capacities that are necessary to retain continuity; he cites the example of an older person who insists on living independently when s/he lacks self-care abilities. The assumption is that it is the functioning of individuals that is pathological or maladaptive, rather than that environmental barriers are preventing older people from realising their aspirations.

Life course theory

A life course approach to ageing draws attention to the connections between an individual's past life, her/his life as currently lived and her/his aspirations for the future (Arber and Evandrou 1993). The emphasis is not so much on preserving continuity as a way of managing the ageing process, but rather on understanding experiences of ageing within the context of the life course as a whole. This perspective is based on the premise that experiences of ageing can only be understood in the context of the whole life course since 'the life lived gives meaning to old age' (Ruth and Oberg 1996: 186). Life course theories do not represent the life course as a series of fixed stages but as characterised by changing and diverse processes, 'a way of envisaging the passage of a lifetime less as the mechanical turning of a wheel and more as the unpredictable flow of a river' (Hockey and James 2003: 5). In terms of the implications of this perspective, it highlights the significance of understanding an older person's past life in order to understand their current needs and plan appropriate service provision. While there is a danger of insufficient attention being given to the significance of social, economic and political factors in shaping life experiences, it is possible to adopt a life course perspective and take account of ways in which a life course has been moulded by structural factors.

Structured dependency theory

The main emphasis of structured dependency, or political economy, theories is that social and economic conditions create conditions of dependency in older people. The focus is shifted from biological/individual to social/structural determinants of ageing:

> Political economy has challenged the idea of older people being a homo-geneous group unaffected by the dominant structures and ideologies within society. Instead, the focus is on understanding the relationship between ageing and economic life, the differential experience of ageing according to social class, gender and ethnicity, and the role played by social policy in contributing to the dependent status of older people.
>
> (Phillipson 1998: 18)

Attention is drawn to compulsory retirement policies that exclude older people from the labour market, pensions policies that relegate older people to lives of poverty and, when they can no longer survive these conditions, to institutional care that segregates and isolates them, creating further dependency (Townsend 1981; Walker 1981).

A criticism of structured dependency theories is that, at least in earlier versions, the emphasis placed on the significance of employment and pensions policies was more relevant to the situations of older men than older women. Structured dependency theories have also been criticised for being too deterministic and not allowing enough scope for the individual and collective agency of older people in challenging and resisting oppressive policies and conditions. For example, some older people take an active role in saving and planning for their future to avoid reliance on a state pension (Roberts and Chapman 2001). Also, retirement and residential care may be positive choices for some older people, rather than outcomes foisted upon them. In other words, it is important to see older people as having the potential to be active agents, rather than simply seeing them as passive victims. Linked with this, it is also argued that structured dependency theories pay insufficient attention to how individuals interpret and give meaning to their situations. For example, there is no direct correlation between objective and subjective assessments of quality of life (George and Bearon 1980; Nolan 2000; Bond and Corner 2004). Individuals in adverse social conditions may evaluate their lives and situations positively and vice versa. For example, 'old older people' have been noted to reconstruct their situations in order to maintain a positive outlook (Johnson, C. and Barer 1997). It is not enough, therefore, to adopt a structural model to understand the experience of ageing; individual and subjective factors must also be included.

Identity management theory

These theoretical perspectives are based on a postmodern understanding of society as complex, rapidly changing and allowing multiple opportunities for individuals to construct and reconstruct identities of their choosing through consumerism. Identity is viewed as fluid, rather than fixed, and individuals are seen as exercising agency in responding to changing social situations and conditions by making particular lifestyle choices (Gilleard 1996: 495). There is recognition that the body places restrictions on the ability of individuals to choose their identity; in later life, the self cannot entirely escape the constraints imposed by an ageing body. There are different views about the nature of the tensions between self, body and social responses and about how these tensions are managed. One view is that a self perceived as youthful is trapped inside an ageing body; society responds to the individual in terms of the visible aged body, or 'mask of ageing', creating tension for the inner youthful self (Featherstone and Hepworth 1989). An alternative view is that in later life, the individual is forced to deny their experience of an ageing self and instead present a youthful façade, or masquerade, because the social space is hostile to and rejects ageing (Biggs 1999). The individual's degree of self-expression depends on their assessment of the particular social situation: 'rather than being seen simply as a form of inauthenticity, masque should be valued as an adaptive response to inhospitable settings' (Biggs 1999: 172). These two interpretations of how identity is managed in later life suggest different social responses. While the 'mask of ageing' indicates the need to recognise the older person's youthful inner self and help them to express this, 'masquerade' suggests the need to create social environments that are accepting and supportive of the ageing self. These understandings and interventions are not, of course, mutually exclusive.

The focus on individual agency in these perspectives can underplay the significance of constraints on choice arising from structural factors, such as restricted access to resources and opportunities. However, in emphasising the fluidity and individuality of experiences of ageing, these theories allow for multiple layers of diversity. Identity management theories also make a valuable contribution in recognising the ways in which the ageing body constrains individual subjectivity and triggers negative social responses.

ACTIVITY 1.9: BILL WATERS

Bill Waters is white British and aged 83. He lives alone in a first floor council flat. He has a heart condition and arthritis in his knees. He walks around the flat holding on to the furniture and uses two sticks when he goes out. He can only walk very short distances and he is finding it increasingly hard to climb the stairs up to his flat. Bill's wife of 51 years, Annie, died eighteen months ago. They had a close companionable relationship, sharing lots of interests, and Bill misses her greatly. They used to enjoy ballroom dancing together and were both keen gardeners who used to enter competitions and often won prizes for their home-grown flowers and vegetables. Bill had to give up his allotment when he moved to the flat six months ago. Having worked for many years as a postman, he misses being in the open air. Bill's only son died in a motorbike accident when he was 25. Bill has one sister still alive but she has dementia and lives in a nursing home. He is not able to visit her often. There is no other close family, though Bill has one or two friends from the allotments who call to see him from time to time.

Bill's GP is concerned that he is sinking into depression and starting to neglect himself. She has asked the social worker to see if s/he can get Bill to go to the local day centre a few days a week so that he can have a hot meal and some company. Bill has never had help from social services and prides himself on his independence. Although he has never been well-off, he says he has never owed anyone anything in his life and he does not intend to start asking for charity now. He says he does not have any problems and can manage just fine. He wants to carry on as he is until it is time for him to join Annie, and he hopes this won't be long in coming.

How do different theories of ageing contribute to your understanding of this situation?

OLDER PEOPLE AS THEORISTS

We have outlined various 'academic' theories of ageing. However, it is important to recognise that older people have their own theories that they use to understand their behaviour and situation, and that of others:

> When we . . . allow the ordinary theoretical activity of the aged (*sic*) and others to become visible, a whole world of reasoning about the meaning of growing old, becoming frail and care-giving comes forth. We find that theory is not something exclusively engaged in by scientists. Rather, there seem to be two existing worlds of theory in human experience, one engaged by those who live the experiences under consideration, and one organized by those who make it their professional business systematically to examine experience.
>
> (Gubrium and Wallace 1990: 147)

This brings us back to the point made at the beginning of the chapter about the need to engage with direct experience. Service user knowledge, or 'ordinary theorising', is a key source of knowledge that must underpin our attempts at generating informed, critically reflective and sensitive theorising. In Activity 1.9, for example, it is important to engage with Bill's own understanding of his situation; what he sees as the strengths, the difficulties and the best ways of addressing them, his hopes and aspirations as well as his fears and concerns. At the same time, the social worker can bring to the encounter additional or alternative ways of understanding and can explore with Bill which 'theories' make most sense in terms of constructing a way forward. Referring back to the dimensions for evaluating theoretical perspectives presented earlier in the chapter, it will be apparent from the theories examined that the strengths offered by one theory often constitute the weaknesses of another. Using a range of theories allows a multi-dimensional understanding of situations, such as Bill's, to develop and enables the limitations of one perspective to be offset by the advantages of another. We need to draw on a plurality of theories so that multiple levels of understanding are addressed – intrapersonal, interpersonal and extrapersonal:

> We maintain that social work's search for one cohesive theory is misplaced. Social workers need a selection of practice principles and values, coupled with a range of theoretical models and methods, as a foundation from which they can respond creatively to the infinite range of situations they will meet. This creativity will enable them to mix and match theoretical ideas, test values and techniques, and be eclectic – making deliberate and rigorous selection, and not merely jumbling ideas together – so that their responses to service users will be individualised rather than routine.
>
> (Milner and O'Byrne 2002: 79)

Milner and O'Byrne argue that the most useful theoretical 'map' in any situation is that which is most helpful and empowering for the service user. The map is produced with service users in an open and reflective way, charting an understanding of the situation and determining how to intervene. At the same time, as discussed earlier, these formulations are treated as working hypotheses, with the social worker adopting 'a position of uncertainty' (Parton and Marshall 1998: 246), always prepared to revisit ideas and change perspective.

KEY POINTS

☐   Social work with older people must start from the experiences, perceptions and perspectives of older people themselves.

☐   Social workers need to be aware of the ways in which 'old age' is constructed socially, culturally and economically and to understand the impact of ageism on policy, practices, attitudes and behaviours. They also need to explore how ageism interacts with other forms of difference, diversity and inequality and to know how to challenge and address these in their practice.

☐   The social category of 'older people' is highly diverse; while there may be certain shared themes between some older people, influenced by wider structural factors and age-cohort experiences, each situation is also unique, affected by individual personalities, life course experiences and individual subjectivities.

☐   Social workers need to draw on a wide range of theories to work effectively with older people. They must be both reflective and reflexive in their practice, building their theoretical understanding in each situation and incorporating as a central component the theories of older people themselves.

☐   Theorising should be regarded as tentative and open to review in the light of new understandings and perspectives.

KEY READING

Milner, J. and O'Byrne, P. (2002, 2nd edn) *Assessment in Social Work*, Basingstoke: Palgrave Macmillan.

Walker, A. and Hagan Hennessy, C. (eds) (2004) *Growing Older: Quality of Life in Old Age*, Maidenhead: Open University Press.

Wilson, G. (2000) *Understanding Old Age: Critical and Global Perspectives*, London: Sage.

CHAPTER 2

THE POLICY CONTEXT OF SOCIAL WORK WITH OLDER PEOPLE

OBJECTIVES

By the end of this chapter you should have an understanding of:

- the historical context of social work with older people;

- the community care reforms of the 1990s and their continuing significance for working with older people;

- recent New Labour policy initiatives and their implications for social work with older people.

Ultimately, the state is the source of social work's legal and moral authority. The state sets out the conditions under which social work is provided and practised through the policies it lays down; social workers implement legislation on behalf of the state, as an arm of social policy. The law sets out the rights, duties and responsibilities of social workers, on the one hand, and of service users, on the other, in those areas of life that have been accorded official recognition as socially problematic. In general terms, the state decides with whom social workers will work, what should be provided for them and how this provision should be made. Policy and legislation embody particular views, attitudes and assumptions and so need to be understood in relation to the social and historical context in which they have been developed and the context in which they are being implemented.

This chapter provides an overview of the policy context of social work with older people. The first part of the chapter reviews policy developments from 1945 to the community care reforms of the 1990s. The second part of the chapter discusses the policy framework from the 1990s onwards in relation to, first, the assessment of older people's needs and, second, the provision of community care and residential services.

The third part of the chapter considers more recent policy initiatives under New Labour. We approach these policy developments not in terms of movement from one clearly defined period to another but as stages in the composition of an increasingly complex legal and policy context within which social workers have to operate in their work with older people:

> Social work is an activity shaped by its institutional context. What social workers do – the practices they adopt, the values they act upon, the outcomes they pursue – are very much the result of *the gradual accumulation of past practices and understandings* . . . which have gradually taken on a (more or less) 'accepted' status.
>
> (McDonald 2006: 3, *our emphasis*)

THE HISTORICAL CONTEXT OF SOCIAL WORK WITH OLDER PEOPLE

Older people only began to be recognised as a social group at the end of the nineteenth century; prior to this, their needs were conflated with those of 'the sick' or 'paupers' under the Poor Law. Although retirement pensions were introduced in 1908 on a non-contributory basis, these provided only meagre help for the poorest older people over the age of 70: 'The terms of the construction of old age are clear: a minimum level of provision but with maximum expectations that this would be seen as sufficient reward by the recipients' (Phillipson 1998: 110). Older people who were able to continue working did so; those who could not, lived in poverty (ibid.). The introduction of the post-war Welfare State was underpinned by different principles – of citizenship, solidarity and mutual responsibility between generations (Estes *et al.* 2003). Citizens were accorded social rights by the state. For older people these principles and rights were manifested primarily in the provision of contributory state pensions through the National Insurance Act (1946), supplemented by means-tested benefits under the National Assistance Act (1948). With increased life expectancy and the introduction of state retirement pensions, retirement itself assumed the status of a recognised life stage. However, intertwined with retirement were notions of older people as dependent, economically unproductive and a 'burden' on others. In their review of provision for older people, Means and Smith (1998) suggest that the longstanding low priority given to older people in social policy is related to the way they have been constructed socially as of little economic or social value (this can also be seen in some of the ideas of both structured dependency and disengagement theories – see Chapter 1).

Whilst the extension of pension provision was clearly an important advance, though much more so for men than for women because of the contributory principle, there was more limited progress in terms of statutory social services for older people. The National Assistance Act (1948, section 29) gave local authorities powers and duties to provide various services to certain categories of people – those who are 'blind, deaf or dumb', 'suffer from mental disorder' or are 'substantially and permanently handicapped' (see discussion in Chapter 3). Older people were thus not specified, though they can receive services if they fall within one or more of these categories. The formulation of section 29 can be understood in its historical context, in the period following World War II. There was a concern to give priority to services for soldiers who had been wounded in the war and people who had been injured in bombings. It has been argued that this prioritisation of the needs of disabled people over those of older people remains a feature of current policy (Clements 2004).

Another continuing strand running through social policy development for older people is the expectation that families, and in particular women, would provide care for their older members (Lewis, J. 2000). There were concerns that extending services to support older people at home would encourage families to relinquish what were regarded as their rightful responsibilities to care for their older relatives (Means and Smith 1998). Domiciliary care was also not seen as effective in supporting more vulnerable older people. Therefore, as an 'add-on', rather than a core service, it could be left to the voluntary sector (ibid.). Accordingly, when the National Assistance Act (1948) was first passed, local authorities merely had powers to arrange for the provision of meals and recreational services by making grants to voluntary organisations. The need for local authorities to assume a more significant role in providing domiciliary services was only gradually accepted and in 1962 the National Assistance Act (1948) was amended to allow the direct provision of mobile meals services by local authorities. Whilst domiciliary services gradually increased from the 1940s to the 1970s, they remained discretionary, were patchy geographically and inadequate to meet need (Means and Smith 1998; Means *et al.* 2002).

The needs of older people were recognised specifically in the Health Services and Public Health Act (1968), implemented in 1971. This Act was concerned with promoting the welfare of older people. It was aimed at older people who were not 'substantially handicapped' but who nevertheless would benefit from the provision of services due to age-related frailty. It enabled local authorities to adopt a preventive – rather than reactive – approach, giving them powers, for example, to make arrangements for 'practical assistance in the home' and for 'meals and recreation'. However, these remained powers, rather than duties, so local authorities were not obliged to provide a service for older people who did not meet the definition of disability contained within Section 29 of National Assistance.

Another key strand that has resonated continuously in policy since the implementation of the National Assistance Act (1948) is the problematic interface between health care for those who are ill and social care for those who are frail. The National Health Service Act (1946), a 'pillar' of the Welfare State, provided for the needs of sick older people to be met through the National Health Service. Part III of the National Assistance Act (1948) imposed a duty on local authorities to arrange residential accommodation for people who were 'aged' and 'in need of care and attention which is not otherwise available to them'. This distinction between those who were 'sick' and those who were 'in need of care and attention' proved problematic from the beginning, with no clear boundary between health and social services responsibilities (Means and Smith 1998). This was and remains significant for service users in that services to meet 'health' needs that are accepted as the responsibility of the NHS are free at the point of delivery, while services to meet 'social' needs can be charged for. So, for example, an older person with 'health' needs occupying a long-term hospital bed would retain their state pension while an older person with 'social' needs accommodated in a residential home would contribute most of their pension towards the cost of care, retaining a small personal allowance.

The vision for residential care according to Aneurin Bevan (health minister for the post-war Labour Government) was that the old Public Assistance Institutions (PAIs) – the former workhouses, which acted as places of last resort for the destitute – would be replaced by 'hotel'-style accommodation. The homes were intended to be small, accommodating 30 to 35 residents. Whereas people admitted to PAIs had lost their pension rights (unless their need was medical), residents of the new-style homes would exercise a positive choice to take up residence, enjoying the status of 'guest' rather than inmate, receiving a pension and paying for their care and accommodation (Johnson, J. 1998). However, many older people were not 'sick' in terms of needing hospital care, but required more than the level of 'care and attention' envisaged in residential homes/ 'hotels'. The necessary increase in the building of small homes did not materialise because of shortages of both building materials and labour and, subsequently, restrictions on local authorities' capital expenditure (Means and Smith 1998). By 1960, nearly half of local authority residential beds were still provided in ex-workhouse institutions rather than the new small residential homes. Shortages in hospital beds led to people with higher levels of health needs being accommodated in residential care. Consequently, 'the idea of residential care available on request for the relatively active, elderly person was abandoned under the overall pressure of demand for such care' (Means and Smith 1998: 171). Problems related to the blurred lines of responsibility between health and social services for those older people who are frail and have health needs, and the shift towards those with increasingly high levels of need being redefined as having primarily 'social', rather than 'health' needs, have continued and intensified in subsequent decades. (We will return to this theme in Chapter 6.)

In sum, therefore, although the National Assistance Act (1948) sought to improve the low status of those accommodated in institutions, it 'did little that was positive to destroy the old Poor Law traditions of institutional care' (Means and Smith 1998: 145). It continued to accept segregated institutions for older people and it did not challenge or change the attitudes of staff or the culture and practices within residential homes. Within local authority welfare departments, there were limited support services available for older people and social work with older people was regarded as low status work, often carried out by unqualified or inexperienced social workers or welfare assistants (Lymbery 1998).

The key themes identified in this review of the legacy of earlier policy for older people – assumptions about family responsibilities to 'care', the dominance of institutional models of care and blurred and shifting boundaries between health and social care – have proved resilient across the decades. The previous chapter discussed 'structured dependency' theories of ageing that see the experience of later life as an outcome of particular social and economic conditions. Townsend points to the connection between policy and service provision for older people and 'the engineering of retirement and mass poverty' (1981: 13). He argues that retirement and poverty restrict the resources, and therefore the opportunities, available to older people and shape the attitudes and expectations of professionals and older people themselves. The social construction of dependence in later life can help to account for the continued reliance on residential care for frail older people and enduring features in the nature of such provision. Thus Townsend writes of residential care:

> Socially, institutions are structured to serve the purpose of controlling
> inmates. The type and level of staffing, amenities and resources have been

developed not only in relation to the characteristics, including the perceived capacities, of inmates but also the roles staff expect inmates to play . . . The majority of residents in homes are placed in a category of enforced dependence. The routine of residential homes, made necessary by small staffs and economical administration, and committed to an ideology of 'care and attention' rather than the encouragement of self-help and self-management, seems to deprive many residents of the opportunity if not the incentive to occupy themselves and even of the means of communication.

(Townsend 1981: 19)

ACTIVITY 2.1: THE IMPACT OF RESEARCH ON POLICIES AND SERVICES

The work of Peter Townsend during the 1950s and 1960s played a significant part in highlighting the need for change in services for older people within the postwar Welfare State, as can be seen in two of his studies in this activity.

First, read the summaries below of two of Townsend's major studies:

The Last Refuge

This study was based on statistical information about homes and residents, visits to 173 residential institutions, resident questionnaires and interviews with welfare managers. It gave a stark and shocking picture of physical conditions in institutions, the lack of training, inadequate staff skills and the abysmal quality of life experienced by residents, with lack of privacy, isolation, boredom and loss of identity being commonplace. The following is an extract from Townsend's account of the conditions observed:

> The impression was grim and sombre. A high wall surrounded some tall Victorian buildings, and the entrance lay under a forbidding arch with a porter's lodge at one side. The asphalt yards were broken up by a few beds of flowers but there was no garden worthy of the name. Several hundred residents were housed in large rooms on three floors. Dormitories were overcrowded, with ten or twenty iron-framed beds close together, no floor covering and little furniture other than ramshackle lockers. The day-rooms were bleak and uninviting. In one of them sat 40 men in high-backed Windsor chairs, staring straight ahead or down at the floor. They seemed oblivious of what was going on around them.
>
> The sun was shining outside but no one was looking that way. Some were seated in readiness at the bare tables even though the midday meal was not to be served for over an hour . . . I was told, in justification of their inactivity, that 'although they sit and vegetate they have company. They can see other people. That's better than solitude

at home in one room. They're less lonely here.' Yet I noticed isolated persons sitting alone in a wash-room, standing in a corridor and one looking out of the staircase window weeping silently. In the day-rooms there was little conversation.

(Townsend [1962], reproduced in Bornat 1998: 10)

The Family Life of Old People

In this study, interviews were carried out with 203 older people in Bethnal Green, London, in the mid 1950s. The research revealed older people as active members of family networks, involved in reciprocal caring. Townsend argued that older people must therefore be seen and responded to by services within the context of their family networks, not as disconnected individuals:

> if many of the processes and problems of ageing are to be understood, old people must be studied as members of families (which usually means extended families of three generations): and if this is true, those concerned with health and social administration must, at every stage, treat old people as an inseparable part of a family group, which is more than just a residential unit. They are not simply individuals, let alone 'cases' occupying beds or chairs. They are members of families and whether or not they are treated as such largely determines their security, their health and their happiness.
>
> (Townsend [1957] reproduced in Phillipson *et al*. 2001: 20–21)

This study revealed that the majority of caring was undertaken by women, especially daughters. Townsend argued that, contrary to the widespread belief that extending support would undermine family responsibilities towards older people, services were needed to support family members who were finding it difficult to care for their older relatives and to support those without families to care for them. The study therefore challenged prevailing assumptions enshrined within policy: first, the notion of older people as passive and dependent and, second, the view that domiciliary services were dispensable and socially and politically inexpedient.

Now consider the following questions:

*   In what ways might these studies have been expected to have influenced policy and practice for older people?
*   What factors might have limited the impact of the research?
*   If the same studies were carried out now for the purposes of comparison, what changes/similarities would you anticipate in the findings and conclusions?

Despite the publication of Townsend's damning evidence in relation to the quality of residential care, Means and Smith comment, 'Perhaps the most striking feature of debates about residential care for elderly people after the publication of *The Last Refuge* was the complacency' (1998: 208). The official view prevailed that 'residential homes were homely places where the lonely and isolated could be brought to end their lives in companionship and friendship' (ibid.: 209). Continued belief in the benefits of residential care, despite evidence to the contrary, was no doubt partly influenced by the view that residential care was more efficient than domiciliary care in economic terms. The need for economic efficiency was located within concerns expressed during the mid- to late 1940s about the declining birth rate and increasing numbers of older people in the population. These arguments about the 'burden of dependency' represented by older people are graphically illustrated by a quotation from a Royal Commission Report (1949): 'The old consume without producing which differentiates them from the active population and makes of them a factor reducing the average standard of living of the community' (Royal Commission on Population 1949: 113, quoted in Means and Smith 1998: 212).

There was, therefore, no willingness within the post-war Welfare State to embark on policy changes that might lead to older people placing an even greater 'burden' on society. This tardiness in initiating and extending services was noted later on by the Seebohm Committee, which sat from 1965 to1968 to review the organisation and responsibilities of local authority social services (Seebohm Report 1968: para. 1). The Committee observed that the 'personal social services for old people in many areas remain underdeveloped, limited and patchy' and that the 'services have been provided though a variety of functions scattered through legislation' (ibid.: para. 293), the latter being an ongoing feature, as we shall see later in this chapter and in subsequent chapters. Although the Seebohm Committee stressed that local authorities should 'play the major part in the provision of the personal social services for old people', albeit with a 'role everywhere for the voluntary organisations' (ibid.: para. 301), even after the Local Authority Social Services Act (1970), which (based on the recommendations of the Seebohm Committee) created large generic social services departments from 1971 onwards, services for older people did not take a great leap forward. However, there were some changes. The NHS Act (1977) imposed a duty on local authorities to provide or arrange for the provision of home help for households where this was required 'owing to the presence of . . . "a person suffering from illness, lying-in, an expectant mother, aged, handicapped as a result of having suffered from illness or by congenital deformity"' (Mandelstam 2005). Despite some expansion in domiciliary support, residential care retained its dominance in social care provision for older people, who continued to be a low political priority and a low status client group (Means *et al.* 2002).

By the mid 1970s, an economic crisis dominated policy-making. High unemployment, low levels of economic growth and high inflation resulted in 'stagflation' (Zifcak 1994: 7–8), leading to public services often being portrayed as non-productive and a drain on the wealth-producing parts of the economy (Flynn 1993: xii). As a result, the post-war Welfare State came under siege and local authorities began looking for ways to achieve cutbacks in their spending (Harris, John 2003: 34–8). In this context, the first Conservative Government under Margaret Thatcher came to power in 1979, committed to radical reform of the post-war Welfare State. Services for older people were swept up in this agenda.

THE RESTRUCTURING OF SERVICES FOR OLDER PEOPLE: THE CONSERVATIVES' COMMUNITY CARE REFORMS

Arguably, it was primarily the economic concerns of the 1970s and 1980s that drove forward the community care reforms that were implemented in the early 1990s (Lewis, J. and Glennerster 1996). Economic pressures from the mid-1970s onwards, coupled with increased demands being made on services particularly by older people, led to increasing resource constraints and cutbacks in services (Walker 1993). In *A Happier Old Age*, a year before the election of the Conservative Government in 1979, the Labour Government reported concern about the increasing proportion of older people in the population, especially those aged over 75, and argued the need for policy to target community services to those in greatest need (Means *et al.* 2002). There were, then, arguments being put forward across the political spectrum about stemming the rising costs of services. These arguments were crystallised in an Audit Commission report, *Making a Reality of Community Care* (Audit Commission 1986), which identified as a particular concern the increased spending on residential care for adult service users, under arrangements introduced by the Conservative Government in 1980. These arrangements meant that the social security system paid the board and lodging costs of people with assets under £3,000. In many circumstances, the easiest service provision to arrange for an older person who needed day-to-day support was a place in a private residential home at central government's expense. As well as opening up this avenue for use by relatives of older people, there was what the Audit Commission described as a 'perverse incentive' for local authorities to place people receiving income support from social security in residential and nursing homes, where their care would be funded by central government, rather than to support them living in the community, when the costs would fall on local authorities themselves. The fragmentation of organisations involved in providing community care and the lack of coordination of resources were other areas of concern.

In response, the Conservative Government commissioned a review undertaken by Sir Roy Griffiths, which was delivered in his report, *Community Care: An Agenda for Action* (Griffiths Report 1988). Griffiths recommended that social services should have the lead role in assessing need and planning and coordinating services, including those provided by the private and voluntary sectors. It was proposed that the perverse incentive to use residential care should be removed by transferring funding from the social security system to social services, and by imposing an assessment 'gateway' for those needing to access this funding. This was intended to establish greater control over the finances committed to residential care and to use the resources transferred to open up greater possibilities for developing community-based alternatives. (The concerns regarding poor coordination of services and resources were to be addressed by means of care management, which will be considered later in the chapter.)

Following on from the Griffiths Report, the White Paper, *Caring for People: Community Care in the Next Decade and Beyond* (Department of Health 1989), was explicit in stating that one of the objectives of community care policy was to secure better value for money. It incorporated the recommendations contained in the Griffiths Report that social services should assess individual need, design tailor-made packages of care and ensure appropriate service provision by acting as enablers rather than care providers. The White Paper also reflected the political objective of restricting the role of local authorities by requiring them to stimulate what became known as the 'mixed economy of care', that is, providing services by a mixture of statutory, private and voluntary sector agencies, alongside support for informal carers. The stated objectives of *Caring for People* were:

- to promote development of domiciliary, day and respite care to enable people to live in their own homes;
- to provide support for carers;
- to make proper assessment of need and good case management 'the cornerstone of high quality care';
- to promote a flourishing independent sector;
- to clarify the responsibilities of agencies, especially between NHS and local authorities;
- to secure better value for money.

(Department of Health 1989)

There has always been a mixture of provision between the state, the market, the voluntary sector and informal carers and in this respect the mixed economy of care was not new. However, the community care reforms reflected a significant shift in the role of the state from an institutional to a residual one (Mayo 1994). In particular, the state's role changed from that of 'provider' to the roles of 'enabler' and 'purchaser' (Wistow *et al.* 1996), mirroring developments occurring in the fields of health, housing and education. Key to achieving this shift in community care provision was the separation of assessment of need from the provision of services. Although neither the legislation nor the policy guidance required local authorities to organise according to what was referred to as 'the purchaser–provider split', it did state that the functions of assessment and direct service provision needed to be clearly distinguished (Department of Health 1990: 37–8). The stated rationale for this distinction was to free the process of determining the appropriate provision to meet need from service considerations and to enable private and voluntary sector providers to compete on equal terms with those provided in-house by the local authority. The 'mixed economy of care' was presented as a way of improving standards through introducing competition. Stimulation of the mixed economy was ensured by the stipulation that 85 per cent of monies transferred to local authorities from central government in the form of a 'special transitional grant' had to be spent on services provided by the independent sector (Department of Health 1992). A further rationale for the reforms was the empowerment of service users and carers through their new status as 'consumers' of services (White and Harris 1999). The care market was represented as enabling them to exercise increased choice and control over the services they received, with the right of redress through new complaints procedures (Department of Health 1990). (The extent to which these objectives have been achieved will be considered in Chapters 3 and 4, which examine practice issues in relation to community care assessment and service provision.)

The NHS and Community Care Act (1990), which followed the *Caring for People* White Paper, was not fully implemented until April 1993. Section 47 of the Act set out the 'gateway' to community care services, namely, the duty of local authorities to assess an individual's need for services. The NHS and Community Care Act (1990) was accompanied by policy guidance, *Community Care in the Next Decade and Beyond* (Department of Health 1990). There were also two further guidance documents, published alongside the Act, one for practitioners and one for managers, detailing how the changes should be implemented locally and, in particular, the arrangements to be made for assessment and care management (Social Services Inspectorate/Department of Health 1991a and 1991b).

Care management

Although assessment and care management were put forward as the processes through which key policy objectives were to be achieved, there was no common understanding in the legislation or policy guidance about what care management meant (Lewis, J. and Glennerster 1996: 42). Originally called case management, care management was based on a model of service provision developed in North America. Research on how the model could be developed and applied in the UK was carried out by the Personal Social Service Research Unit (PSSRU) at the University of Kent. The PSSRU evaluated a number of pilot projects. These included a project in Kent concerned with evaluating intensive home-based care as an alternative to the admission of older people to residential care (Challis and Davies 1986) and a project in Darlington concerned with evaluating schemes to facilitate the discharge of older people from hospital (Challis *et al.* 1990). There were also a further 28 community care projects focused on the discharge of people from long-stay hospital care and their resettlement in the community. Common to all of the projects was the use of care management as a process for matching needs with resources. A quasi-experimental design was used in the studies, with a comparison of individuals receiving the care management approach with matched control groups. Evaluation encompassed both cost-effectiveness and care process issues. The overall framework of the projects was the 'production of welfare' model, adopted and adapted from economic theories of production (Knapp 1984; Challis and Davies 1986; Davies and Knapp 1988; Davies *et al.* 1990). Within this production model, care management is a process that is explicitly concerned with managing the tension between need, on the one hand, and limited resources, on the other. It is defined as

> the point at which welfare objectives and resource constraints are closest together. Therefore care management has a pivotal role as the setting where the integration of social and economic criteria must occur at the level of service provision, where the balancing of needs and resources, scarcity and choice must take place.
>
> (Challis 1994: 1–2)

Understanding care management in these terms helps to make sense of the conflicts and constraints that social workers experience at the level of practice. (These issues will be discussed in Chapters 3 and 4.)

ACTIVITY 2.2: REALISING GAINS FROM SPECIAL PROJECTS

Read the following information about the Kent Community Care Scheme, one of the pilot schemes evaluated by PSSRU.

The aim of the intervention was to prevent admission of frail older people to residential care and the outcomes of the pilot project were compared with a comparison group receiving a standard service. Key features of the project were:

- a carefully selected target group of older people – those on the threshold of residential care;
- experienced workers with continuing responsibility for small caseloads;
- decentralised budgets managed by care managers and based on up to two-thirds of the costs of residential care;
- a knowledge by care managers of service unit costs and costing of care packages;
- individually constructed care packages that interwove formal and informal care.

A number of positive findings were reported from the project:

- Reduction of the need for institutional care: the older people receiving case management showed a lower rate of admission to both residential care and long-term hospital care after twelve months. This reduction was found to remain over the subsequent three years. The project was taken as indicating that 'at least for some cases, the new approach should be more cost-effective than the usual range of services' (Challis and Davies 1986: 219).
- Closer matching of resources to needs: in the case managed group, resources were seen to be more closely matched to needs than in the comparison group, with those individuals deemed most dependent receiving higher levels of provision.
- Improvements in quality of life: various measures were used to demonstrate that there were also improvements in quality of life and subjective well-being for both older people and carers receiving case management.
- Synthesis of 'care' and 'management': case management was seen as facilitating a synthesis of social work roles and tasks, encompassing both 'indirect activity', for example, the coordination and monitoring of care, as well as 'direct work' in the form of tasks such as assessment, support and counselling. One reported outcome of the scheme was the building of social support through the close confiding relationships developed between older people, their community care helpers and social workers.
- Flexibility: the approach allowed a variety of responses to different problems, though both individual worker and organisational obstacles to innovative intervention were noted.
- Support for care networks: the case management approach was found to be more sensitive to the care network as a whole, with formal services provided through the project complementing, but not substituting for, informal care.
- Meeting of new needs: it was also reported that case management enabled new needs to be met. There was found to be an improvement in 'horizontal target

efficiency' (ibid.: 13), that is, more proactive 'reaching out' of the service so that needs were met that would not have been addressed by a standard service response. In addition, under case management workers made efforts to do more than provide basic services but focused also on enhancing subjective well-being and meeting therapeutic objectives.

Now think about these questions:

- Based on your reading and/or experience of care management practice, to what extent are the gains that were reported from the Kent project achieved in current community care practice with older people?
- In areas where you think the reported gains are not being realised in practice, why do you think this is? Think about the conditions of, and criteria for, the project, as well as barriers in current practice that were not faced by the pilot project.

The PSSRU's positive findings from the pilot projects were taken as evidence that similar gains could be achieved if care management was adopted nationally. However, this seems questionable given key differences in the circumstances pertaining to the pilot projects and those in mainstream care management practice (Petch 1996). As outlined above, older people included in the experimental group were carefully targeted and questions have been raised about whether too many frail people – the very people at whom care management was primarily directed after the community care reforms – were filtered out (Means et al. 2003). Equally, one criterion for excluding cases from the community care project in Kent was that the older person was 'insufficiently needy' (Challis and Davies 1986: 17). This suggests the positive findings emanated from a tightly defined sample of candidates deemed suitable for care management. Indeed, the need for careful targeting of intensive care management was emphasised by the projects. While care management could reduce the use of residential care for certain service users, for others with lower level needs it was pointed out that it could lead to increased costs (Challis and Davies 1986).

After the implementation of the NHS and Community Care Act (1990), rather than being a targeted response to particular types of need and situations, care management tended to be applied to all adult service users accessing services. In 1997, the Annual Report of the Chief Social Services Inspector noted that local authorities were failing to differentiate between different levels of intervention, with all service users in need of services receiving care management in many authorities. The report recommended three distinct types of care management: administrative, where the need was for advice or information; coordinating, where a single service or straightforward response was required; and intensive, where planning and coordination of services needed to be combined with supportive or therapeutic objectives. The latter was seen as a response that would apply to a small number of service users with complex or changing needs (Department of Health 1997a: para. 3.4).

In addition to the lack of targeting of care management as a process, there are other differences between the features of the pilot projects and mainstream care management practice. The pilot projects tended to involve highly motivated staff given preferential workloads and extra resources, features not typical of the general care management system introduced after the implementation of the NHS and Community Care Act (1990). Considerable emphasis was given in reports of the PSSRU research to the significance of care managers having control over resources in the pilot projects:

> It is the capacity to influence both the type and content of service available that permits genuine individualisation of care . . . The devolution of budgets to individual case managers would seem to be a crucial element of the development of more responsive patterns of care.
>
> (Challis 1994: 14–15)

The pilot project reports struck some notes of caution about whether devolving control of resources to the level of front-line workers could be achieved in mainstream local authority structures, without the introduction of controls that would lead to 'excessive routinisation and loss of flexibility' (Challis and Davies 1986: 224).

In summary, then, while the PSSRU projects demonstrated the effectiveness of care management, this was under particular conditions, not all of which were characteristic of care management as later developed in community care practice after the Conservatives' reforms. The researchers themselves emphasised that care management would benefit certain types of users in certain types of situations with certain conditions in place. These included: careful targeting of older people on the margins of residential care; trained and experienced workers with continuing case responsibility, small caseloads and devolved budgets; the clear costing of care packages; and close working relationships with health services (Chesterman et al. 1994). A later reanalysis of the care management model in the pilot projects found strong support for its effectiveness, but subject to the preconditions of staff having sufficient time to implement it, being trained in the requisite skills and being given adequate control of budgets to allow flexibility and the best use of resources (Davies et al. 1996).

THE MAINSTREAM MODEL OF CARE MANAGEMENT

As we have seen, the NHS and Community Care Act (1990) was accompanied by detailed guidance for managers and practitioners that contained a shared summary (Social Services Inspectorate/Department of Health 1991a and 1991b). This guidance emphasised that care management is a process for tailoring services to individual need:

> Care management and assessment constitute one integrated process for identifying and addressing the needs of individuals within available resources, recognising that those needs are unique to the individuals concerned. For this reason, care management and assessment emphasise adapting services to needs rather than fitting people into existing services, and dealing with the needs of individuals as a whole rather than assessing needs separately for different services.
>
> (Social Services Inspectorate/Department of Health 1991a and 1991b: para. 3)

Two key components within this description of the assessment and care management process are first, that assessment is to focus holistically on the unique individual needs of the person concerned; and second, that assessment of need is to be kept distinct from preoccupation with what services might be available. A contribution at the time of the reforms explains what was to be involved in a shift away from what was described as 'the traditional view of assessment':

> Assessment has, for many years, been the method used by professionals to determine whether people meet the criteria for a particular service. Different assessment formats exist, but essentially they all act as a 'sifting' process, by identifying those most vulnerable. The focus, therefore, was to use assessment as a gatekeeper to the resources, be it home help, meals on wheels and residential accommodation.
>
> The emphasis of the National Health Service and Community Care Act is on moving away from this service-led assessment, where the assessor begins with a set of criteria for services and decides how the person fits in. This approach to assessment begins by taking a look at the needs of the individual. The assessment ensures that the individual client is placed at the centre of the process in order for their needs to be met.
>
> (Myers and Crawford 1993: 125)

(The central concept of 'need' within assessment will be discussed further in Chapter 3.)

The assessment and care management process is described as circular and comprising seven distinct stages: the publishing of information, determination of the level of assessment, assessment, care planning, implementation of the care plan, monitoring and review.

The stage of determining the level of assessment, along with that of publishing information, occurs outside of the circular process formed by the other five stages, as shown in Figure 2.1 (Social Services Inspectorate/Department of Health 1991a and 1991b). At the stage of determining the level of assessment, some referrals will be screened out of the process altogether, if the referred need is seen as not requiring social work assessment. How need is defined and interpreted at this stage of the process is therefore of crucial significance in terms of the eventual service response. (Specific issues regarding screening and assessment in practice will be discussed in Chapter 3.)

ACTIVITY 2.3: FRAGMENTING THE PROCESS OF ASSESSMENT AND CARE MANAGEMENT

As we have seen, assessment and care management guidance outlined the need to distinguish the different stages of the care management process, in particular to keep assessment separate from consideration of what services might be available. As care management practice has developed over time, the functional distinction of tasks has tended to lead to increasing organisational separation. The tasks of assessment, care plan implementation, monitoring and review have become increasingly fragmented in terms of the worker, team and/or agency responsible for carrying them out. For example, many councils have separate teams of reviewing officers who review care plans.

What are the implications of the responsibility for different stages of the care management process being carried out by different workers, teams and, perhaps, agencies? Consider this from the perspectives of:

- the council with social services responsibilities;
- the social worker/care manager;
- the older person using the services.

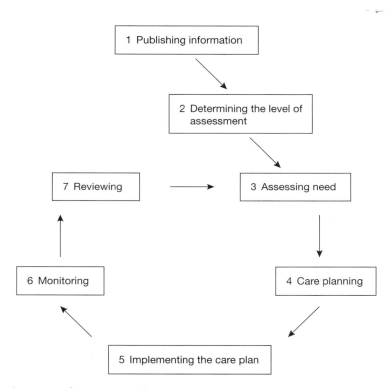

FIGURE 2.1 The process of assessment and care management

The Conservatives' reforms of community care had been in operation for four years when the Labour Government came to power in 1997.

POLICY FOR OLDER PEOPLE UNDER NEW LABOUR

It has been argued that 'there can scarcely have been a time when policy interest in the quality of provision of health and social care services for older people has attracted greater interest' (Reed *et al.* 2004: 170). This is, of course, related to the intensification of existing concerns about demographic factors and the potential demands that the increasing proportion of older people in the population, particularly those aged 85 and over, will make on society in the coming decades. For example, it is projected that while there will be overall population growth of 10 per cent in the next 20 years in England, the number of people aged 85 and over will increase by two-thirds (Wanless 2006). In this context, New Labour's policy in respect of older people will be discussed in relation to three themes: the exercise of central control over standard setting and monitoring of outcomes; promotion of the need to intervene in ways that will maximise older people's independence in order to reduce the need for high cost services in the longer term; and the introduction of organisational and procedural arrangements to ensure that organisations work together to provide a coherent and coordinated response to older people's needs.

Standards and outcomes

The 'top down' imposition of standards, targets and requirements to direct organisations to the delivery of defined objectives has been one of the hallmarks of New Labour (Jordan and Jordan 2000; Harris, John 2003: Ch.5). It has placed great emphasis on seeking to control policy outcomes as one of its key strategies in seeking 'modernisation' of services. Specific policy initiatives are intertwined with, and evaluated by, audit, inspection and review, resulting in a high level of regulatory activity. In effect, civil servants and central government ministers dictate priorities at the local level in order to ensure that social services organisations deliver New Labour's agenda, with detailed stipulations about the management of practice. The proliferation of regulation since New Labour came to power has resulted in a high degree of uncertainty and instability as local authorities await judgements on their performance through rating systems and league tables, especially in relation to the annual publication of their overall level of performance as measured by the 'star ratings' awarded by the Commission for Social Care Inspection. The pressures of being constantly accountable in this way are amplified by changing demands and indicators. What were previously seen as questions of professional standards, are now seen as management processes (Jones, C. 1999: 4), which need to be subjected to the 'independent evaluative practice' of audit (Clarke *et al.* 2000: 253).

The increase in direction from central government can be seen in the publication of the *National Service Framework for Older People* (Department of Health 2001a).

BOX 2.1   NATIONAL SERVICE FRAMEWORK FOR OLDER PEOPLE (DEPARTMENT OF HEALTH 2001A)

The National Service Framework (NSF) sets out eight standards for the care of older people across health and social services, applicable in all settings. It specifies the aims, the standard, rationale, key interventions, milestones and targets in relation to each standard.

Standard 1: Rooting out age discrimination

NHS services will be provided, regardless of age, on the basis of clinical need alone. Social care services will not use age, in their eligibility criteria or policies, to restrict access to available services.

Standard 2: Providing person-centred care

NHS and social care services treat older people as individuals and enable them to make choices about their own care. This is achieved through the single assessment process, integrated commissioning arrangements and integrated provision of services, including community equipment and continence services.

Standard 3: Intermediate care

Older people will have access to a new range of intermediate care services at home or in their designated care settings, to promote their independence by providing enhanced services from the NHS and councils to prevent unnecessary hospital admission and effective rehabilitation services to enable early discharge from hospital and to prevent premature or unnecessary admission to long-term residential care.

Standard 4: General hospital care

Older people's care in hospital is delivered through appropriate specialist care and by hospital staff who have the right set of skills to meet their needs.

Standard 5: Stroke

The NHS will take action to prevent strokes, working in partnership with other agencies where appropriate. People who are thought to have had a stroke have access to diagnostic services, are treated appropriately by a specialist stroke service, and subsequently, with their carers, participate in a multidisciplinary programme of secondary prevention and rehabilitation.

Standard 6: Falls

The NHS, working in partnership with councils, takes action to prevent falls and reduce resultant fractures or other injuries in their populations of older people. Older people who have fallen receive effective treatment and, with their carers, receive advice on prevention through a specialised falls service.

Standard 7: Mental health in older people

Older people who have mental health problems have access to integrated mental health services, provided by the NHS and councils to ensure effective diagnosis, treatment and support, for them and for their carers.

Standard 8: The promotion of health and active life in older age

The health and well-being of older people is promoted through a coordinated programme of action led by the NHS with support from councils.

This sets out national standards for the health and social care of older people in England (see Box 2.1) and a ten-year programme for improving services. (National Service Frameworks have also been developed for a number of other service areas, including mental health and children's services.) Although some of the standards relate more directly to health services, the standards concerning tackling age discrimination, the provision of person-centred care and the promotion of health and active life in older age are important for social work with older people in all contexts. A mid-way review of progress in meeting the NSF standards noted that although there had been progress, there was a need for continued improvement in certain areas. In particular, the progress report drew attention to the need for health and social care services to do more to address age discrimination within services and to increase their sensitivity to issues of diversity. A number of recommendations were also made concerning the need for improvements in partnership working between the different services involved with older people's well-being (Healthcare Commission *et al.* 2006). Following the progress review, a document setting out the 'next steps' in implementing the *National Service Framework* was published (Department of Health 2006a). The programmes to be developed are located under three themes: promoting dignity in care (including end of life care); enhancing 'joined-up' care, for example, in the areas of stroke care, falls services and mental health services; and promoting healthy ageing. These areas are related to targets (Public Service Agreement Targets) that are set by the government for health and social care.

Whilst the *National Service Framework for Older People* can be seen as an attempt to improve older people's access to services and the quality of services, it has been argued that the standards emphasise equity of access at the expense of responsiveness to diverse needs (Estes *et al.* 2003). The agenda for change presented is both fixed and restricted:

> There is . . . a focus on the distribution of existing resources within systems. This has the dual disadvantage of tacitly accepting the parameters of what is already available, and tending to overlook the micro interactions of power and hierarchy that perpetuate the daily realities generated by the systems themselves.
>
> (Estes *et al.* 2003: 83)

Promoting independence

Throughout the 1990s, the pattern in community care services was to focus increasingly on supporting those with high levels of need, as evident from Department of Health statistics. Since 1993, that is, just prior to full implementation of NHS and Community Care Act (1990), the number of home care contact hours provided by councils has doubled (National Statistics 2006a). However, there has also been a steady decrease in the number of households receiving home care since 1993. In other words, the increase in the number of home care hours provided combined with the decrease in the number of households receiving help indicates that a smaller number of people overall are receiving help but this involves higher levels of input. There has been a steady increase in the proportion of households receiving six or more visits and more than five hours of home care contact per week from 12 per cent in 1993 to 48 per cent in

2005. On the other hand, there has been a decrease in the proportion of households receiving just one visit of two hours or less per week from 37 per cent in 1993 to 12 per cent in 2005. This trend continues year on year. In 2005, the average number of contact hours per household per week was 10.1, compared with 9.4 in 2004 and 7 hours in 2000 (ibid.) These trends reflect the priority placed by councils on supporting those with high level needs to live at home, as required by central government targets, but this is achieved at the expense of those with lower levels of support needs.

There has been growing recognition of the need for a shift in policy and practice towards more proactive preventive intervention in order to avert the continuous 'vicious circle' resulting from the focus on those in crisis (Audit Commission 1997). The White Paper, *Modernising Social Services*, set out its vision that social services are 'for all of us' (para. 1.1) and not just for 'a small number of social casualties' (para. 1.3) (Department of Health 1998a). It announced a new prevention grant to enable people to 'do things for themselves as long as possible, in their own home' (para. 2.12). However, prevention is an ambiguous concept; there are multiple perspectives on what exactly is to be prevented, how this is to be achieved and the desired outcomes (Godfrey 2001). One facet of prevention, and arguably the concern on which prevention grants were founded (Nolan 2000), is preventing the need for more costly services. Another facet is promoting the quality of life of older people and their engagement in communities (Wistow and Lewis 1997). More recent policy initiatives appear to embrace a more positive understanding of prevention as promoting well-being and quality of life. For example, standard eight of the *National Service Framework for Older People* is concerned with the promotion of health and active life in old age (Department of Health 2001a – and see above). A report by the Association of Directors of Social Services argues for 'radical steps, rather than tinkering round the edges' if significant improvements in older people's quality of life are to be achieved (Association of Directors of Social Services 2003: Foreword). The Association of Directors of Social Services (ADSS) proposals are based on shifting from a concentration on acute services for a smaller number of people with severe needs to a wider community focus on universal services to promote well-being in order to 'invert the triangle of care' (see Figure 2.2).

Similarly, an Audit Commission summary of five reports relating to older people and independence highlights the need for 'a fundamental shift in the way we think about older people, from dependency and deficit towards independence and well-being' (2004: 3). It argues for a strategic approach based on increasing older people's choice and control, proactively promoting health and well-being, adopting a whole-person approach and building a whole-systems response (p. 17).

As we have already noted, within the policy discourse on prevention there has been a shift from the language of prevention – a concern to stop negative events or situations from happening – to a more positive approach based on promoting well-being. This involves identifying the factors that are significant to older people in maintaining a good quality of life and building on the strengths and resources contained in their personal, family and community networks (Joseph Rowntree Foundation 2004). One aspect of this emphasis on strengths is that consultation with service users formed part of the process in formulating the Green Paper on Adult Social Care, *Independence, Well-being and Choice: Our Vision for the Future of Social Care for Adults in England* (Department of Health 2005a). The Green Paper, which concerned all adult social care users, not just older people, reinforced the shift in policy from a focus on dependency

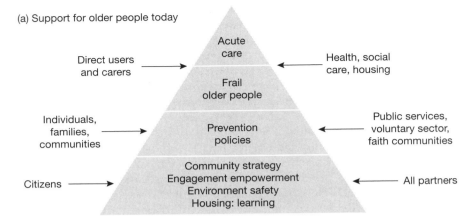

(a) Support for older people today

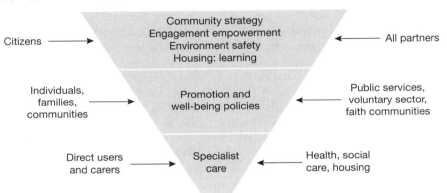

(b) Support for older people tomorrow

FIGURE 2.2 Inverting the triangle of care

Source: Local Government Association/Association of Directors of Social Services 2003: 9

and need to broader concerns with well-being and quality of life. It set out 'a radical vision for the future of adult social care in England':

> we want to move from a system where people have to take what is offered to one where people have greater control over identifying the type of support or help they want and more choice about and influence over the services on offer. We plan to do this by giving everyone better information and signposting of services, putting people at the centre of the assessment process and creating individual budgets that give them greater freedom to select the type of care or support they want.
>
> (Department of Health 2005a: para. 4.2)

A number of key areas were outlined in the Green Paper:

- Setting clear outcomes for social care: improved health; improved quality of life; making a positive contribution; exercise of choice and control; freedom from discrimination or harassment; economic well-being; and personal dignity.
- Putting people in control by making greater use of self-assessment, introducing individualised budgets (where the local authority holds the budget but the individual chooses how to spend it) and increasing the use of direct payments. (These schemes are discussed in Chapter 4.)
- Providing better support for people accessing services, for example through a care navigator, a care broker, a person-centred planning facilitator, and/or a care manager.
- Improving access to universal services.
- Shifting the balance from meeting high level needs to earlier preventive interventions.
- Improving integrated partnership working between agencies.
- Strengthening engagement in local communities and building capacity in the voluntary and community sectors, for example through time banks.
- Improving the design and delivery of services and developing or building on new models of care, for example extra care housing, homeshare and telecare.
- Appointment of a director of adult services with a key strategic and leadership role in ensuring that the social care needs of local communities are managed in a way that coordinates services provided by a wide range of agencies.

However, the Green Paper's stance – that the proposed changes did not require additional funding but could be financed by making better use of existing funding – was seen as unfeasible by a number of commentators and interest groups (see, for example, Local Government Association 2005). The subsequent White Paper, *Our Health, Our Care, Our Say: A New Direction for Community Services* (Department of Health 2006b) takes forward the Green Paper's emphasis on prevention and earlier intervention, though the document as a whole is more oriented towards health than social care. A series of pilot projects to test and develop approaches to delivering the White Paper's objectives have been established and will be evaluated (Department of Health 2006c). One set of projects are the *Partnerships for Older People Projects*, designed to explore how different partnership arrangements can lead to improved outcomes for older people (see Box 2.2).

BOX 2.2 PARTNERSHIPS FOR OLDER PEOPLE PROJECTS (POPPS)

In 2005, the Department of Health announced ring-fenced funding available for pilot projects that would 'provide truly integrated preventative approaches for local older people across the whole system' (Department of Health 2006d: 2.1). The first round of projects came into

continued

operation in 2006, with a second round of applications and funding for projects to commence in 2007. Councils with Social Services Responsibilities are appointed leads of the projects but their applications must reflect full partnerships with Primary Care Trusts and other health partners, the voluntary, community and independent sectors and older people. The aim of the projects (second round) is to:

- provide person-centred and integrated responses for older people; and
- encourage investment in approaches that promote health, well-being and independence for older people and thereby prevent or delay the need for higher intensity or institutionalised care.

(Department of Health 2006d: 4.1)

A requirement of any application for funding is that older people are involved in developing the proposals and in delivering and evaluating the projects. Proposals are asked to comment on how projects will address the needs of those older people who are often excluded from services.

The application guidance makes clear that projects should be oriented to delivering 'large scale, systemic reform with the aim of releasing funding from across the whole system for reinvestment in preventative approaches to care' (Department of Health 2006d: 4.2). There is an emphasis on establishing partnership mechanisms and sustainability. The projects run for up to two years and it is expected that after this time successful approaches will become part of mainstream provision.

(Department of Health 2006d)

Closely linked with the policy goal of promoting the independence and well-being of older people is the objective of reducing costs. This raises some of the same conflicts that were inherent in the contradictory objectives of the Conservatives' community care reforms, discussed earlier in the chapter, that is the aim of carrying out assessments that were 'needs-led' at the same time as containing resources. The conflation of well-being and cost-effectiveness objectives is apparent, for example, in the report setting out the 'next steps' for the *National Service Framework* (discussed earlier). The introduction to the report spells out the dual and related objectives that underpin New Labour's policy for older people: 'Not only can we improve outcomes for older people's health, independence and well-being. We can also save money by reducing the overall demand for expensive hospital and long-term care services' (Department of Health 2006a: 3).

However, the idea that it is possible to improve the independence and well-being of older people at the same time as achieving cost savings, at least in the short and medium terms, is questionable. It is more likely that if there is a substantial investment in resources to improve well-being now, then this may reap benefits in terms of reducing the need for high cost services several years later. In the meantime, investment in well-being *and* at the same time continued investment in services for those with 'high level' needs would be required. Referring back to the diagrams in Figure 2.2, this means that in the short term, at least, resources would need to be directed at all levels of the triangle before any gradual inversion of the triangle could be achieved. A review by

Derek Wanless concluded that the evidence base for the cost-effectiveness of preventive services for older people is weak (Wanless 2006). However, there is substantial evidence of the potential of community care services to enhance subjective well-being (Quilgars 2000). Wanless argued that considerable additional resources are needed to fund good quality care for the growing number of older people in the population and he proposed different models of funding social care. He pointed out that decisions about levels and methods of funding are essentially value-based choices (Wanless 2006). In a climate where the social and economic 'burden' of providing for older people is often stressed, this is an important reminder that restrictive policies are not inevitable. Policies reflect values and the choices made are based on those values.

Developing a coordinated strategy and joined up services

One of the important themes to emerge from New Labour's *Better Government for Older People* programme was the need for greater coordination of strategy and services (Better Government for Older People 2000). One aspect of this that is of particular relevance to social work with older people has been the range of changes under New Labour that have sought to facilitate more effective working relationships between health and social services. It is only possible to provide a brief summary of the key dimensions of these extensive changes here. The Health Act (1999) Section 31 introduced 'flexibilities' whereby health and social services could pool their budgets, designate a lead commissioner for particular services and share resources, including staff, in meeting their statutory obligations. Further impetus for joint working came in the Health and Social Care Act (2001), which provided for the setting up of joint Health and Social Care Trusts. (More detailed discussion of these changes can be found in Glasby and Littlechild [2004]. Specific examples of the interface between health and social work at the level of practice will be discussed in Chapter 6.)

A central theme within New Labour's health and social care policy is the need for a coordinated and joined up strategy between all key agencies, not just health and social services (Better Government for Older People 2000; Hayden and Boaz 2000). There are at least seven different governmental departments with responsibility for services that are highly significant for older people (Department for Work and Pensions 2005). An overarching strategy to meet the needs of an ageing population structure is set out in the Labour Government's *Opportunity Age* document (ibid.). Like the initiatives mentioned previously, this also stresses 'active ageing' and measures to support older people's independence. It sets out a comprehensive programme that encompasses a range of measures to improve the lives of older people, addressing, for example: age discrimination; employment, learning and leisure opportunities; welfare benefit reforms; crime reduction programmes; housing standards; access to public transport; public health; tackling inequalities, for example, those associated with rural living and with ethnicity. The report outlines a coordinated strategy for the whole of the UK but it is accepted that there will be differences of policy and practice in England, Scotland, Wales and Northern Ireland. For example, while leadership on the strategy in England rests with the Department for Work and Pensions, in Wales the Commissioner for Older People (Wales) Act (2006) legislates for the appointment of an Older People's Commissioner. As well as indicating an overall national direction, *Opportunity Age* sets out arrangements to provide local strategic direction, for example, through Local Area Agreements that allow relevant agencies to work together flexibly in providing integrated services.

The need for a holistic 'joined up' approach to enhance older people's social participation and well-being is addressed further in a Social Exclusion Unit report on inequalities and older people, *A Sure Start to Later Life* (Office of the Deputy Prime Minister 2006). Drawing on work by Barnes *et al.* (2006), the report considers seven areas of exclusion faced by older people:

- **social relationships,** for example, with family or friends;
- **cultural activities,** for example, going to the cinema or theatre;
- **civic activities,** for example, carrying out voluntary work or voting;
- **access to basic services,** for example, shops and health services;
- **neighbourhood,** for example, feelings of safety in the local area;
- **financial products,** for example, having a bank account or savings;
- **material consumption,** for example, being able to afford certain household goods or an annual holiday.

(Office of the Deputy Prime Minister 2006: 26)

The report sets out a model and principles based on the Sure Start approach already developed in children's services. This involves creating a single gateway to access a wide range of services in a local area:

> It will not be just about better social services, which is often seen as the service responsible for older people, but comprehensive services that can empower older people and improve quality of life. The Sure Start approach is designed to address this and is part of building inclusive communities where older people themselves are leading change.
>
> (ibid.: 9)

A range of services is seen as relevant to this agenda (see Figure 2.3).

ACTIVITY 2.4: REALISING THE VISION?

- What are the main features of New Labour's vision of services for older people?
- What are some of the main obstacles to achieving this vision?

Taking stock

New Labour thinking and policies have extended and developed, rather than radically changed, aspects of the reforms instituted by the previous Conservative Governments (Jordan and Jordan 2000; Harris, John 2003: ch. 5). In particular, a belief in the 'mixed economy of care' has been retained, but with a new emphasis on central regulation and

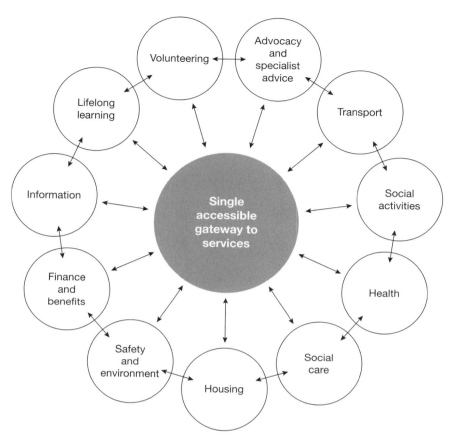

FIGURE 2.3 Sure Start for older people
Source: Office of the Deputy Prime Minister 2006: 26

control to monitor and enforce standards. There has also been a shift in the way individual service users are constructed, from consumers with limited, largely procedural, rights in the welfare market, to citizens with responsibilities as well as rights (Harris, John 1999; 2002), as can be seen in policy documents such as *Building a Better Britain for Older People* (Inter-Ministerial Group on Older People 1998). An example of this shift is provided by New Labour's preventive agenda's insistence that 'the primary responsibility for keeping active and participating in communities lies with older people themselves' (Department for Work and Pensions 2005: 30). These changes are significant for both service users and social workers, when set against the context of the historical development of services for older people, outlined earlier:

> A new and individualized approach to welfare policy and service delivery has emerged where the *primary* responsibility for managing social and economic risks facing individuals and families is devolved from the . . . state to the individual and his or her social worker or welfare worker . . . As a consequence of this devolution, the outcome of policies are now dependent,

more than ever before, on how they are implemented by those responsible
for working with service users.

(McDonald 2006: 22, *emphasis original*)

The drive for individuals to take responsibility for their own welfare, rather than
relying on the state, is compounded by the throwing into question of the former
'intergenerational contract' (Walker 1996), based on assumptions that younger people
would, through their taxes, support older people, and then, in their turn, would be
supported by the next generation. In the same way that the advent of state retirement
pensions and the Welfare State in the 1940s affirmed the categorisation and status of
'old age', such fundamental changes now pose new challenges to older people, making
their identities more fluid and uncertain (Estes *et al.* 2003). However, Biggs *et al.* (2006)
argue that in recent social policy, such as *Opportunity Age*, there is evidence of identities
becoming fixed in new ways. In particular, they argue that a specifically 'old age' identity
is being eroded by policies such as *Opportunity Age*, which refer to those in their 50s
as 'older people'. Accordingly, old age is amalgamated with other stages of the adult
life course, with an assumption that, for older people as for others, work is the central
source of personal meaning and social engagement:

> In policy terms, a picture is painted of a sameness of quality and aspiration
> across different age-groups, a tendency to assume that adults of different ages
> desire the same forms of social participation and self-development, plus,
> a levelling down of the diversity of social experience to the workplace.
>
> (Biggs *et al.* 2006: 248)

This echoes the argument presented in Chapter 1 that denial of age-based differences
is in itself ageist, creating barriers, limiting opportunities and constraining self and
social identities in much the same way as occurs when older people are seen only in terms
of their age.

As well as an underlying concern with employment, New Labour policy also
reflects a continuing concern with what is seen as older people's potential drain
on financial resources. There is a contradiction between these two discourses, one
concerned to promote an 'active ageing' view of the ever-youthful older person and the
other preoccupied with the costs associated with 'dependent' and frail older people.
As we saw in Chapter 1, neither view captures the complexity and diversity of older
people's experiences and perspectives. Both constructions are ageist; indeed, it seems
that ageism remains rife within social policy. Despite the emphasis in New Labour's
policy initiatives on improving services for older people, they remain a low priority
group within health and social care provision overall. While there have been a plethora
of policy developments concerned with enabling older people to remain in their own
homes, these have yet to have a significant impact on the lives of many older people with
health and social care needs who, as we shall see in the next two chapters, too often
experience difficulty accessing the support services they require.

One of the criticisms Means *et al.* (2002) put forward of policy developments in
respect of older people since New Labour came to government in 1997 is that the central
political concern driving developments is with resources, in particular protecting acute
hospital services, rather than a central focus on the quality of life of older people. Others
support the view that cost-effectiveness concerns overwhelm the emphasis on older

people's quality of life (Nolan 2000). Means *et al.* (2002) argue that the objectives set for social care services for older people are unrealistic without significant increases in funding. The Social Policy on Ageing Information Network (SPAIN) has examined progress in relation to the under-funding of social care for older people. It makes a number of important points:

- Even though older people constitute the largest group of users of social services, less is spent on their care than on other service user groups. In 2001–2002, older people represented 62 per cent of social services service users but local authorities spent 47 per cent of their social services budgets on older people.
- It is not the case that growth in the older population is responsible for social services overspending. The biggest overspend in social services budgets in 2001 was on children's services (64 per cent), whereas overspending on older people's services accounted for only 21 per cent of the total overspend.
- Within adult services, younger service user groups account for most of the increase in social services expenditure for the period 2000 to 2003.
- Older people's services are the area where most local authorities are seeking to restrict services.
- Although between 2000 to 2003 there was a 22 per cent increase in spending on older people's services, most of this expenditure increase was taken up in increasing demands and rising costs, rather than improved services.

(Social Policy on Ageing Information Network 2005)

SPAIN argues that the under-funding of older people's services reflects age discrimination. Despite the fact that 'rooting out age discrimination' is Standard 1 of the *National Service Framework for Older People*, SPAIN argues that age discrimination is evident in policies and practices, citing examples. For example, lower rates are paid for residential care for older people than for other adult service user groups. In 2004, the average weekly cost of residential care for younger adult service users was between £447 and £734, while for older people it was £377. Since the 'ceilings', or upper limits, for domiciliary care packages are often based on a proportion of the costs of residential care, this means that older people receive less care hours than other adult service users. As a consequence, older people are more likely to be compelled to enter residential care as the permitted cost of the domiciliary care package will be lower. Another example cited is that older people over the age of 66 are not eligible to apply to the Independent Living Fund (ILF) for funding to 'top up' a social services care package (though people who are already in receipt of ILF by the time they are 66 can continue to receive the funding, regardless of age, for as long as they remain eligible). Finally, SPAIN argues that the National Minimum Standards for care homes (see Chapter 4) are less stringent for older people than for younger adults in respect of their involvement in the running of homes and participation in local communities.

There is a need for substantial additional funding to address these existing shortfalls as well as new funding to address effectively more recent policy objectives concerned with the promotion of independence and well-being. However, although significant, funding is not the only issue hampering the delivery of quality support and services for older people. Other factors include lack of information about services and how to access them; managerial procedures and processes that run counter to 'person-centred' assessment and services; confusion and inconsistency concerning the funding of long-term care; lack of participation and choice in decision-making and a lack of dignity and respect experienced by older people in the services they receive. These and other issues concerned with assessment and care provision in practice will be discussed in the next two chapters.

KEY POINTS

- ☐ Policy concerning social services for older people was not a central considera-tion in the post-war Welfare State.
- ☐ The community care reforms of the 1990s introduced a system of assessment and care management into social work with older people.
- ☐ Although a range of policy initiatives have been introduced by New Labour, the central political concern driving policy is with resources, rather than with the quality of life of older people.
- ☐ The objectives set for services for older people are unrealistic without significant increases in funding.

KEY READING

Harris, John (2003) *The Social Work Business*, London: Routledge.
Means, R., Morbey, H. and Smith, R. (2002) *From Community Care to Market Care? The Development of Welfare Services for Older People*, Bristol: The Policy Press.
Means, R. and Smith, R. (1998) *From Poor Law to Community Care? The Development of Welfare Services for Elderly People*, Bristol: The Policy Press.

CHAPTER 3

ASSESSING THE NEEDS OF OLDER PEOPLE

OBJECTIVES

By the end of this chapter, you should have an understanding of:

- the importance of assessment in social work with older people;

- key issues relating to the use of the law in assessing the needs of older people;

- key concepts underpinning assessment policy and practice;

- the impact of relevant policy, in particular, the *Single Assessment Process* and *Fair Access to Care Services.*

This chapter focuses on a key area of social work practice with older people: the process of assessing their needs for services. Particular attention is given to clarifying the legal framework pertinent to assessment. As we saw in the previous chapter, legislation and policy embody particular views, attitudes and assumptions and so they need to be understood in relation to the social and historical context in which they have developed and the current context in which they are implemented. The present chapter follows on from the wider discussion of policy developments in Chapter 2, as we refine the focus by providing detailed analysis of how legislation and policy relate to the practice of assessment. Having considered assessment, the next chapter will move on to the significance of legislation and policy for the processes of planning and providing community and residential services for older people.

WHY FOCUS ON ASSESSMENT?

Assessment is 'the foundation for all effective intervention' (Baldwin and Walker 2005: 36). It is a significant stage in the social work intervention process but it is also a process in itself, with a number of key features:

> Assessment is an ongoing process, in which the client participates, whose purpose is to understand people in relation to their environment; it is a basis for planning what needs to be done to maintain, improve or bring about change in the person, the environment or both.
>
> (Coulshed and Orme 1998: 21)

Thus, assessment is rooted in understanding people in their social and environmental context. Understanding, in turn, depends upon engaging with or making meaningful connections with the individual and other appropriate people in their social network. This is a task that requires both skill and sensitivity. Key Role 1 of the *National Occupational Standards for Social Workers* states that social workers must be able to 'Prepare for, and work with individuals, families, carers, groups and communities to assess their needs and circumstances' (Training Organisation for the Personal Social Services 2002). This includes:

- preparing for social work contact and involvement;
- working with individuals, families, carers, groups and communities to help them make informed decisions; and
- assessing needs and options to recommend a course of action.

Assessment, therefore, requires the capacities to plan ahead, work with people to maximise their involvement in the process and to analyse the information gathered so that a way forward is indicated. The assessment of need constitutes a significant component in the care management process (see Figure 2.1, Chapter 2). Assessment links directly with the stage of care planning but it is also part of the continuous cycle of the care management process as a whole – monitoring and review feed back into reassessment and further care planning. Research that explored the amount of time care managers in England spent on different aspects of their role estimated that assessment activities took up about 27 per cent of their time (Weinberg *et al.* 2003). As far as older people are concerned, assessment has been described as 'the single dominant element' of a social worker's role (Lymbery 2005: 152). Assessment is important, as it determines not just what services are received at the care planning stage but whether services are received at all, as will be explored later in this chapter. However, assessment is presented in policy as a service in its own right, as well as the gateway to other services. The general principles of assessment contained within the *Fair Access to Care Services* guidance (discussed in detail later in the chapter) state that assessment should enable individuals to:

- gain a better understanding of their situation;
- identify the options that are available for managing their own lives;
- identify the outcomes required from any help that is provided;
- understand the basis on which decisions are reached.

(Department of Health 2002b: para. 36)

This implies that even if assessment does not result in the provision of services, it may produce a positive outcome if it helps an older person to understand their situation better and increases their knowledge and awareness of different options for meeting their needs. It is important for social workers to have this broader understanding of the purpose of assessment and not see it simply as an instrumental process for determining eligibility for the services that the local authority is responsible for arranging. The way in which health and social care professionals carry out assessment – their exercise of knowledge, skills and commitment to working in partnership with service users – can make a crucial difference to the outcome of the assessment and to people's lives. (Particular aspects of social work skills will be considered further in Chapter 5.)

ACTIVITY 3.1: THE IMPACT OF THE QUALITY OF ASSESSMENT ON OUTCOMES

Mr A. has dementia. He has not been taking his medication and has shown a marked deterioration over the last few days. He has been admitted to hospital for an assessment. Tests show a recent stroke and damage to his brain. On the ward he is clearly disorientated – after two weeks he still cannot find his way around. Mr A. is also very agitated and continuously attempts to leave the ward. The consultant informs you that the medical assessment is completed and asks you to assess for discharge.

Scenario 1

You have spoken with Mr A. on the ward on two occasions – he still fails to recognise you. You attempt to elicit information from him but all he says is he wishes to return home. He shows no insight as to his dementia. An occupational therapist's assessment on the ward has shown that Mr A. is unable to manage in the kitchen, not even being able to make a cup of tea without prompts. Family members tell you that Mr A. is now much worse and they feel he could no longer cope at home alone. A discharge planning meeting decides that, in the interests of Mr A.'s safety, a residential placement is the only solution. Mr A. is not happy with this but the assessment has demonstrated his inability to make an informed choice or assess risk.

Scenario 2

You have spoken to Mr A. on a number of occasions about who you are and your role in planning with him for his discharge. Mr A. has been adamant throughout that he wishes to return home. A kitchen assessment in the hospital showed Mr A. as unable to cope. However, on a home visit, after some initial disorientation, Mr A. was able to find his way around and make tea. Family members tell you that Mr A. is now much worse and they feel he could no longer cope alone at home. You are able to reassure them that Mr A. manages much better in his own home. A discharge planning meeting discusses the various options. Mr A.'s disorientation within a strange environment precludes the use of external resources such as day care and, at this time, residential care. His own coping mechanisms within a known environment suggest that a return home is viable. However, his memory and recognition problems suggest that the fewer strange faces the better; the home care organiser will try to get the seven mornings covered by only two home care assistants. They will check that he has taken his medication. A graduated discharge is discussed but it is felt inappropriate as this would disorientate Mr A. further. Mr A. is to be discharged home after visits from the home care assistants. The home care organiser will be the key worker. The situation will be reviewed after two weeks.

Identify the factors that seem to have contributed to the different outcome achieved in Scenario 1, compared with Scenario 2.

(Case example adapted from Littlechild and Blakeney 1996: 77)

Before considering in detail the legal framework pertinent to the assessment of older people's needs, more general points about the relationship between community care law and social work practice will be considered.

THE RELATIONSHIP BETWEEN COMMUNITY CARE LAW AND PRACTICE

Mandelstam (2005) makes a number of key points about the nature of community care legislation that it is important for practitioners to understand. First, the legislation relevant to community care, and therefore social work with older people, is highly complex and fragmented. To understand the current legal framework, it is necessary to go as far back as 1948; since this time there have been numerous pieces of legislation that have built up the community care legal edifice, some of which have been subsequently amended. Some services, for example home care for older people, may be provided under a number of different pieces of legislation. The interface between social services, health and housing in the provision of community care contributes further to the legal uncertainties and complexities.

This complexity leads on to a second important point. It is not only a matter of 'knowing' the law, which can sometimes be difficult in itself, but also that legislation has to be interpreted and applied in practice. Thompson (2005) outlines four main levels at which the law is interpreted:

- *Guidance:* A vast amount of guidance relating to community care is issued by the Department of Health. Policy guidance and practice guidance have a slightly different legal status. Policy guidance is issued by the government under the Local Authority Social Services (1970, Section 7[1]). Policy guidance sets out how the law should be interpreted. For example, *Community Care in the Next Decade and*

Beyond (Department of Health 1990 – see Chapter 2) was published as guidance alongside the NHS and Community Care Act (1990); *Fair Access to Care Services* (Department of Health 2002b) provides guidance on assessment and the basis on which decisions about access to care services should be made. Local authorities should follow policy guidance unless they have clear reasons for departing from it. However, whereas policy guidance specifies what an authority, in effect, 'must' do, practice guidance advises on how it 'might' function (Clements 2004). Local authorities should have regard to practice guidance, but do not have the strong obligation to adhere to it that exists with policy guidance. An example of practice guidance is the *Practitioners' Guide* issued alongside the NHS and Community Care Act (Social Services Inspectorate/Department of Health 1991a – see Chapter 2).

- *Local policies:* policies and procedures are developed by local authorities and other agencies that represent their interpretation of legal requirements, taking account of their own local context. Mandelstam (2005) comments on the wide scope for local authority interpretation of legislation that results from the uncertainties in community care law. Indeed he argues, 'these uncertainties are so prevalent as to be an integral and essential part of the system' (ibid.: 36). Uncertainties are described as 'essential' because they allow local authorities scope for flexibility, particularly in relation to how they deploy and manage scarce resources. At the same time, uncertainties create problems as they leave areas of law unclear and enable local authorities to exploit this lack of clarity when formulating their polices and procedures. As a consequence, legislation is often interpreted in a way that serves and protects the local authority's interests, for example, the need to remain within budget, rather than in a way that promotes the interests of older people.

- *Precedent:* current interpretation of the law has recourse to how the law has been interpreted in previous cases. Carers and service users can seek judicial review of acts and decisions by local authorities and health authorities; judges examine whether authorities have acted unreasonably, illegally or unfairly. When a case goes for a full hearing, the decision of the court sets a precedent for the future that must be observed by other local authorities. Examples of significant case law decisions relating to social work with older people are the Gloucestershire case (discussed later in this chapter) and the Sefton case (considered in Chapter 4).

- *Direct practice:* social workers have a certain amount of discretion to interpret both the law and local policies and procedures in their practice (Evans and Harris 2004b). Such discretion is often necessary for practitioners to be able to do their jobs; they need a degree of freedom of movement to deal with uncertainty and unpredictability.

The scope for interpretation of the legislation at these four levels contributes to the possibility of yawning gaps in social work with older people between the stated objectives of community care and reality, at the level of practice:

> On its face, community care is about assisting people with social care needs, and enabling them to remain living at home, as independently as possible for as long as possible . . . This apparently straightforward aim of community care seems at times to have evaporated and been replaced by constant

anxiety about resources, cost shunting between statutory services, ever stricter eligibility criteria, waiting times for services, and attempts by local authorities to evade or continually to reinterpret legal duties. Local authority staff and managers seem, in many areas at least, to be as concerned about how to say no to meeting people's needs as to say yes.

(Mandelstam 2005: 39)

Mandelstam argues that as a consequence of the complexity of community care legislation, lack of legal knowledge by local authority managers and other staff and the conflicting pressures caused by resource shortfalls, many local authorities are probably acting unlawfully in some of their practices. This view is upheld by other community care law experts:

Local authorities are breaking the law and social workers do not know whether they are making legal errors when deciding community care issues, according to a leading community rights lawyer. Luke Clements told Oxfordshire Community Care Rights Group last week that social services departments were not equipping their staff with the skills to make decisions about eligibility for, and access to, services. He said he knew no other area of public law where there are so many breaches of the law by local authorities. 'Social workers know they are walking on thin ice but they don't know how thin because they've not had the training', he added.

(*Community Care* 2003: 15)

As we shall see in relation to assessment, a sound knowledge of the law enables social workers not only to identify and contest illegal policies and practices but also to appreciate the scope to interpret the law in ways that advance service users' interests.

THE LEGAL AND POLICY FRAMEWORK FOR ASSESSING OLDER PEOPLE'S NEEDS

The following pieces of legislation relate to duties to assess the needs of older people: the Disabled Persons Act (1986) applies to older people who are disabled; the NHS and Community Care Act (1990) contains a general duty to assess the need for community care services; and the Mental Health Act (1983) applies to older people who are 'mentally disordered' under the terms of this Act. Older people may also be entitled to an assessment under the Carers Acts (1995; 2000; 2004) if they are undertaking substantial caring responsibilities. (Legislation relating to carers will be considered in Chapter 6.) The legal duties concerning assessment set out in the Disabled Persons' Act (1986), the NHS and Community Care Act (1990) and the Mental Health Act (1983) are described below.

Disabled Persons (Services, Consultation and Representation) Act (1986: Section 4)

The Chronically Sick and Disabled Persons Act (1970, Section 2) imposes duties on local authorities to provide services for disabled people. The definition of disability is to be found in the National Assistance Act (1948, Section 29 – see Chapters 2 and 4). Although the duty to assess is implied in the duty to provide services, this is not explicit (Clements 2004). However, Section 4 of the Disabled Persons Act (1986) does include a specific requirement for local authorities to assess the needs of a disabled person (who may, of course, be an older person) for services provided under the Chronically Sick and Disabled Persons Act (1970), upon request by the disabled person or their representative. The local authority's role is, therefore, reactive to requests by disabled people, but there is also a duty under this Act to inform disabled people of their right to an assessment.

NHS and Community Care Act (1990: Section 47)

This section widens the duty to assess need, or more accurately, need for services. Under this legislation, the duty to assess applies not only to people who may need services provided under the Chronically Sick and Disabled Persons Act (1970), but also to anyone aged 18 years or over for whom the local authority believes it may have a power or duty to provide services. This would include older people who may have a need for 'welfare' services provided under the Health Services and Public Health Act (1968 – discussed in Chapter 2). Unlike Section 4 of the Disabled Persons Act (1986), the duty does not depend upon a request for assessment by the person concerned (or their representative) but is triggered when the local authority believes the person *may* be in need of services it has a power or duty to provide. Clements (2004) points out the implications for local authorities. If knowledge of potential need comes to light in another part of the authority (for example, housing services), this still triggers the duty to assess under Section 47:

> authorities should ensure that they have the necessary internal organisational networks so that the needs of vulnerable individuals are automatically referred to the relevant community care team irrespective of the point at which the first local authority contact with that individual occurs. A failure to make such arrangements may amount to maladministration.
>
> (Clements 2004: 63)

Section 47 triggers duties under Section 4 of the Disabled Persons Act (1986). It states that if it appears that the person receiving an assessment is a disabled person, the local authority has a duty to inform her or him of the rights provided by the Disabled Persons Act (1986) and must decide (regardless of whether this is requested) whether s/he requires services provided under the Chronically Sick and Disabled Persons Act (1970). The Chronically Sick and Disabled Persons Act (1970) contains strong duties to provide services and decisions are more open to challenge if this Act is involved (Mandlestam 1998). Section 47 of the NHS and Community Care Act (1990) should make it unnecessary for an older disabled person to request an assessment of the need for services under the Chronically Sick and Disabled Persons Act (1970), since the local authority is under a duty to carry this out anyway. However, if for some reason, a community care assessment under the NHS and Community Care Act (1990) is not forthcoming, a disabled person remains entitled to request an assessment under Section 4 of the Disabled Persons Act (1986), rather than needing to wait for the local authority to recognise that she or he may be someone who may be in need of its services.

Mental Health Act (1983)

Assessment under the Mental Health Act (1983) may be relevant to older people who are suffering from 'mental disorders' according to the terms of Section 1 of the Act, that is, 'mental illness, arrested or incomplete development of mind, psychopathic disorder and any other disorder or disability of mind'. An older person could, therefore, be assessed under the Mental Health Act (1983) if her/his behaviour or situation is causing concern *and* this seems to be associated with mental disorder (for example, depression, schizophrenia, bipolar disorder or dementia) *and* it is thought that detention in hospital might be necessary for the purposes of assessment and/or treatment. Under Section 13 of the Mental Health Act (1983), specially trained social workers who are approved to carry out functions under the Act (approved social workers) have a duty to make an application to admit people to hospital or guardianship, if they are satisfied that the application should be made. This will be decided after the social worker has carried out a mental health assessment, interviewing the person 'in a suitable manner' and considering all the circumstances of the case. The approved social worker has a duty to make the application for compulsory admission to hospital for assessment (Section 2) or treatment (Section 3), if the criteria for admission to hospital are met (including the completion of relevant medical recommendations) and if the approved social worker believes it is necessary to make an application. The Mental Health Bill (2006) includes provisions for widening the definition of mental disorder and extending the approved social worker role to other mental health practitioners, who would become approved mental health professionals (see Department of Health 2006e).

These are the main legal provisions under which social workers are likely to be carrying out assessments with older people, unless the older person is a carer (see Chapter 6). In addition to legal duties concerning assessment, there are specific policy guidance documents that comprise a significant part of the framework for the assessment of older people's needs. These are the *Single Assessment Process* guidance (Department of Health 2002c) and the *Fair Access to Care Services* guidance (Department of Health 2002b).

The *Single Assessment Process*

The *Single Assessment Process* (SAP) was introduced in the *National Service Framework for Older People* (Department of Health 2001a) and implemented in April 2004. It is concerned with making assessment and care planning in respect of older people 'person-centred, effective and co-ordinated' (Department of Health 2002c: 1). The aim is to coordinate the different elements of an assessment so that an older person has one assessment, which becomes more comprehensive as it is added to over time, as opposed to there being separate assessments by a number of professionals. The intention is to avoid duplication and facilitate holistic assessments that are shared between different agencies. The SAP does not replace, as such, the general assessment and care management guidance (referred to in Chapter 2), but is another layer of prescription that specifically relates to the assessment of older people. Whereas the assessment and care management guidance emphasises social work as the lead agency in assessment, with contributions invited as appropriate from health and housing agencies, SAP requires agencies to agree local protocols about responsibilities for coordinating assessments and requires that a single assessment summary is produced. SAP also introduces the concept of 'case finding' and talks explicitly about a stage concerned with determining eligibility. The stages of SAP are:

- *Publishing information about services:* this is also the first stage of the assessment and care management process. Local authorities do, in any case, have legal responsibilities to provide information about their services for disabled people (which may, of course, include older people) under Section 2 of the Chronically Sick and Disabled Persons Act (1970).
- *Case finding (seen as 'optional'):* this relates to older people who have not been referred for assessment but who might benefit from assessment, according to health and social care professionals. The aim is to identify potential risk factors early in order to trigger preventive interventions. There is clearly a tension between this stage and the emphasis in adult services on targeting services on those with high level needs.
- *Completing an assessment:* this may be one of four types – a contact, overview, specialist or comprehensive assessment (see below).
- *Evaluating assessment information:* this involves 'weighing up' the information gathered with a focus on 'the risks to independence that result from the needs' (Department of Health 2002c: Annex E, 21).
- *Deciding on what help should be offered (including eligibility decisions):* the distinction between presenting and eligible needs is described here in the same way as in *Fair Access to Care Services*, discussed later in the chapter.
- *Care planning:* this will be undertaken by relating eligible needs to the 'statements of purpose' developed by services to help determine appropriate provision:

> At the care planning stage, services are matched to eligible needs through the use of 'statements of purpose', which all service providers should prepare. These statements should set out the objectives and philosophy of care underpinning the service, the nature of services, facilities, physical and geographical access and likely charges. They should also describe the types and circumstances and the people for whom the service is designed.
>
> (Department of Health 2002c: Annex E, 23)

- *Monitoring and review.*

(Department of Health 2002c: Annex E)

The four types of assessment that may be carried out under the *Single Assessment Process* are described as follows.

Contact assessment

This refers to contact with an older person where significant needs are first described or suspected. The level of assessment involves collecting basic personal information, establishing the nature of the presenting problem and exploring whether there may be wider health and social care needs. The *Single Assessment Process* guidance states that there are seven key issues to be addressed at this stage:

- the nature of the presenting need;
- the significance of the need for the older person;
- the length of time the need has been experienced;
- potential solutions identified by the older person;
- other needs experienced by the older person;
- recent life events or changes relevant to the problem;
- the perceptions of family members and carers.

It is important to note the emphasis here on the older person's views, both about the significance of the need, other needs and potential solutions. Equally, it is expected that the views of those in the informal network will be obtained. This is consistent with the 2004 statutory directions to involve service users and carers in assessment (Department of Health 2004a).

SAP guidance states that contact assessment should be carried out by 'trained but not necessarily qualified staff'. It is not clear in the guidance what 'training' staff undertaking contact assessments are expected to have. Practice experience suggests that this involves training in screening calls, taking basic information, understanding bureaucratic and managerial processes and completing agency requirements in terms of computerised recording. The skills in establishing connections with people, and working with them in empowering ways to establish the sort of help they feel they need, appear to be given much less emphasis. (These and other skills in working with older people will be discussed in Chapter 5.) As Nolan *et al.* argue, it is not enough for services to be provided in a technically competent way, in terms of adhering to particular standards and processes; they must also 'incorporate a consideration of interpersonal dynamics and personal meanings' (2001: 166). Arguably these are skills that require professional training. While this 'lower order' assessment at the point of contact may be seen as less important, and therefore a stage that can be delegated to staff who are not professionally qualified, what happens at these early junctures may be crucial in determining the nature and level of support someone receives subsequently.

Overview assessment

This type of assessment is carried out if a 'more rounded' assessment is needed. Different 'domains' of assessment are listed within the SAP guidance (see Box 3.1) and some or all of these must be explored in an overview assessment. Assessment tools and scales may be used. An overview assessment may be completed by a social services or NHS professional, though a qualification is regarded as not essential if the person is 'professionally competent'.

Specialist assessment

The purpose of specialist assessment is to explore specific needs in detail: 'As a result of a specialist assessment, professionals should be able to confirm the presence, extent, cause and likely development of a health condition or problem or social care need, and establish links to other conditions, problems and needs' (Department of Health 2002c, Annex E: 17). This type of assessment should be carried out by 'the most appropriate qualified professional'. This may be, for example, a social worker, nurse, occupational therapist, physiotherapist, consultant in old age or old age psychiatry, dietician, or housing or welfare benefits professional.

Comprehensive assessment

A comprehensive assessment is carried out when a specialist assessment indicates that all or most of the domains within the SAP guidance (see Box 3.1) are involved. It should be completed where the level of support and treatment is likely to be 'intensive or prolonged'. A comprehensive assessment involves a range of different professionals or specialist teams. It is likely that a lead role will be played by geriatricians and old age psychiatrists and their teams.

BOX 3.1 THE DOMAINS AND SUB-DOMAINS OF THE *SINGLE ASSESSMENT PROCESS*

User's perspective

- Needs and issues in the user's own words;
- user's expectations, strengths, abilities and motivation.

Clinical background

- History of medical conditions and diagnoses;
- history of falls;
- medication use and ability to self-medicate.

Disease prevention

- History of blood pressure monitoring;
- nutrition, diet and fluids;
- vaccination history;
- drinking and smoking history;
- exercise pattern;
- history of cervical and breast screening.

continued

Personal care and physical well-being

- Personal hygiene, including washing, bathing, toileting and grooming;
- dressing;
- pain;
- oral health;
- foot care;
- tissue viability;
- mobility;
- continence and other aspects of elimination;
- sleeping patterns.

Senses

- Sight;
- hearing;
- communication.

Mental health

- Cognition and dementia, including orientation and memory;
- mental health including depression, reactions to loss and emotional difficulties.

Relationships

- Social contacts, relationships and involvement in leisure, hobbies, work and learning;
- carer support and strength of caring arrangements, including the carer's perspective.

Safety

- Abuse and neglect;
- other aspects of personal safety;
- public safety.

Immediate environment and resources

- Care of the home and managing daily tasks such as food preparation, cleaning and shopping;
- housing – location, access, amenities and heating;
- level and management of finances;
- access to local facilities and services.

(Department of Health 2002c: Annex F)

Health and social care agencies are required to produce a shared current summary record that covers basic personal information, needs and health and a summary of the care plan (Department of Health 2002c: Annex I). A worked example specifies that the summary should include information about the following areas:

- personal demographics;
- other people involved;
- the older person's perspective of her or his current needs;
- clinical background;
- disease prevention;
- assessment of individual needs;
- evaluation of needs and risks;
- a note of validated tools and scales used;
- a summary of the current care plan;
- any additional personal information;
- administrative details.

(Department of Health 2002d)

The guidance recommends that records are held by the older person in their own home. A good practice guide produced in the West Midlands makes specific recommendations about person-held records (see Activity 3.2).

ACTIVITY 3.2: PERSON-HELD RECORDS

Read these good practice points about person-held records:

- Person-held records should be considered in all localities as a way of sharing information between agencies and empowering the person as keeper of their own record.
- An easily recognisable folder should be used that is similar to those used in neighbouring localities.
- The ambulance service should be informed of the format and purpose of the record.
- The person-held record should contain a copy of the contact assessment, overview assessment and the care plan (as minimum requirements).
- A recently signed 'consent to share information' form should be signed by the older person and included in the record.
- The record should include guidance for the older person on its purpose, how to use it and who might need to read it.
- An emergency action or contingency plan should be clearly located in the record.
- It would be helpful to include a table of contents and separate section dividers.
- There should be sections for summaries of any specialist assessments and sections for service providers to add their notes.
- The information should remain with the older person even if the service is no longer being provided.

- A system should be agreed with the older person for updating the person-held record.
- The use of person-held records should be formally evaluated with service users and professionals.

(West Midlands Regional Single Assessment Process Group 2004: 5)

Consider what problems and issues may arise from using person-held records in practice.

The *Single Assessment Process* places considerable emphasis on the use of assessment tools: 'An assessment tool is a collection of scales, questions and checklists that have been brought together for specific assessment purposes' (Department of Health 2002c: Annex E, 15). The use of such tools can supplement and enhance assessment information, in particular, providing frameworks for an assessment and enabling comparison between an individual's functioning in specific areas and general indicators of need and risk. However, a key part of assessment is evaluating or making sense of the information obtained. Simply gathering more or additional types of information does not in itself lead to a 'better' assessment if the measure of 'good' assessment is 'the one that leads to the most useful understanding and to an intervention that achieves the service user's goals' (Milner and O'Byrne 2002: 77). While the use of tools and scales can supplement and enhance assessment information, it cannot substitute for the understanding gained from 'tuning in' to the service user's own perspective on their situation. Although the collection and recording of information is a key focus of SAP, it is important to bear in mind the *purpose* of this process:

> The Single Assessment Process is not about the kind of forms you fill in, but about delivering person-centred care. The documentation is only the means of recording and sharing information, in order that people can get the help they need.
>
> (West Midlands Regional Single Assessment Process Group 2004: 7)

A number of concerns have been expressed about SAP (Glasby 2004). For example, social care dimensions may be eclipsed by medical perspectives; some of the suggested tools for collecting and recording information are more medical in their orientation and this is reflected in the assessment domains (see Box 3.1). Given the historically problematic relationship between social care and health personnel, there are also significant barriers to achieving the understanding and trust between the professions that is required for effective collaborative working. Aside from ideological differences, there are more practical obstacles such as organisational and technological barriers to cooperation. For example, the sharing of information between agencies is fundamental to the *Single Assessment Process* but shared systems for recording and accessing information are not well developed and would require a substantial investment of additional resources. (These and other issues related to interprofessional working will be discussed further in Chapter 6.)

Fair Access to Care Services

As shown above, deciding on what assistance should be offered to an older person is one of the stages within SAP, occurring after information has been gathered about presenting need and after the 'the risks to independence that result from the needs' have been weighed up. Risks to independence are codified in eligibility criteria. Local authorities originally had considerable discretion to set their own local eligibility criteria. This resulted in widespread geographical variation, with some local authorities having different criteria for different service user 'groups' as well as different criteria for access to different services. From April 2003, a standard framework for eligibility criteria has been set out under *Fair Access to Care Services* (FACS) guidance (Department of Health 2002b). This imposes one set of criteria for all adult service users and for access to all types of service. SAP guidance states that councils should make decisions about eligibility for services with reference to the FACS guidance. Social workers are expected to assess need comprehensively, then to evaluate the presenting needs that are identified in terms of the risk they present to independence if help is not provided and, finally, to compare these risks to the council's eligibility criteria (Department of Health 2002b: para. 42). In essence FACS guidance retains the significance of eligibility criteria for service provision but seeks to distance the criteria from the process of assessment of need. Thus, FACS guidance states that eligibility criteria should not be used to determine the type of assessment offered (ibid.: para. 34) but clarifies that assessment information is to be evaluated and only then should this lead on to decisions about eligibility. This is essentially the same process envisaged within the legal duty contained in Section 47 of the NHS and Community Care Act (1990) – a low access threshold for assessment followed by, as a separate stage, a decision about service provision. The assessment process, as outlined in FACS, is shown in Figure 3.1.

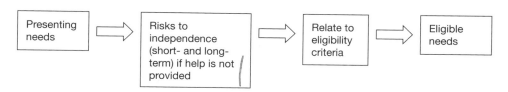

FIGURE 3.1 The process of assessment in *Fair Access to Care Services*

In providing a national approach to assessment and eligibility criteria, FACS not only imposes a framework for decisions about service provision for individual service users but also advocates using eligibility criteria as a tool for regulating service provision in line with resources. The document explains the assessment process in terms of:

- assessing *presenting needs*;
- evaluating these needs in terms of *risks* to autonomy, health and safety, ability to manage daily routines and involvement in family and community life;
- comparing risks to independence with the council's *eligibility criteria*;
- identifying *eligible needs*, that is, risks that fall within the eligibility criteria.

There are four bands within the eligibility framework set out in FACS, representing 'the seriousness of the risk to independence or other consequences if needs are not addressed' (Department of Health 2002b: para. 16): critical, substantial, moderate and low categories of needs (see Box 3.2).

BOX 3.2   ELIGIBILITY FRAMEWORK AS SET OUT IN THE *FAIR ACCESS TO CARE SERVICES* GUIDANCE

Critical – when:

- life is, or will be, threatened; and/or
- significant health problems have developed or will develop; and/or
- there is, or will be, little or no choice and control over vital aspects of the immediate environment; and/or
- serious abuse or neglect has occurred or will occur; and/or
- there is, or will be, an inability to carry out vital personal care or domestic routines; and/or
- vital involvement in work, education or learning cannot or will not be sustained; and/or
- vital social support systems and relationships cannot or will not be sustained; and/or
- vital family and other social roles and responsibilities cannot or will not be undertaken.

Substantial – when:

- there is, or will be, only partial choice and control over the immediate environment; and/or
- abuse or neglect has occurred or will occur; and/or
- there is, or will be, an inability to carry out the majority of personal care or domestic routines; and/or
- involvement in many aspects of work, education or learning cannot or will not be sustained; and/or
- the majority of social support systems and relationships cannot or will not be sustained; and/or
- the majority of family and other social roles and responsibilities cannot or will not be undertaken.

Moderate – when

- there is, or will be, an inability to carry out several personal care or domestic routines; and/or
- involvement in several aspects of work, education or learning cannot or will not be sustained; and/or
- several social support systems and relationships cannot or will not be sustained; and/or
- several family and other social roles and relationships cannot or will not be undertaken.

Low – when

- there is, or will be, an inability to carry out one or two personal care or domestic routines; and/or
- involvement in one or two aspects of work, education or learning cannot or will not be sustained; and/or
- one or two social support systems and relationships cannot or will not be sustained; and/or
- one or two family and other social roles and responsibilities cannot or will not be undertaken.

(Department of Health 2002b)

Local authorities are instructed to prioritise the meeting of critical needs, then those assessed as substantial and so on. In practice, this means that the threshold for needs that will be met is, in many authorities, set at the critical and substantial levels.

We will now consider further the implications of these legal and policy provisions for assessment practice.

ASSESSMENT OF WHAT?

Baldwin and Walker (2005: 36) state that the starting point for assessment is the question, 'What does this person need in order to maximise well-being in all key areas of his or her life?' This sees the objective of intervention as the maximisation of well-being and assessment as identifying what is required for this objective to be achieved. The previous section has shown that central concepts within legal and policy constructions of assessment are needs, risks and independence, rather than well-being. As discussed in Chapter 2, part of the rationale for care management was that it would be 'needs-led', separating assessment from service considerations. How 'need' is defined is critical, as this constitutes the dividing line between the responsibilities of the state, on the one hand, and those of the market, informal carers and the individual, on the other (Wetherly 1996). Need is a slippery concept (Godfrey and Callaghan 2000), as its definition is influenced by the particular social, cultural and historical context:

> Historical and cultural variations in what is seen as 'need' are interesting because they are the result of contested processes of social construction . . . These differences are important because they are the visible points – the outcomes – of processes of contestation, conflict and negotiation around what counts as 'need' and who is allowed, or required, to have needs.
>
> (Clarke and Langan 1998: 270)

It is not simply that there are historical and cultural variations in concepts of need. Ways of defining need within a specific cultural and historical context also vary. Bradshaw (1972) developed a 'taxonomy of need' that distinguished four different ways of defining need:

- *'Felt' need* refers to need that an individual experiences (but does not necessarily express). It should not be assumed that if a need is not expressed, the need does not exist. For example, there have been erroneous assumptions in the past that the low take-up of services by Black and minority ethnic communities was because 'they look after their own'. Simplistic assumptions about the availability of social support within Black and minority ethnic communities have been challenged by research that highlights the disruptive impact of migration on kinship networks and the detrimental effects of social exclusion on access to sources of support (Nazroo *et al.* 2004). Moreover, the picture is diverse within and between ethnic groups (Moriarty and Butt 2004). There are many reasons why felt need may not be expressed. For example, older people from Black and minority ethnic communities may not seek help with difficulties they experience because of lack of information about services available, language barriers or because services are seen as culturally insensitive or inappropriate to their needs (Butt and O'Neil 2004). When considering 'expressed need' (see below) for certain types of support, therefore, it is always worth considering the nature and level of 'felt' need that may not be expressed in the form of requests for help. Whose felt needs are under-represented in expressed need and why might this be?
- *'Expressed' need* is need that an individual publicly acknowledges; it may or may not be the same as felt need. For need to be expressed in the form of a request for help, the individual has not only to experience it but to perceive it and be able to translate it into service terms: 'people's conceptions of their needs relate to their expectations, their view of what the agency can and should provide, what it is legitimate to ask for and their knowledge of the services that are available' (Godfrey and Callaghan 2000: 9). Need may not be expressed if it is believed that the service will not be provided. For example, this could account for a decline in referrals following publicity about social services budget shortfalls or tightened eligibility criteria (Parry-Jones and Soulsby 2001). When older people do express their needs they may be obstructed in getting these needs heard and understood by, for example, restricted assessment agendas or 'tick-box' style formats that adopt a narrow focus on physical needs (Stanley 1999; Richards 2000). Equally, there may be obstacles for practitioners in hearing and understanding expressed need. For example, practitioners may lack the time, knowledge or skills to address particular communication difficulties, such as the loss of verbal communication that may be experienced by someone with dementia (Killick and Allan 2001).
- *'Normative', or 'prescribed', need* is defined according to an agreed standard established by an expert or professional; it may differ significantly from an individual's felt and expressed needs. Care management explicitly states that need will be determined according to a normative definition; need refers to 'the requirements of individuals to enable them to achieve, maintain or restore an acceptable level of social independence or quality of life, *as defined by the particular care agency or authority*' (Social Services Inspectorate/Department of Health 1991a: para. 11, *our emphasis*). This is reinforced by FACS in its distinction between 'presenting need', which equates with Bradshaw's expressed need, and 'eligible' need, the normative definition of need that the local authority accepts as being necessary to meet. Normative definitions of need change over time, as shown in the historical review of policies for older people in Chapter 2. Within this policy

context, the provision of home helps to assist with cleaning and tasks around the house was widely accepted up until the mid-1980s. While 'home care' support, normally for personal care needs, is still arranged, the sort of 'low level' assistance previously given by home helps now falls outside of local authorities' normative definition of need. Assistance with household tasks is seen as need that can be met privately through the independent and informal care sectors.

- *'Comparative' need* refers to what is perceived as a need relative to that of other groups or individuals; it is likely to influence an individual's felt and expressed need as well as how normative need is defined. When deciding whether to seek help, older people will be influenced by their evaluation of their own perceived need compared with that of others. There is some evidence that making positive comparisons between themselves and others is one of the strategies used by older people to maintain a sense of their own coping ability and quality of life (Bury and Holme 1991; Beaumont *et al.* 2002). This, in turn, may deter them from expressing need and seeking assistance. Comparative need also influences the normative definition of need in the care management and FACS guidance. This is because what is defined as a need is decided by reference to eligibility criteria and these criteria are set with reference to the local authority's resources in relation to current demand. The level of need expressed by other potential service users is, therefore, a factor in determining the threshold to be met before an individual receives help. At practitioner level, decisions about an individual's level of need and risk will inevitably be made in the context of awareness of the needs and circumstances of other service users and potential service users.

It is primarily *normative need* that forms the basis of assessment as outlined in care management guidance. In the guidance, as we have already seen, need is defined primarily by 'the particular care agency or authority' (Social Services Inspectorate/ Department of Health 1991a: para. 11). Despite the many statements in the original care management guidance and, more recently, in the SAP and FACS guidance, to the effect that service users should be involved in the assessment process and treated as experts on their own needs, it is clear that, ultimately, normative need prevails when determining 'need for services' and that social workers are expected to be the arbiters of normative need:

> The practitioner has to define, as precisely as possible, the cause of any difficulty. The same apparent need may have many different causes . . . having weighed the views of all parties, including his/her own observation, the assessing practitioner is responsible for defining the user's need.
> (Social Services Inspectorate/Department of Health 1991a:
> paras 3.32 and 3.35)

Although Section 47 of the NHS and Community Care Act (1990) echoes these concerns in framing the duty to assess in terms of 'need for services', the SAP and FACS emphasise basing decisions about service provision on evaluation of 'risks to independence if care is not provided'. Independence is interpreted broadly and both of these guidance documents use identical wording in stating that the assessment of risks to independence should focus on the following dimensions:

- autonomy and freedom to make choices;
- health and safety including freedom from harm, abuse and neglect, and taking wider issues of housing circumstances and community safety into account;
- the ability to manage personal and other daily routines; and
- involvement in family and wider community life, including leisure, hobbies, unpaid and paid work, learning and volunteering.

(Department of Health 2002b; 2002c)

The inclusion of 'autonomy and freedom to make choices' and 'involvement in family and wider community life' suggests a view of assessment that is congruent with the concern with maximising well-being that is central to definitions of assessment contained in the social work literature. The underpinning principles set out in the SAP guidance state that assessment should focus on: an older person's strengths and abilities, as well as needs; any external or environmental factors that impact on needs; and promoting health and well-being, not just reacting to existing needs (Department of Health 2002c: Annex D). This broader emphasis on independence and well-being is consistent with the messages contained in polices such as the Social Exclusion Unit report, *A Sure Start to Later Life* and the White Paper, *Our Health, Our Care, Our Say* (both discussed in Chapter 2). The well-being approach requires that older people are seen as citizens with rights, rather than as dependent people in need of services, and this in turn means addressing the barriers that prevent their full participation in the society of which they are members (Joseph Rowntree Foundation 2004). A shift in the agenda from meeting the needs of individuals in crisis to promoting independence and well-being has obvious implications for the focus and process of assessment, the range of services that are relevant to achieving this broader objective and the working relationships between agencies and with older people themselves. However, there remains a fundamental tension between the well-being objectives expressed in policy and the narrow risk-based assessments that characterise much social work practice.

ACTIVITY 3.3: ASSESSMENT OBJECTIVES

Assessment in community care policy and practice is variously presented as concerned with:

- identifying needs;
- evaluating risks;
- promoting independence and well-being.

Consider the differences between these three approaches to assessment in terms of the sorts of questions a social worker carrying out an assessment would ask.

Review your understanding of older people's concerns and perspectives from Activity 1.1, Chapter 1. Which of the approaches to assessment do you think would be most likely to address the needs and concerns of older people?

ACCESS TO ASSESSMENT

There are three key points to note from the wording of the legal duty to assess need contained in Section 47 of NHS and Community Care Act (1990). First, the duty is to carry out an assessment 'where it appears to a local authority that any person for whom they may provide or arrange for the provision of community care services may be in need of any such services'. The phrase used is 'may provide', not 'will provide'. This means that the duty to assess applies wherever it seems as though it might be the case that someone may need services that the local authority has a power or duty to provide – not that, according to current policy, they will necessarily provide the service. The gateway to assessment is, therefore, legally speaking, wide (Clements 2004). However, in practice it appears that even at the stage of 'screening', the gateway narrows, with service availability influencing decisions about entitlement to assessment. Social workers have been found to make decisions about eligibility for assessment on the basis of their understanding about eligibility for services so that assessment itself becomes a service that is rationed (Ellis *et al.* 1999). However, a judicial review (Bristol City Council ex parte A. Penfold 1998) ruled that the scope to refuse assessment is very limited. The duty to assess is triggered by the appearance of need for any service that could (in theory) be provided, not what is actually likely to be provided, making the threshold for access to assessment very low (Brammer 2003).

Second, although the rationale underpinning care management was that it was to be 'needs-led', the wording of the duty to assess contained in Section 47 of NHS and Community Care Act (1990) makes clear that the assessment is about determining 'need for services'. The need for care or support can be distinguished from the need for services. Older people's need for care or support has to be considered in relation to the forms of help already available to them; only then can 'need for services' be determined (Patsios and Davey 2005). Having assessed need for services, a separate stage within the assessment process is involved in deciding whether it is necessary to provide services to meet the assessed need. To have had a truly 'needs-led' service based on the expressed need of individuals would have undermined a principle objective of the community care reforms, the curtailing of public expenditure: 'The potentially risky ambiguity inherent in the concept of need had to be eliminated at the outset if the primary objective of cost-effectiveness was to be accomplished' (Ellis *et al.* 1999: 269). Thus, the second part of the definition of the duty to assess – 'having regard to the results of that assessment, shall then decide whether his (*sic*) needs call for the provision by them of any such services' – clarifies that assessment of need does not necessarily imply the provision of services. Decisions about service provision will be made by the local authority on the basis of the 'necessity of meeting the need'. As already discussed, this is decided by reference to eligibility criteria: local authorities' decisions about the 'level' of need that it is necessary to meet are made with regard to resources. Implicit within the legal definition of the duty to assess is the merging of the focus on individual need with considerations of service availability. In effect, this is 'a masterpiece in the art of circle-squaring' (Lewis, J. and Glennerster 1996: 15) that effectively re-entangles the strands of 'needs' and 'services' that the policy declared should be clearly distinguished (Richards 1994), thus creating a number of difficulties for practitioners trying to carry out 'needs-led' assessments. A study based on semi-structured interviews with health and social care practitioners and managers in North Wales between 1994 and 1999 noted a number of problematic issues in relation to assessing need. In general terms, practitioners felt that the new system increased their workloads and made heavy administrative demands. Social workers experienced difficulty in extricating the assessment of 'need' from knowledge of service restrictions and budget constraints. There was uncertainty about how to respond to and record needs that were expressed by service users but that did not meet eligibility criteria for service provision. There were difficulties in the 'grey areas' of responsibility between health and social care agencies, with lack of clarity about whether a need should be met by health or social care providers. Practitioners also felt that their professional autonomy was undermined by resource panels that scrutinised their assessments and made decisions about care funding (Parry-Jones and Soulsby 2001).

Third, the financial circumstances of individuals are irrelevant to whether or not they can access a community care assessment. The FACS guidance stipulates that someone's financial situation is only relevant after needs have been assessed and it has been decided that s/he is eligible to receive services (Department of Health 2002b). At this point a financial assessment will determine whether and how much they should contribute towards the costs of services. Older people with capital above the prescribed capital limit for financial assistance with residential accommodation (see Chapter 4) are entitled to have their needs assessed. Even if they will be self-funding, they are entitled to have assistance with arranging accommodation, if this is needed. In sum, an individual's financial resources are relevant to determining the charge levied for any services arranged to meet assessed needs; they should not be a consideration in relation to accessing an assessment.

UNMET NEED

The distinction between unmet need as expressed need or 'wants', outside of normative definitions, and unmet need as normative need that cannot be met is critical to the legal status of unmet need and how it is dealt with in social work with older people. When carrying out assessments, practitioners have been nervous about recording unmet need, fearing this may create a legal obligation to meet the need identified (Parry-Jones and Soulsby 2001). This has been summed up as: 'do not tell clients what their real needs are and make sure you do not write them down in case you get found out and have to provide for them' (Lewis, J. and Glennerster 1996: 15). The legitimate recording of 'wants' that fell outside normative definitions of need became confused with the legal obligation to meet normative need that fell within eligibility criteria. This contributed to a culture of concealment and 'learning to be economical with the truth' (Hadley and Clough 1997: 186). A significant legal case in 1997, the Gloucestershire judgment (see Chapter 4), confirmed that local authorities can act lawfully in taking into account resources when deciding whether it is necessary to meet need and this is confirmed in the FACS guidance (Department of Health 2002b). However, such decisions must be taken on the basis of an assessment or reassessment of need and they must be made in relation to general eligibility criteria; resources cannot be the sole consideration, and decisions must be reasonable, taking account of the right to life and right to family life and home under the Human Rights Act (1998) (Brammer 2003). As already noted, the FACS guidance distinguishes between presenting needs and eligible needs. While it is entirely legitimate to identify and record unmet need in the sense of presenting needs that are not eligible needs, all needs assessed as eligible must be met.

The FACS guidance stipulates that where services are not provided following assessment, the reasons for the decision should be communicated in writing and information and advice about alternative sources of support should be given (Department of Health 2002b: para. 67). It also states that local authorities should monitor presenting needs that are not assessed as eligible needs. Failure to record this unmet need has significant implications for service development: 'The risk of ignoring data from individual assessments is that service development is not rooted in local issues and needs and, instead, may be driven by "top-down" organisational factors such as budgets and the preferences of managers' (Parry-Jones and Soulsby 2001: 424). One inspection report noted that even where authorities did have systems for recording unmet need, these were often not utilised and there was no sense of the information being used to inform the planning and development of services (Department of Health 1999a). A study of the commissioning of care services for older people carried out between August 2000 and May 2001 in seven local authorities found a lack of services available to meet assessed need and lack of systems to record this unmet need; in three of the sample authorities, there was either no system for recording unmet need or the process had been abandoned (Ware *et al.* 2003). In addition to fear about the legal obligations invoked by recording unmet need, another explanation for the lack of its recording is that it is simply not identified in the first place. If, as some studies suggest (for example, Baldwin 2000), care managers restrict the needs they consider to those they know can be met, such 'service-led' practice will inevitably not uncover unmet need.

The FACS guidance does, then, clarify issues around legal responsibilities in respect of unmet need. In short, unmet need in terms of presenting needs that do not fall within eligibility criteria should be recorded and monitored. On the other hand, failure to meet need that has been assessed as eligible in terms of the local authority's criteria constitutes a breach of statutory duty. If the preferred means of meeting the need is not available, other avenues to meet the need should be pursued. Clarity about the legal status of unmet need and about the broader purpose of assessment – helping individuals to reach a better understanding of their situation and to identify options for dealing with difficulties – are important for individual practitioners and their employing authorities. This broader purpose should encourage them to be concerned with need as perceived and expressed by older people ('presenting needs') rather than just need for which they know help will be provided ('eligible needs'). It should also reinforce the identification and recording of unmet need as a key mechanism for monitoring the nature and level of need so that this can be used to inform the planning and commissioning of services.

With regard to unmet needs, it appears that certain types of need are frequently overlooked or given low priority by social services. One example, the needs of older people with visual impairments (Department of Health 1998b), can be used to illustrate how needs remain unmet, despite the legislation and policy relating to assessment that we have examined. Interviews and focus group discussions carried out with over 400 visually impaired people over the age of 55 in Plymouth, London and Birmingham highlighted the lack of early detection of support needs and failure to deliver proactive and holistic assessment (Percival and Hanson 2005). Just over half of the people interviewed reported that they were not in touch with any formal services even though half of them were registered blind or partially sighted. There are a number of possible reasons for this. First, as discussed at the beginning of the chapter, people may experience 'felt' need but not express it, if they do not know that services are available or do not feel that services will help them. Second, there may be poor communication between and within agencies responsible for providing support. When people who are blind or partially sighted see a consultant ophthalmologist, a form is completed that triggers the person's registration with the local authority. Through this process, the local authority should become aware that the person is someone who falls within the definition of disability contained in Section 29 of National Assistance Act (1948), and therefore is someone who 'may be in need of services', and thereby someone in respect of whom they have a duty to carry out an assessment under Section 47 of NHS and Community Care Act (1990). The implementation of the *Single Assessment Process* aims to address difficulties associated with inter-agency coordination and should, in theory, ensure that needs identified by one professional or agency are communicated to others who may be able to provide support. Third, it may be that assessment is triggered through the process of registration but that the 'presenting' needs of older people with visual impairments are not 'eligible' needs in terms of FACS criteria. Yet small amounts of low-cost services can make a crucial difference to well-being. Percival and Hanson's research identifies the need for information about social services, disability benefits and low-vision equipment to be much more available and accessible to people with low vision, especially people from minority ethnic groups. Only one in five of the sample had received any rehabilitation following the onset of sight loss. Support with household tasks and access to home carers to help with correspondence and bills, for example, was found to be particularly important for people with sight loss. Problems of social isolation and the need for psychological and emotional support and social contact to promote mental well-being were also noted. As mentioned previously in this chapter, the FACS guidance states that the assessment of risks to independence should encompass autonomy and freedom to make choices, the ability to manage personal and other daily routines and involvement in family and wider community life. However, despite this broad understanding of 'independence', the areas of need experienced by people with low vision are likely to be regarded as 'moderate' or 'low', and therefore not eligible for services. A key message from the study is that the unmet needs of older people with low vision contribute to their social marginalisation. The authors argue that timely and more comprehensive assessments and better support services can play a key role in promoting the social inclusion of older people with low vision. Specific recommendations are that systems should be put in place to provide earlier detection and support for older people with sight loss and that holistic assessments should be undertaken. The study proposes greater use of peer support groups, offering social contact and support, and resource centres to provide a 'one-stop shop' for information, advice, equipment and access to home visitors.

ACTIVITY 3.4: ASSESSING TO PROMOTE CITIZENSHIP

Refer back to the components for well-being set out in the Social Exclusion Unit Report, A *Sure Start to Later Life* (Office of the Deputy Prime Minister 2006) in Chapter 2, Figure 2.3. Draw up a list of headings and prompts that could serve as a framework for an assessment aimed at promoting older people's citizenship and well-being.

Now revisit the description of the domains and sub-domains of the *Single Assessment Process* presented earlier in this chapter (Box 3.1).

- To what extent do the domains and sub-domains of the *Single Assessment Process* cover the headings that you have identified?
- Are any issues in your list neglected or underplayed in the *Single Assessment Process*?
- What are your conclusions about the extent to which the *Single Assessment Process* supports a citizenship and well-being agenda?

On the basis of the discussion thus far, we can conclude that older people's access to community care services is based on professional assessment of need or risk (negative concepts), rather than their rights or entitlements (positive concepts). Rights depend on a means of enforcement; if receipt of services depends on discretion exercised by someone else, there is no 'right'. In terms of their access to social care services, older people have procedural rights, such as the right to be involved in decisions and the right to complain, but few clear-cut substantive rights. What help they are entitled to will depend largely on professional assessment (Evans and Harris 2004b), which in turn is influenced by factors such as interpretation and application of legislation, national and local policies and resource availability. The next chapter will continue discussion of these issues in relation to the planning and provision of care services.

KEY POINTS

- ☐ There is no coherent legal framework underpinning social work with older people but instead a complex myriad of different pieces of legislation, some of which date back to 1948.

- ☐ It is important for social workers to be aware of the practice issues raised by the legal framework for assessment.

- ☐ The process of assessment also takes place within the guidance provided by the *Single Assessment Process* and *Fair Access to Care Services*.

- ☐ There are tensions between expressed need and normative need (as set out in eligibility criteria), between needs-led and service-led assessment.

- ☐ It is important to be clear about the nature of unmet need and how it can be dealt with in social work practice.

- ☐ Good practice would indicate that assessment should focus on promoting individuals' well-being and this seems to be reflected in recent policy relating to older people. However, there are conflicts within policy and contradictions at the level of practice.

KEY READING

Department of Health (2002b) *Fair Access to Care Services*, London: Department of Health.

Department of Health (2002c) *The Single Assessment Process for Older People*, London: Department of Health.

Mandelstam, M. (2005, 3rd edn) *Community Care Practice and the Law*, London: Jessica Kingsley Publishers.

CHAPTER 4

PLANNING AND PROVIDING SERVICES

OBJECTIVES

By the end of this chapter you should have an understanding of:

- the nature and significance of the stages of planning, implementing and reviewing services within the assessment and care management process;

- the legal and policy framework relevant to the provision of services, both non-residential and residential;

- requirements and procedures for regulating care provision;

- the changing nature of the 'care market' and the implications for older people.

Key messages in the previous chapter – about the disjunctions between what the law appears to state, the objectives set out in policy and what actually happens at the level of practice – apply as much to care planning and service provision as they do to assessment. The nature of the service responses that follow from assessment will be influenced by whether the assessment is framed in terms of meeting professionally defined need, evaluating narrowly defined risks or promoting independence and well-being, as seen from the older person's perspective.

In Chapter 2, Figure 2.3 identified the different dimensions to be addressed in a holistic assessment concerned with promoting well-being and social inclusion. To respond effectively to the needs and issues identified by such an assessment, social workers need to work collaboratively with a range of different agencies and individuals in planning and providing services. Examples of the range of services that may be needed to promote older people's independence and well-being are shown in Figure 4.1.

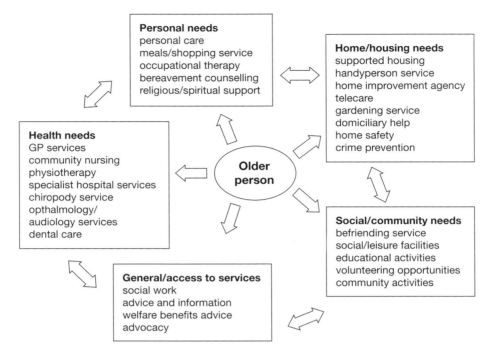

Personal needs
personal care
meals/shopping service
occupational therapy
bereavement counselling
religious/spiritual support

Home/housing needs
supported housing
handyperson service
home improvement agency
telecare
gardening service
domiciliary help
home safety
crime prevention

Health needs
GP services
community nursing
physiotherapy
specialist hospital services
chiropody service
opthalmology/
audiology services
dental care

Older person

Social/community needs
befriending service
social/leisure facilities
educational activities
volunteering opportunities
community activities

General/access to services
social work
advice and information
welfare benefits advice
advocacy

FIGURE 4.1 Examples of services to support well-being, as is relevant to the individual needs of the older person

Figure 4.1 highlights the potential complexity of care planning and provision for older people, if a well-being remit is adopted. The different forms of support are likely to be provided through a mix of statutory, private or voluntary sources and through informal relationships with family and friends and within the community more broadly. As far as older people are concerned, what matters is that the support they need is available, accessible, appropriate to their specific needs and provided in a way that is acceptable to them (see, for example, Age Concern 2006c). Furthermore, where people have complex needs, they require services to be coordinated or 'joined up' to minimise gaps between them and to provide smooth interrelationships, or 'seamless care', between the different providers. Chapters 2 and 3 have highlighted the emphasis in policy on a coordinated approach between organisations in order to avoid duplication between agencies. (Issues concerning the working relationship between social workers and others involved in supporting older people will be considered in Chapter 6.) The first part of this chapter will outline the policy framework relevant to planning services for older people. The second part of the chapter will discuss the legal and policy framework of providing services, both in the community and in residential settings. The final part of the chapter will consider processes for reviewing the care plan.

CARE PLANNING

Care planning is undertaken at the level of planning services for individual service users and at the level of planning the services required to meet the needs of whole communities. This section concerns care planning for individual service users. (Strategic planning for whole communities will be discussed in Chapter 6.) As we saw in Chapter 2, the community care reforms of the early 1990s separated out assessment of need from the provision of services and promoted the 'mixed economy' of care as a way of improving the quality of services and increasing consumer choice. Since services were now to be provided not by one organisation – the local authority – but by an individually tailored amalgam from private, voluntary and informal sources, coordinated by the local authority social worker, it was essential that there were adequate mechanisms in place to plan and coordinate care arrangements.

Care planning is one of the key stages within the process of assessment and care management identified in the practitioners' guidance (Social Services Inspectorate/ Department of Health 1991b – see Figure 2.1 in Chapter 2). Clements (2004) argues that the guidance on care planning needs to be understood and adhered to, as it has been accorded considerable weight in legal challenges. The guidance states that the care plan should be: 'set out in concise written form'; accessible to the service user in terms of the language and form of communication used; shared with the service user; and, subject to confidentiality considerations, shared with other contributors to the care plan (ibid.: para. 4.37). The guidance also specifies the information that should be contained within the care plan (see Box 4.1).

BOX 4.1 THE CONTENTS OF A CARE PLAN

The practitioners' guidance states that the following information should be contained in a care plan:

- the overall objectives;
- the specific objectives – for service users, carers and service providers;
- the criteria for evaluating the achievement of objectives;
- the services to be provided by different agencies/personnel;
- the costs to the service user and other organisations;
- the other options considered during the process of care planning;
- any points of difference between the service user, carer, care manager or other agency;
- any unmet needs with reasons stated as to why needs remain unmet;
- the name of the person responsible for implementing, monitoring and reviewing the care plan;
- the date planned for the first review.

(Social Services Inspectorate/Department of Health 1991b: para. 4.37)

Under the *Community Care Assessment Directions* (Department of Health 2004a), local authorities are required to take all reasonable steps to reach agreement with individuals and, if appropriate, their carers, about services that are being considered. These directions also require the local authority to provide information to individuals and carers about any charges that are payable for the services.

Whereas the practitioners' guidance and the assessment directions relate to work with all adult service users, the *Single Assessment Process* guidance (see Chapter 3) contains additional requirements for care plans for older people:

> Care planning involves users and professionals discussing the support and treatment that can best meet identified/eligible needs and achieve agreed goals . . . Care planning should build on the strengths and abilities of individuals and the part they can play in addressing their needs. It should address external or environmental factors that have caused the needs to arise, or will hamper the resolution of needs if not addressed. All agencies providing or commissioning services that are part of an individual's package of care should have been involved in planning the care.
>
> (Department of Health 2002c: Annex E, 23)

It is envisaged that a single care plan is produced, shared by all relevant agencies, subject to the older person's agreement. The required contents of the care plan as set out in the SAP guidance are shown in Box 4.2.

BOX 4.2   THE CONTENTS OF A CARE PLAN ACCORDING TO *SINGLE ASSESSMENT PROCESS* GUIDANCE

A single care plan should be produced containing the following information:

- a summary of eligible needs (i.e. those that fall within eligibility criteria), indicating 'the intensity, instability, predictability, and complexity of needs, the associated risks to independence, and the potential for rehabilitation';
- a note on whether the older person has agreed the care plan and, if not, a reason for this;
- a note on whether the older person has agreed for the care plan to be shared with relevant agencies and reasons if this consent was not obtained;
- the objectives of providing help and the outcomes that this is anticipated to achieve;
- a summary of how the services provided will impact on needs and risks;
- the role to be played by the older person in addressing needs, including their strengths and abilities;
- details on how any risks will be managed, including a written note if the older person has agreed to accept certain risks;
- details of the help that carers are willing to provide and their own support needs;

- a description of responsibilities of different agencies and the level and frequency of help they will provide;
- details of care costs to be met by the older person;
- the integration of a nursing plan into the care plan, if appropriate;
- the level of Registered Nurse Care Contribution for older people to be admitted to care home providing nursing care (this is discussed later in the chapter);
- the name and contact number of the person responsible for coordinating the care plan;
- a contact number in case of emergencies and a contingency plan if things go wrong;
- arrangements for monitoring the care plan and a date for a review.

(Department of Health 2002c: Annex E, 24–5)

As shown in Boxes 4.1 and 4.2, key requirements of the care plan are that: objectives for the intervention are clearly articulated; the services to be provided by different agencies are specified; there is clarification of how the achievement of objectives (i.e. the changes that are anticipated) is to be evaluated; the service user is given fundamental information about costs and contact points; and a review date is agreed. Additional components required under the *Single Assessment Process* are that: risks and how they are to be managed have to be detailed; the contribution of carers and their support needs have to be included; and nursing input has to be integrated as part of the plan.

ACTIVITY 4.1: DRAWING UP A CARE PLAN

Ada, aged 87, is a single white British woman who lives alone in an isolated bungalow in a rural area. Ada has been struggling to manage for the last three years since the death of her sister, who lived with her. She has found it very hard to manage on only her pension. She is afraid to use the heating because of the cost and the bungalow is in need of repairs, in particular improved insulation to the roof, doors and windows. Ada has been neglecting to eat properly as she does not bother to cook just for herself. She has become very frail and has been having increasingly frequent falls. She has no close family and she rarely goes out. She has a friend in the village who does her shopping but this friend is also in her 80s. Ada worries about her friend's health and thinks that she is being a burden. Ada has become depressed over the last few months and admits that everything is getting on top of her. She misses her sister's companionship and has no one to talk to about her worries. Her problems only came to light when she visited the nurse for her flu injection and broke down in tears when the nurse asked how she was. The nurse completed a contact assessment under the SAP guidance and has passed the information to the social worker linked to the surgery to complete an overview assessment and draw up a care plan.

Imagine that you are drawing up a care plan for Ada. Referring back to Figure 4.1, think about some of the services that might be helpful to her. Assume for the purposes of this exercise that your assessment has been completed, that

Ada is in agreement with the resulting plan and that all of the services you want to put in place are available. Draw up an outline care plan specifying:

- a summary of Ada's needs and any risks present in the situation;
- the objectives of the intervention with Ada;
- the services that are to be provided and by which personnel/agencies;
- the anticipated outcomes in terms of the changes that you will expect to see if the care plan is successful.

Once needs have been assessed, eligibility has been determined and objectives have been clarified, it is likely that there will be different intervention options. For example, assistance to obtain adequate nutrition might be an eligible need for an older woman who is unable to prepare food for herself. The objective might be to ensure that she has one main meal every day. The outcomes might be weight gain and improved physical health. There could be a number of different services that would meet the objective. For example, a home carer could visit daily to prepare a meal; a home carer could visit daily to work alongside the woman, assisting her to prepare a meal; frozen meals could be stored in the woman's freezer for her (or a family member) to heat up; mobile meals could be delivered daily; transport could be arranged for the woman to attend a day centre or a lunch club; a support worker/befriender could assist the woman to go to a local pub or café for her lunch; a family member or neighbour could visit every day to bring or prepare a meal. A number of these or other options could potentially address the objective and facilitate achievement of the desired outcome. However, looking at the needs of the older woman and the needs of those in the support network holistically, it is likely that not all of the options would meet all of the needs. For example, relying on input from family members might place unacceptable strain on the informal network; providing frozen or mobile needs might not address the woman's wider need for social contact and activity.

For a social worker planning services to meet needs, the prime requirement in legal terms is that the help provided meets the individual's (eligible) needs. If all options meet the need equally well, case law (the *Lancashire judgment*[1]) has established that local authorities are allowed to take cost into account in deciding which option will be pursued (Clements 2004). Thus, if an assessment indicates that a person needs 24-hour care, the local authority can legitimately elect to arrange for the provision of residential care, rather than an intensive domiciliary care package, if the former is less costly. However, if the physical needs could be met equally well by either option but the social, emotional or psychological needs could only be met by the domiciliary care option, the local authority would have to proceed cautiously (as demonstrated in the *Avon judgment*). The duty to meet eligible needs includes needs that are social and emotional in nature, as well as physical.

This brings us back to some of the tricky issues around determining 'need' versus 'want', discussed in Chapter 3. Ultimately, there is a difficult balancing act between legal, policy and practice directives to, on the one hand, consult and involve service users and carers and, on the other hand, seek cost-effectiveness. (This issue is discussed further in Chapter 7.) As already mentioned, directions issued in 2004 require that local authorities take all reasonable steps to reach agreement with individuals and, if appropriate, their carers, about care services that are being considered (Department of Health 2004a). To select care options based on rigid rulings, such as 'we only provide domiciliary packages up to a maximum of "x" level and, beyond this, we provide residential care', would constitute a fettering of the local authority's discretion and a failure to consider individual needs, circumstances and wishes (Mandlestam 2005). To depart legitimately from the service user's wishes, the local authority would need to demonstrate that: it had taken 'all reasonable steps' to reach agreement with the individual(s) concerned; *and* that the care package it was offering or providing met the assessed eligible needs (defined broadly, not just in terms of physical needs); *and* that the care package it was offering or providing was more cost-effective (see *Southwark judgment*). In addition, if the local authority was pursing a residential, rather than a domiciliary option, it would need to be mindful of, first, the strong emphasis in policy and legislation on supporting people to live in the community; and, second, the potential for challenge under Article 8 of Human Rights Act (1998), 'the right to respect for private and family life, home and correspondence' (Clements 2004).

The next part of the chapter moves on to legislation, policy and practice issues in relation to the provision of services. These are discussed, first, in terms of the provision of community care (non-residential) services and, second, in relation to care home provision.

COMMUNITY CARE (NON-RESIDENTIAL) SERVICES

It is important to note that, in addition to the specific laws concerned with the provision of services to be considered in this chapter, local authorities also have general powers under the Local Government Act (2000, Section 2) to promote or improve the economic, social or environmental well-being of their area. This includes the well-being of all or part of the area or of any individual resident within it (Clements 2004). As local authorities cannot do anything that the law does not empower them to do, this is an important legal tool, allowing them flexibility to act creatively in responding to the needs of communities and individuals. Innovative initiatives to address the well-being objectives set out in some of the policies discussed in Chapter 2 could potentially be provided under this section. However, the section cannot be used to act in any way that is prohibited or limited by other legislation (ibid.).

Non-residential community care services for older people may be provided under five different pieces of legislation: the National Assistance Act (1948); the Health Services and Public Health Act (1968); the Chronically Sick and Disabled Persons Act (1970); the National Health Service Act (1977); and the Mental Health Act (1983). The assessment of need that provides access to these services will be carried out (primarily) through the duty to assess contained within the NHS and Community Care Act (1990, Section 47), discussed in the previous chapter.

National Assistance Act (1948)

Section 29 of National Assistance Act (1948) gives local authorities various powers and duties to provide services. The section defines the people to whom it applies, that is, those aged 18 or over who are blind, deaf or dumb, or who suffer from mental disorder of any description and other persons aged 18 or over who are substantially and permanently handicapped by illness, injury or congenital deformity or such other disabilities as may be prescribed.

Despite its outdated and oppressive language, this is an important definition and one that still provides the foundation for the provision of services by setting out the definition of disability to be used when deciding who falls within the terms of the legislation. Older age is not in itself grounds for service provision under this piece of legislation but older people may, and often do, fall within the Section 29 definition of disability because they are 'substantially and permanently handicapped'. Guidance issued to local authorities instructs them to be inclusive and flexible in the way they interpret such phrases (Department of Health 1993). The duties and powers contained within the National Assistance Act (1948) Section 29, are as follows.

Duties

The local authority has the following general duties in respect of people who are ordinarily resident within the area it serves and who meet the section 29 definition of disability:

- maintaining a register of disabled people;
- providing a social work service, advice and support;
- providing facilities for social rehabilitation and adjustment to disability;
- providing facilities for occupational, social, cultural and recreational activities.

These are general 'target' duties, rather than specific duties to individuals. Whereas target duties are broad, allow scope for interpretation and are, in part, aspirational, specific duties are precise and intended to give rights that are enforceable (Clements 2004). Target duties such as those contained in Section 29 of the National Assistance Act (1948) are framed in general terms that are difficult to enforce legally in the event of any of the services covered not being provided to a particular person. These duties also only have the status of powers (that is, the legislation is permissive rather than mandatory) for disabled people who are not ordinarily resident in the local authority's area (Mandelstam 2005).

Powers

The local authority has powers to arrange other services for both people who are ordinarily resident in the area and those who are not. These are powers to:

- inform disabled people about services available to them under Section 29;
- instruct people about overcoming the effects of their disabilities;
- provide workshops so that people can engage in suitable work;
- provide suitable work and help people dispose of the produce of their work;
- provide holiday homes;

- provide free or subsidised travel for people who do not qualify for other forms of free or subsidised travel;
- assist people to find accommodation to enable them to take advantage of arrangements under Section 29;
- contribute to the cost of employing a warden in housing schemes with warden assistance or provide a warden in private housing.

Section 47 of the National Assistance Act (1948) contains powers to remove people from their homes in specific circumstances. These are now rarely used and may conflict with the Human Rights Act (1998).

Health Services and Public Health Act (1968)

So far the legislation considered has concerned adult service users generally, including older people, rather than older people specifically. In contrast, under Section 45 of the Health Services and Public Health Act (1968), local authorities have powers and duties specifically for promoting the welfare of 'old people', though how this category of people is to be defined is not clear. (There is no clear legal definition of an older person in community care legislation, unlike children's legislation where a child is defined as someone under the age of 18 [Brammer 2003].) As mentioned in Chapter 2, the purpose of this legislation is to enable local authorities to arrange services for older people who are not 'substantially and permanently handicapped', and so do not fall within Section 29 of the National Assistance Act's (1948) definition of disability. This Act could, therefore, constitute the legal underpinning for the development of preventive services for older people with lower level needs. The services that may be arranged under this section are:

- meals and recreation, whether in the home or elsewhere;
- information about the services available to older people and about older people who are in need of services;
- assistance with travel to enable older people to use services;
- help in finding accommodation;
- visiting, advisory and social work support services;
- practical assistance in the home, including help with adaptations or facilities that will help increase safety, comfort or convenience;
- help with the costs of employing a warden or providing a warden in private housing.

Under the Act, the Secretary of State may give directions making the provision of these services a duty but, to date, no directions have been given, only approval:

> Despite the potential value of providing such services for older people, no government in over 30 years has had the financial courage to issue such directions and thereby create a duty. Instead the approvals issued in 1971 make the provision of these services merely a power.
>
> (Mandelstam 2005: 234)

Although there are no duties to provide services under Section 45 of the Health Services and Public Health Act (1968), social workers should be aware of the powers available under this Section for promoting older people's welfare:

> It is possible that if, in developing its community care policies and services, a local authority could be shown not even to have taken account of the approvals and guidance in respect of s.45, then a case might be arguable in the law courts. Local authorities should at least have regard to guidance; and even in respect of powers, should beware of fettering their discretion.
>
> (Mandelstam 2005: 235)

The Immigration and Asylum Act (1999, Section 117) amended Section 45 of the Health Services and Public Health Act (1968) to the effect that older asylum seekers are not eligible for services under this section solely on the basis that they are 'destitute' (Clements 2004). Asylum seekers who require community care services because of 'destitution' come within the remit of National Asylum Support Service.

Chronically Sick and Disabled Persons Act (1970)

Section 2 of this Act gives local authorities duties to arrange services for disabled people who are ordinarily resident in their area. There is a duty on local authorities under Section 2 to make arrangements for the following services to be provided, if the local authority is satisfied that this is necessary to meet the person's needs:

* practical assistance in the home;
* provision of or help obtaining recreational facilities such as a television or library access;
* provision of recreational facilities outside the home such as lectures, games or outings or helping the person to use educational facilities;
* provision of or help with travel to enable the person to participate in any services provided under Section 29 of the National Assistance Act (1948);
* help in arranging for adaptations to the home or providing any other facilities to increase the person's safety, comfort or convenience;
* helping the person to take holidays, whether or not these are provided through the local authority;
* provision of meals, in the home or elsewhere;
* provision of, or help in obtaining, a telephone and any special equipment necessary to enable the person to use a telephone.

The duties in this Act are 'stronger' than those in the National Assistance Act (1948) in that this section sets out specific duties towards individual disabled people, rather than general duties toward the local population. As mentioned previously, individuals are more likely to be able to enforce these specific local authority duties than the general duties contained in Section 29 of the National Assistance Act (1948).

In deciding whether someone is 'disabled' for the purpose of Section 2 of the Chronically Sick and Disabled Persons Act (1970), the definition of disability given in the National Assistance Act (1948) Section 29 applies (see above). Section 2 of the Chronically Sick and Disabled Persons Act (1970) states that a local authority has a duty to make arrangements for the provision of the services outlined above, if it is satisfied that it is necessary to make those arrangements in order to meet the person's needs. A key issue here is whether a service is 'necessary to meet needs'. This decision is taken by relating assessed need to eligibility criteria, as set out in the *Fair Access to Care Services* guidance (Department of Health 2002b). As discussed in Chapter 3, this provides a national framework for determining eligibility for services, based on four levels of risk: critical, substantial, moderate and low. Once a local authority has established that it is necessary for it to make arrangements for services to be provided in order to meet the needs of a disabled person who is ordinarily resident in its area – in other words, it is satisfied that the assessed need is 'eligible need', according to its criteria – then it has a legal duty to arrange for those services to be provided.

The question of whether 'assessed need' constitutes 'eligible need' has been a contested area and was central to a significant legal ruling, the *Gloucestershire judgment*. Mr Barry was a disabled man, aged 79. He had been receiving help with cleaning and laundry from Gloucestershire local authority. However, when Gloucestershire was under financial pressure, it withdrew or reduced home care services to 1,500 service users. It reduced Mr Barry's help with laundry and withdrew the cleaning service. Mr Barry's case went to judicial review in 1995 on the grounds that the service should not have been reduced as his needs had not changed. The Court of Appeal's decision was that the local authority's resources were not a relevant consideration and Mr Barry should receive the service he was originally assessed as needing. However, on further appeal to the House of Lords, the final ruling (based on a majority view) in 1997 was that the local authority could take account of its financial resources when deciding what is a 'need'. However, once it has established that there is a need, it must meet that need, regardless of its financial resources.

Key principles established by the Gloucestershire case are that:

- Local authorities must define 'need' in individual cases against general eligibility criteria set by the department (these now have to fall within the FACS framework – see Chapter 3).
- The local authority's resources can be taken into account when determining the level at which these eligibility criteria should be set.
- If a person's needs meet the local authority's eligibility criteria, this signifies that it is 'necessary' for it to make arrangements for the provision of services to meet the need under Section 2 of the Chronically Sick and Disabled Persons Act (1970). However, this 'absolute' duty to meet eligible need may not apply in the same way to the weaker general duties under other legislation, such as Section 29 of the National Assistance Act (1948) (Mandelstam 2005).
- In satisfying themselves that it is necessary to meet need, local authorities can change their threshold of what counts as a need that it is necessary for them to meet by changing their eligibility criteria. This is likely to happen when there are resource shortfalls.
- Eligibility criteria must be applied consistently to individual service users, both those whose needs are being assessed for the first time and existing service users who are already receiving services.
- Local authorities must always make decisions based on reassessment of the needs of individual service users and not make blanket decisions to reduce or stop services.

- In making decisions about what counts as a 'need', resources should not be the only consideration. Guidance issued following the *Gloucestershire judgment* clarified that local authorities must be 'reasonable' in their behaviour. 'Unreasonableness', for example, would be tightening their eligibility criteria so much that only those at imminent risk of death or serious injury were regarded as having a 'need' that it was necessary to meet. Local authorities must also not be unreasonable by breaching human rights. For example, they must respect life and not subject people to degrading treatment (Human Rights Act 1998).

ACTIVITY 4.2: LAWFUL PRACTICE?

On the basis of your understanding of the legislation and the principles established in the *Gloucestershire judgment* (see above), which of the following actions are lawful/unlawful? Give a brief explanation for your answer.

All of the people in the following exercise are 'older people'.

1   Mrs A. is partially sighted. She phones adult services for help with cleaning, shopping and maintaining social activities. The call centre worker receiving the call informs her that her needs are 'low' and that she does not meet the criteria for services to be provided. He sends Mrs A. a list of private domiciliary care agencies.

2   Mrs B. is partially sighted. She phones adult services for help with cleaning, shopping and maintaining social activities. These needs would normally be assessed as 'low'. The local authority concerned is currently only providing support to people with critical or substantial needs. However, it is the end of the financial year and some of the budget is unspent. The manager agrees that help can be provided to Mrs A.

3   Mr C. is disabled and needs assistance with personal care. He is assessed as having eligible needs in the 'substantial' category. However, it is nearing the end of the financial year and the budget is overspent. Mr B. is put on a waiting list for two months so that his care package will be funded from the next year's budget.

4   A local authority has had to review its provision in the light of a significant budget deficit. It decides to cease providing support to those with 'moderate' needs and that only those with needs in the 'critical' and 'substantial' categories will receive assistance. Miss D. has been receiving help for two years but her needs were assessed as 'moderate'. The local authority writes to tell her that her care will be ceasing in view of the change to their eligibility criteria.

5   A local authority has had to review its provision in the light of a significant budget deficit. It decides to cease providing support to those with 'substantial' needs and that only those with needs in the 'critical' category will receive assistance.

National Health Service Act (1977, Schedule 8)

This Act gives local authorities a general duty (rather than specific duties) to arrange, at an adequate level for their area, home help 'for households where help is required owing to the presence of a person who is suffering from illness, lying in, an expectant mother, aged, handicapped as a result of having suffered from illness or by congenital deformity'. There is also a power to arrange laundry services for households who are eligible to receive home help. Help may be provided to 'households' (so, for example, to benefit carers living in the house), rather than just to the individual. Similar to the target duties contained in the National Assistance Act (1948), the general duty to arrange home care may be difficult to enforce in individual cases (Mandelstam 2005). Following the Immigration and Asylum Act (1999, Section 117) people who are asylum seekers are excluded from receiving community care services under the NHS Act (1977, Schedule 8), if their need for community care services arises solely because they are 'destitute' (Clements 2004).

Mental Health Act (1983)

We saw in Chapter 2 that older people may be assessed and detained under the Mental Health Act (1983). Section 117 of the Mental Health Act 1983 may be relevant to the provision of services for older people. This section places a duty on health and social services, in cooperation with voluntary organisations, to provide aftercare in the community for people who have been compulsorily detained under certain sections of the Act. This includes those who have been detained under Section 3 for treatment, but not those detained under Section 2 for assessment or as informal patients, though people who are discharged from a relevant section and remain in hospital as informal patients are still covered by the duty on their discharge from hospital. The duty to provide aftercare services is a 'strong' duty to individuals. It continues until health and social services are satisfied that the services are no longer required. The services covered under Section 117 are not defined and as such there is considerable scope for a range of services, both residential and non-residential, to be provided under this section.

The legislation considered so far in this chapter has been concerned with the legal framework under which services to support older people in the community may be provided. Also relevant to planning and providing services is the form in which that support is provided. In particular, help can be provided by local authorities in the form of specific services, whether provided directly by the local authority or commissioned from the private or voluntary sectors. It may also be provided by way of a 'direct payment' to the service user to enable them to purchase their own care. The next section considers direct payments and their implications for supporting older people in the community.

Direct payments

The Community Care (Direct Payments) Act (1996) introduced direct payments, that is, payments made by local authorities to individuals with assessed social care needs to enable them to purchase their own services, rather than having services arranged by the local authority. Initially, people over the age of 65 were excluded from receiving direct payments and local authorities only had a power, rather than a duty, to make such payments to them. New regulations extended direct payments to older people in 2000. The Health and Social Care Act (2001, Sections 57–58) superseded the Community Care (Direct Payments) Act (1996). It places a duty on local authorities to make direct payments to service users who fulfil the criteria and consent to receiving a direct payment. The payment made must be 'equivalent to the reasonable cost of securing the provision of the services concerned' (Health and Social Care Act 2001, Section 57). Regulations issued in 2003 state that no limit should be set on either the amount of care that can be purchased via a direct payment or the value of the direct payment (Department of Health 2003a). As well as the regulations, there is practice guidance concerning direct payments (Department of Health 2003b).

The duty to make a direct payment applies where:

- the person has an assessed eligible need for community care services. Direct payments do not therefore bypass a community care assessment, but are a potential outcome of such an assessment (Lyon 2005). An assessed eligible need has to be established before a direct payment can be made;
- the service(s) must be likely to meet the assessed need(s);
- the person must consent to receiving a direct payment;
- the person must be capable of managing the direct payment, either on her/his own or with the assistance of someone else.

There are some restrictions on what a direct payment can be used for.

- Direct payments can be used for domiciliary care services and for community equipment. They can only be used for residential accommodation if this does not last for more than four continuous weeks or amount to more than 120 days a year.
- Direct payments cannot be used to buy services that the local authority is not responsible for providing (for example, NHS services).
- Direct payments cannot be used to purchase services directly provided by the local authority, although it is possible for someone to receive both a direct payment and a local authority provided service.
- A direct payment cannot be used to pay specified relatives living in the same household, unless there are particular reasons why this is necessary to meet the person's needs. However, there are no legal restrictions on a direct payment being used to pay close relatives who do not live in the same household.
- Other restrictions may be specified, for example that the direct payment may not be used to purchase services from certain individuals.

Access to and take-up of direct payments is not just a matter of law and policy but also of practice. Glasby and Littlechild emphasise the key role played by front-line social workers in giving information, advice and support in relation to direct payments. They suggest that the necessary knowledge, resources (particularly time) and attitudes to undertake these roles are often lacking, so that it is not people 'making informed decisions to reject the idea of a direct payments package, but their social workers effectively depriving them of access to direct payments by failing to provide support and information' (2002: 138). They argue that the success of direct payments depends on social workers being well informed about direct payments, having the time to talk through the options and implications with service users and ensuring that those who wish to use the scheme have access to effective support, including peer support. Consultations with people who use direct payments, local and central policy makers and researchers highlighted the low level of awareness and understanding of direct payments by staff and the lack of information, advocacy and support for direct payments users. Other barriers identified included the negative beliefs and attitudes of staff about the capabilities of service users and their own reluctance to relinquish power. Difficulties were also noted in recruiting, employing and retaining personal assistants to provide good quality support (Commission for Social Care Inspection 2004a). It seems that additional barriers are faced by Black and minority ethnic people, who are considerably underrepresented amongst direct payment users, despite the potential of direct payments to deliver a more culturally responsive service (Butt *et al.* 2000).

Research specifically with older people (Clark *et al.* 2004) identified similar issues. The research, conducted in three local authority areas in England, involved in-depth interviews carried out with 41 older people in their own homes and/or in discussion groups. Some senior managers, team managers, care managers and direct payments support workers were also interviewed. Direct payments were found to increase older people's sense of choice, continuity and control over their support arrangements. This had 'added value', having a positive impact on older people's social, emotional and physical health. Direct payments gave opportunities for flexibility and choice regarding support arrangements, for example allowing the use of personal assistants to support social activities. However, as these tended not to be assessed as 'eligible needs', this often meant creative juggling of 'care' hours allocated and/or the older people having to pay additional costs themselves. For Somali women in the study, direct payments enabled them to access culturally relevant services. Having someone who spoke the same language was very important in enabling them to be in control and maintain independence in family relationships. Older people in the study experienced some problems in recruiting personal assistants. Help with advertising, drawing up contracts and interviewing was important in enabling them to deal with these issues. As noted in the research discussed previously, support to manage the financial and administrative demands associated with direct payments was crucial to making the scheme work for older people and easy access to support to deal with queries and difficulties was valued. In terms of care managers, the factors they identified as important to the success of direct payments were: adequate training; supportive managers; time to think and work creatively; feeling confident and enthusiastic about direct payments; a clear understanding of the support available; and easy access to direct payment support services. The study concluded that direct payments were not a central part of care management culture but were usually offered in response to particular problems, such as the breakdown of relationships between service users and existing providers.

The Adult Social Care Green Paper, *Independence, Well-Being and Choice* (Department of Health 2005a – see Chapter 2) proposed increasing the use of direct payments as well as introducing individualised budgets. Consultation on the Green Paper's proposals indicated wide general support for the extension of direct payments but particular concerns were expressed by older people and organisations representing them. Concerns included: anxieties about the potential for physical and financial abuse;

the need for effective support and advice in organising services; changing abilities that might make it difficult to manage a direct payment; and fears that some older people would not want the level of responsibility involved in managing a direct payment (Department of Health 2005b).

The Green Paper's proposals were taken forward in the White Paper, *Our Health, Our Care, Our Say* (Department of Health 2006b), which announces the intention of increasing the take-up of direct payments. Local authorities are to be proactive in their promotion of direct payments: 'direct payments should be discussed as a first option with everyone, at each assessment and each review' (para. 4.25). In addition to measures to increase the take-up of direct payments, plans to develop individual budgets are presented. Individual budgets are sums of money allocated to individuals that bring together different sources of funding to which they are entitled, not just an allocation for eligible social care needs. This allocated sum can be taken as a cash payment or used for services, or a mixture of the two. This is seen as offering the advantages of direct payments but without the potential difficulties inherent in becoming a budget manager and employer:

> Individual budgets offer a radical new approach, giving greater control to the individual, opening up the range and availability of services to match needs, and stimulating the market to respond to new demands from more powerful users of social care.
>
> (Department of Health 2006b: para. 4.30)

A two-year programme to pilot individual budgets commenced in November 2005 and 13 local authorities are taking part in this at the time of writing. The programme is being evaluated and a website has been created to offer support and disseminate good practice (www.individualbudgets.csip.org.uk). The pilots are testing out individual budgets with different service user 'groups', including older people.

Clark *et al.*'s findings (see above) indicate that it is important that assumptions are not made about what older people might, or might not, want. Some may prefer direct payments or individual budgets while others may prefer to have services provided for them. Direct payments and individual budgets should not be the only route to services: 'Rather than using direct payments to justify avoiding service development, the challenge for local authorities is to support service developments that incorporate principles of flexibility, choice and control as the norm for all styles of service provision' (Lyon 2005: 250). Good social work practice should include giving clear information and advice to older people about the options available, providing access to effective support and building in opportunities for them to review decisions in the light of changing circumstances.

ACTIVITY 4.3: THE IMPLICATIONS OF DIRECT PAYMENTS

Refer back to the situation of Ada (see Activity 4.1, page 97). Ada was assessed as having 'substantial' needs on the basis of her frailty, self-neglect and low mood. Her care package includes a half-hour visit once a day to help her prepare a meal. The agency providing the service has difficulty recruiting staff who can travel to

Ada's rural location, and visits are often late or cancelled. Ada's friend has introduced her to someone, who has just moved into the village, who would be willing to provide support for her.

You are visiting Ada to advise her about direct payments. Write out a list of points that you would want to cover or questions you would want to ask during your visit.

Charging for non-residential services

Local authorities have a power (not a duty, as is the case for charging for residential accommodation) to make reasonable charges for non-residential services. This power is contained in the Health and Social Services and Social Security Adjudication Act (1983, Section 17). As shown earlier in the chapter (see Boxes 4.1 and 4.2), local authorities are expected to give service users clear information about charges and to write this into their care plans. Policy guidance on charging for non-residential services was issued in 2001 (Department of Health 2001b). This lays down certain rules in an attempt to address the national variation in charging polices and establish greater fairness and consistency. The guidance was reissued in 2003, with examples of how the rules apply in practice (Department of Health 2003c). This guidance states that people receiving direct payments should make the equivalent contribution to the cost of their care package as if they were receiving services. Practice guidance concerning charging for home care services was published in 2002 (Department of Health 2002e). This recommends separating out the assessment of need from financial assessments.

It is important to note that whereas residential and non-residential services arranged by the local authority are charged for, services provided by the National Health Service are free at the point of delivery. The shifting boundaries between health and social care have had significant implications for the costs of care borne by individual service users, as well as the respective resources of health and social services (Twigg 1998). For example, individuals are now charged for services associated with intimate personal care provided by 'home care' staff, whereas some of these services were once provided free of charge, either through the community nursing service or in hospital. Similarly, the relocation of people once accommodated in long-stay hospital care to nursing or residential care has shifted financial responsibility from the NHS to social services and/or individual residents and their families. There are, however, services provided under specific provisions that local authorities cannot charge for. Intermediate care services (see Chapter 6), provided to help prevent admission to hospital or long-term care or to facilitate speedy discharge from hospital, must be provided free of charge up to a maximum of six weeks. Community equipment, that is aids or minor adaptations to property that cost £1,000 or less, must be provided free of charge under the Community Care (Delayed Discharges) Act 2003 (see Chapter 6 for discussion of this legislation). It is also unlawful for a local authority to charge for any aftercare services, whether community or residential services, provided under Section 117 of the Mental Health Act (1983).

We now turn to the legal and policy framework for the provision of residential services.

RESIDENTIAL PROVISION

This section outlines legal provisions concerning residential care for older people.

The National Assistance Act (1948)

Section 21 of the National Assistance Act (1948) places a duty on local authorities to arrange residential accommodation for 'persons aged 18 or over who by reason of age, illness, disability or any other circumstances are in need of care and attention which is not otherwise available to them'. This is sometimes referred to as 'Part Three' accommodation as Section 21 comes under Part Three of the Act. Points to note from the wording of Section 21 are that the duty to arrange residential accommodation applies where:

- the person is over 18 years of age;
- s/he has a need for care and attention;
- the need for care and attention arises from age, illness, disability or any other circumstances. Here, 'any other circumstances' should be interpreted widely (Mandelstam 2005: 178);
- the need for care and attention can only be met by providing accommodation under Section 21.

Residential care is to be provided, therefore, only when supporting people to live in their own homes is not possible. The duty does not apply if it is possible to arrange other types of support since in this case care and attention is 'otherwise available'.

As far as asylum seekers are concerned, Section 21 of National Assistance Act cannot be used to provide accommodation for people whose need for accommodation has arisen 'solely' because of destitution or the physical effects of destitution (Clements 2004). This is the same exclusion as that noted earlier in the chapter in relation to Schedule 8 of the National Health Service Act (1977) and Section 45 of the Health Services and Public Health Act (1968).

The duty to arrange residential accommodation applies to people who are 'ordinarily resident' in the area served by the local authority or to those in urgent need. 'Ordinary residence' refers to the geographical area a person has adopted as their permanent place of living. The question of where people are 'ordinarily resident' can cause disagreements between local authorities because it implies taking financial responsibility for any arrangements that are made. Even if someone has only lived in a certain area for a short time, this will still be deemed their ordinary residence if they intend to settle long-term in that place. When someone enters residential care, their place of residence immediately prior to the admission is taken to be their ordinary residence. So, for example, financial responsibility for providing residential accommodation for an older person, who needs 'care and attention not otherwise available', and who wishes to enter a care home in a different authority to be near her/his son or daughter, would rest with their own local authority, not that of the son or daughter (Clements 2004). The local authority also has powers (rather than duties) to arrange residential accommodation for people who are not 'ordinarily resident' in its area. The local authority can provide residential accommodation itself or, under Section 26 of the

Act, can make arrangements with private and voluntary sector organisations to provide residential accommodation. Since the community care reforms in the early 1990s and the promotion of the 'mixed economy of care' (see Chapter 2), many local authorities have closed some or all of their residential homes or transferred them to the private sector or to non-profit making trusts.

Government directions state that prospective residents should be given a choice of care homes. This is set out in the *National Assistance Act (1948) – Choice of Accommodation Directions (1992)* and subsequent guidance (Department of Health 2004b). The guidance states, 'As with all aspects of service provision, there should be a general presumption in favour of individuals being able to exercise reasonable choice over the service they receive' (ibid.: para. 2.1). However, choice is subject to considerations of suitability, cost and availability. The home chosen must meet the person's assessed needs, be available, be within the normal rates that the local authority pays for such accommodation, meet the local authority's standards and be located within England, Scotland or Wales. If an older person chooses to live in a home that is more expensive than the local authority's usual rates, the fees may be 'topped up' either by the older person or by her/his family. This arrangement is permitted under the Health and Social Care Act (2001). In such cases, the local authority retains responsibility for payment of the fees, collecting the 'top up' payment from the older person or her or his family. Problems are created when the rate paid by local authorities to care homes is so low that the 'topping up' of fees is almost inevitable, if there is to be any choice of home at all:

> the principle of topping up appears to have been seriously undermined in those local authorities that offer such a low usual cost level that there is little choice (if any) of a care home at that cost. In which case, it seems that families are pressured into topping up, in order to meet not additional preferences but those basic needs that should properly be met by the local authority. Such practices are likely to be unlawful.
>
> (Mandelstam 2005: 190)

Indeed, the guidance states:

> residents should not be asked to pay more towards their accommodation because of market inadequacies or commissioning failures. Where an individual has not expressed a preference for more expensive accommodation, but there are not, for whatever reason, sufficient places available at a given time at the local authority's usual costs to meet the assessed care needs of supported residents, the local authority should make a placement in more expensive accommodation. In these circumstances, neither the resident nor a third party should be asked to contribute more than the resident would normally be expected to contribute and local authorities should make up the cost difference between the resident's assessed contribution and the accommodation's fees. Only when an individual has expressed a preference for more expensive accommodation than a council would usually expect to pay, can a third party or the resident be asked for a top up.
>
> (Department of Health 2004b: para. 2.5.5)

This seems to be an example of the issue discussed at the beginning of Chapter 3, that is, a discrepancy between what happens in practice and the strict letter of the law. Although in practice top-up fees are sometimes used to off-set low rates paid to homes by local authorities, in legal terms if no accommodation is available to meet the person's needs at the level normally paid by the local authority, then the local authority should pay a higher rate in order to fulfil its duty to provide 'care and attention not otherwise available'.

Charging for residential care

Section 22 of the National Assistance Act (1948) imposes a duty on local authorities to charge people for the residential accommodation it arranges for them. Detailed guidance about charging for residential accommodation, the *Charging for Residential Accommodation Guide* (known as CRAG guidance), is issued to local authorities and periodically updated. This section of the National Assistance Act (1948) requires that charges for residential accommodation are means-tested and that every resident retains a minimum weekly personal allowance. CRAG guidance (Department of Health 2007) sets the personal allowance rate and this is regularly reviewed. To give an indication, the rate for 2007 is £20.45 per week (ibid). This is for residents' personal use, for example, for treats, outings or buying presents for family or friends. The guidance stipulates that residents should not be pressurised into using their personal allowance in particular ways and that it should not be claimed by homes to cover expenses related to eligible needs that should be detailed in the person's care plan (for example, continence supplies).

A capital threshold is set by government and capital above this limit is regarded as a source that is available to the person for purchasing 'care and attention'. Again, to give an indication, the upper capital threshold for 2007 is £21,500 (Department of Health 2007). If the person has capital above this threshold and is capable of making their own arrangements for residential accommodation, the local authority can leave the person to make their independent arrangements on a self-funding basis. At some point in the future if their capital falls below the given threshold at that time, the local authority becomes responsible for assessing whether they are in need of care and attention that can only be provided to them through residential provision. If the local authority has assessed someone as needing residential care and subsequently arranges it for them, it will pay the home provider and then recover from the resident the amount she or he has been assessed as liable to pay. The assessment of charges is made according to a sliding scale of capital. According to 2007 allowances, any capital above £13,000 was taken into account when assessing the resident's contribution; capital above the upper threshold (£21,500 in 2007) means that the person is likely to have to pay the total cost of their care (Brayne and Carr 2003: 501). In all cases, except fully self-funding arrangements, residents retain the prescribed personal allowance.

The question of a local authority's responsibility to provide 'care and attention' when someone is already resident in a care home but their capital falls below the threshold was the issue at the heart of the Sefton case (R v Sefton MBC ex parte Help the Aged [1997]). Residents who were funding their own residential care were referred to Sefton social services for an assessment when their capital fell below the threshold.

This meant that, subject to an assessment determining that they were in need of residential accommodation, they were eligible for local authority assistance with the fees. Sefton Council tried to deal with its resource problems by refusing to assess self-funders until their capital assets fell to £1,500, significantly below the capital threshold at that time. Sefton Council argued that residents who had made private self-funding arrangements and were already in a home had the necessary care and attention otherwise available to them and that, therefore, it had no duty under Section 21 of the National Assistance Act (1948). The Court of Appeal rejected Sefton Council's policy as unlawful, holding that care and attention were not to be treated as 'otherwise available' in circumstances where residents were unable to pay for it according to the financial assessment arrangements provided for in Section 22. The case also established that once a local authority has concluded that the care and attention needed by an individual is not 'otherwise available', the authority has an absolute duty to provide the accommodation, regardless of its resources (Schwehr 2000). Legislation passed subsequently (Community Care [Residential Accommodation] Act [1998]) makes clear that when the capital of an individual who is paying their own residential care home fees falls below the given capital threshold at that time, local authorities must undertake an assessment and, if necessary, assume responsibility for funding so that the person is not obliged to draw upon their capital. These arrangements must be made without 'undue delay' (see Spiers 2004: 38).

This section has illustrated the ways in which a social worker's sound understanding of the law can help to ensure that older people's rights in relation to residential accommodation are protected. To sum up, the areas that have been highlighted here are ensuring: choice of care home; that top-up fees are not used unlawfully; that personal allowances are protected; and that duties to assess the need for 'care and attention' are triggered when capital falls below the prescribed limit.

REGULATING RESIDENTIAL AND DOMICILIARY SERVICES

Legislation and national standards are in place to promote the quality of residential and domiciliary care and to protect people receiving these services from abuse or neglect. Responsibility for the registration and inspection of health and social care residential establishments and domiciliary care providers lies with the Commission for Social Care Inspection (CSCI). The CSCI was established by the Health and Social Care (Community Health and Standards) Act (2003), replacing the National Care Standards Commission and Social Services Inspectorate.

The Care Standards Act (2000) replaced the Registered Homes Act (1984) and extended the sphere of regulation from residential accommodation to include domiciliary care. The same standards and requirements now apply to local authority providers as to independent sector providers. Registration is based on three key criteria: the fitness of the premises to provide the service; the fitness of the persons running and managing the service; and the fitness of the services and facilities. To be registered, providers must demonstrate that they meet the legal requirements and National Minimum Standards that relate to the service in question (Mandelstam 2005).

Care homes are defined as establishments providing accommodation for people who are or who have been ill, disabled, infirm or dependent on drugs or alcohol and which provide 'assistance with bodily functions'. There are various requirements that have to be met for care homes to be registered. These are set out in the *Care Home Regulations* (2001). There are also national minimum standards that have to be upheld by registered care homes and failure to comply with these requirements can lead to cancellation of registration (Department of Health 2003d). There are currently 38 standards in all, grouped into seven areas: choice of care home; health and personal care; daily life and social activities; complaints and protection; environment; staffing; and management and administration (Department of Health 2003d).

While the intention of minimum care standards is to improve the quality of care for residents, some homes, particularly smaller homes, have been unable to afford to meet the requirements. Between 2000 and 2001, approximately 5 per cent of residential and nursing homes for older people closed. There was a similar rate of closures in 1999–2000. Contributory reasons for home closures are financial losses and concerns about inadequate profits, the financial implications of meeting the National Minimum Standards, difficulty in recruiting staff and meeting staffing costs and a reduction in demand for permanent care (Williams *et al.* 2002). The impact of registration and inspection requirements and low fee levels paid by local authorities have been felt by smaller homes in particular. The closure of smaller homes and an increasing monopoly of the care home market by large providers diminish choice for service users and reduce the likelihood that the 'care market' is responsive to diversity and minority needs. Another consequence of home closures is that some residents have to be moved to new homes. Home closures have been challenged under the Human Rights Act (1998), including on the grounds that this interferes with residents' right to private and family life and right to life, since the stress and upheaval of a move can lead to the death of transferred residents. Although most of the legal challenges to homes closures have not been successful, they have drawn attention to the responsibilities of local authorities in the event of home closures. They should carry out individual assessments of the residents affected to determine whether their needs will be met by the alternative care arrangements and they must consult with residents, giving them adequate notice and time to object (Mandelstam 2005).

ACTIVITY 4.4: IMPROVING STANDARDS

This extract is taken from a chapter written by an inspector of residential care homes in the 1990s, prior to implementation of the Care Standards Act (2000) and the establishment of Commission for Social Care Inspection in 2004.

> It is impossible to say the number of occasions when I observed staff handling residents roughly, almost dragging the older people out of easy chairs into wheelchairs. This practice has been done in front of me. Some homes stink of urine and faeces; can you imagine how you would feel, eating your meals in a room that stinks of faeces? . . .
>
> Food is another concern; several homes use cheap brands of food and give little choice. I have seen potatoes, cabbage and meat

all liquidised together and served to residents as a green mess on a plate.

Imagine retiring to bed at night and being expected to sleep on stained bed linen, dried-out urine on a damaged mattress, with black bin liners used as bed protectors. This is not uncommon practice either. The most common bad practice I see is residents with ill-fitting teeth, stained, damaged glasses and hearing aids that buzz non-stop. The other common bad practice is the restraining of residents; many older people's homes have the door locked for most of the day and night. Furthermore, it is not uncommon for some homes to lock bedroom doors to restrict residents having access to their rooms during the day.

(Griffin 1999: 118–19)

Consider the seven areas of the National Minimum Standards for care homes, outlined earlier. If you were appointed manager in such a home, how would you attempt to improve standards within the home and enhance the quality of life of residents?

Often the main interface between social workers and care homes will be when they are carrying out an assessment of an older person whose needs indicate that this form of care may be required. For many older people, this is likely to be a time of social, psychological, emotional and financial loss, associated with feelings of uncertainty, apprehension and sadness (Dwyer 2005). A report based on research carried out by the Office of Fair Trading (2005) emphasises the significance of this transition for older people and their families:

For older people, moving into a care home is usually a lasting decision taken under very difficult circumstances. They may often be in poor physical or mental health, under pressure to make a decision quickly, and typically have little previous experience of choosing a care home. In this situation, even with help from friends and relatives, it can be difficult to make a considered decision on care. Yet entering a care home is a major decision that will have an on-going effect on the older person's daily quality of life; and for some older people and their families, it will require a large financial commitment.

(Office of Fair Trading 2005: para. 1.3)

The research highlights a number of concerns about the information and support available to older people at this critical time. In particular, it notes: the lack of clear information about processes and procedures for entering a care home and about the responsibilities of local authorities; lack of information about fees, services, terms and conditions; unfair and complex contracting processes that were hard for people to understand; and lack of information and support regarding the making of complaints (ibid.). A well-informed, accessible and supportive social worker can play a crucial role in addressing some of these deficits and helping to ease this often difficult stage in an older person's life.

Like care homes, all domiciliary agencies providing personal care services are required to register with the Commission for Social Care Inspection. Registration requirements for domiciliary care agencies are set out in the *Domiciliary Care Agencies Regulations* (2002). As with care homes, there are minimum standards for domiciliary care agencies (Department of Health 2003e). These consist of 27 standards grouped under the following headings: user-focused services; personal care; protection; managers and staff; organisation and running of the business.

Recent changes have been made to the system for inspecting care providers, including care homes and domiciliary care agencies. From April 2006, greater flexibility was introduced in the frequency with which inspections have to be carried out. All care services have to be inspected at least once every three years but the frequency of additional inspections is determined by assessment of the quality and safety of the service. There are key inspections that are comprehensive, involving scrutiny of documents, visits to homes and interviews with staff, residents and families. These inspections contribute to a quality rating of the service and this helps to determine the frequency of future inspections. Random inspections may be carried out to assess or review a particular aspect of the service. There may be themed inspections, relating to a particular issue that is being inspected at a given time, for example nutritional standards or administration of medication. There is also a requirement for providers to produce an Annual Quality Assurance Assessment (AQAA), giving data and information about the home and an evaluation of its performance. A programme of involving 'experts by experience' in the inspection process is being introduced (Commission for Social Care Inspection: 2005a).

The review of inspection processes was partly triggered by concern about the impact of detailed and stringent regulation requirements and standards on service providers, particularly smaller organisations. The aim was to make the requirements more focused on the outcomes of services for service users and to make the system less burdensome on service providers, whilst not jeopardising concerns with quality and safety. There is a potential conflict between the needs of service providers for less onerous inspection requirements and service users' concerns about attaining and retaining quality. A national survey of the sorts of social services and inspections people want in later life found strong support for rigorous inspection systems, with eight in ten people believing that services should be inspected at least twice a year and over a third saying inspections should be monthly (Commission for Social Care Inspection: 2004b).

A more fundamental issue relating to quality and accountability in relation to services provided by independent sector agencies is that they are not subject to the provisions of the Human Rights Act (1998). Currently, the Act only applies to 'public authorities' and case law has set out a narrow interpretation of what this means, not regarding independent sector organisations as 'public authorities'. Therefore, they are not obliged to comply with the Act, even when they are providing services on behalf of local authorities (Age Concern: 2005a). Government guidance advocates the use of conditions and specifications in contracts agreed with independent sector providers to clarify requirements in respect of human rights issues (Department of Constitutional Affairs 2005). However, organisations such as Age Concern argue the need for independent care providers to be brought clearly within the remit of the Human Rights Act (Age Concern 2005b).

THE CHANGING CARE MARKET

We have seen that a key change since the implementation of the community care reforms of the early 1990s relates to who provides services. As discussed in Chapter 2, one of the objectives of the reforms was the promotion of a 'mixed economy of care'. This has been achieved in that the role of local authorities in directly providing services has decreased significantly while that of the independent sector has increased. In relation to domiciliary care, the number of home care hours provided by independent sector agencies has increased dramatically, from 2 per cent in 1992 to 73 per cent in 2005 (Commission for Social Care Inspection: 2006a). With regard to care homes, there has been a decrease in the number of people resident in local authority-run homes (a decline of a third between 2002 and 2006), and an increase in the number who are supported by the local authority in independent sector homes (National Statistics: 2006b). At 31 March 2006, 89 per cent of residents supported by local authorities were living in independent sector homes (either residential or nursing homes). This compares with 50 per cent in 1995 and only 20 per cent in 1993 (the year the NHS and Community Care Act was implemented) (ibid.). The number of residents supported (temporary and permanent) during 2005/6 fell by 3 per cent on the previous year to 256,900 (ibid.).

This fall reflects another change – in the nature of services provided for older people. Again reflecting the objectives of the reforms, older people with 'high level' needs are being supported to live at home with intensive packages of care, while admission rates to care homes have declined. Since 1992, the number of home care contact hours funded by local authorities has doubled. In 1992, the average number of home care hours provided to each household per week was 3.2, compared with 10.1 in 2005 (Commission for Social Care Inspection: 2006a). (However, as highlighted in Chapter 2, the increase in home care contact hours has been paralleled by a decrease in the number of households receiving help, as older people with 'lower level' needs are deemed ineligible for home care support.) This trend is encouraged by Government targets set for local authorities to increase the numbers of older people assisted to live at home and to increase the proportion of intensive home care. Over time the savings derived from the reduction of spending on care home costs should enable savings that can be reinvested in low-level, preventive services, addressing the objectives outlined in recent policy (see Chapter 2). However, despite the increase in spending on home care, this still only accounts for around 21 per cent of local authorities' expenditure on services for older people, compared with 56 per cent spent on care homes (Commission for Social Care Inspection: 2006a – based on figures for 2004–5).

Although the statistics considered above suggest that considerable progress has been made in relation to two key objectives of the community care reforms – promoting a 'mixed economy of care' and supporting people to live in the community – it is important to examine outcomes for older people. Some argue that the growth in the 'quasi-market' of care, and recurrent crises in it, have not been in their interests. For example, Scourfield (2006) suggests that home care services capable of significantly improving older people's lives need to be stable, flexible and better placed to integrate more effectively with health agencies and that such services can only be achieved by expanding local authorities' in-house provision. With regard to the expansion in private sector residential care, Drakeford (2006) traces changes in the pattern of ownership and regulation and concludes that regulation has proved of limited effectiveness in securing the interests of older people in homes under private ownership.

A study that examined the extent to which the current and predicted future care market meets the needs and preferences of older people was carried out in London by the King's Fund in 2004 (King's Fund 2005). This inquiry sheds light on resource issues and, although focused on London, the researchers see the findings as of national significance. There were a number of key findings. First, older people were found to have poor access to information and practical support, especially concerning the meeting of lower level needs. Second, older people were noted to have limited choice and control over care services. New types of services, such as extra care housing, were very limited; 'older people with care needs have limited options, dominated by care homes or conventional home care services' (ibid.: 5). Certain groups, such as older people with mental health problems and Black and minority ethnic older people, were found to have even less choice than others. Third, older people were placed at risk because of untrained and unqualified staff. The high turnover of staff and staff vacancy rates in both care homes and home care services were compromising the quality of care. Fourth, the inadequate funding of long-term care and the lack of clarity about who pays for it were causing considerable hardship for older people. Confusion over entitlement to free NHS continuing care was found to be particularly problematic. (This issue is considered in Chapter 6.) The inquiry sees the problems in the care system as falling into three areas:

- Failures in the care market that restrict choice and control and prevent services from being responsive to individual need. These factors include: older people's lack of information and lack of purchasing power; the lack of resources of small care providers to compete; and insufficient capital investment in care homes and extra care housing.
- Policies based on ageist attitudes and negative views of older people. These focus on need and dependency rather than on rights and treat older people less favourably than other service user groups. (This is discussed further in Chapter 7.)
- Insufficient public resources, which mean that access to support is restricted, with complex funding systems making service entitlements confused and confusing.

The report makes thirty recommendations to improve care services. These fall within four areas: reforming policy; investing in market development; improving services for specific groups, for example, older people with mental health problems and older people from Black and minority ethnic communities; and mobilising more public and private resources to support older people.

The bulk of this chapter has been concerned with issues that are pertinent to care planning; issues concerned with accessing non-residential and residential services for older people in response to needs identified by assessments. Of course, the access to these two kinds of services are linked. Research with 99 health and social care staff, using focus groups and semi-structured interviews, indicated that their decision thresholds regarding admission to residential care were influenced by the level of funding available for non-residential services, the availability of home care workers and workload pressures on primary care services (Taylor and Donnelly 2006).

We have now considered assessment, in the previous chapter, and care planning, in this chapter. As we saw in Chapter 2 (Figure 2.1), after assessment and care planning, the remaining stages in the assessment and care management process are monitoring and reviewing.

MONITORING AND REVIEWING THE CARE PLAN

Monitoring and review are recognised stages within the assessment and care management process. As noted earlier in the chapter, practitioners' guidance and the *Single Assessment Process* guidance require that the care plan records the arrangements for a review (see Boxes 4.1 and 4.2). The SAP guidance states that arrangements should be put in place to monitor the older person's needs and the effectiveness of the services being provided. It notes that monitoring may be undertaken by service providers, who should be commissioned to 'keep a watching brief for marked changes' (Department of Health 2002c: Annex E).

A review goes beyond the on-going checking involved in monitoring. It is a more formal and comprehensive mechanism for checking whether there have been any changes in need and for evaluating the effectiveness of the care plan. The SAP guidance states that a review should be carried out within three months, either of services first being provided or of major changes being put in place. After this, reviews should be carried out at least annually and when there are major changes. The purposes of the review according to the SAP guidance are: to determine how far the support being provided is achieving the outcomes specified in the care plan; to reassess the needs of the older person; to establish continuing eligibility; to confirm or change the care plan, or terminate involvement; and, if appropriate, to check how the older person is managing direct payments. The care plan should be updated following the review. If the review determines that an older person is no longer eligible for services, the reasons should be recorded and shared with the individual concerned (Department of Health 2002c: Annex E). This is consistent with the guidance on reviews given in *Fair Access to Care Services* (FACS), although FACS offers more detail. FACS states that reviews may be held at the request of service users. It suggests that reviews are coordinated by independent and competent local authority professionals, rather than by service providers. It also specifies who should be involved in the review: the service user, carers or representatives of the service user; agencies that have purchased services for the service user; and key service providers. It envisages that the review is normally a face-to-face meeting but states that 'in exceptional circumstances' a review may be carried out without face-to-face contact with the service user (Department of Health 2002b: para. 62). As a result of the fragmentation of the assessment and care management role, discussed in Chapter 2, many local authorities now have separate reviewing teams who carry out care plan reviews. This means that the professional reviewing the care plan will be a different person from the one who drew it up and implemented it. As shown in Activity 2.3, this may pose issues for older people with regard to the lack of continuity of personnel.

The purposes of the review, set out in the SAP and FACS guidance, highlight that part of the review function is to determine continuing eligibility for service provision. Clearly if the older person's situation has improved and their level of assessed need has changed they may no longer be entitled to a service. For example:

> Mrs A.'s needs were originally assessed as in the 'substantial' category of need. At a review one year later, her situation has improved and her needs are reassessed as in the 'moderate' category. The local authority has publicised its criteria and made clear that it only provides assistance to those

with critical or substantial needs. Mrs A is therefore no longer eligible to receive a service.

It is also possible, and lawful, for services to be withdrawn if the older person's needs have not changed. This could be the case if, in line with budget shortfalls, the local authority has reviewed its eligibility criteria since the original assessment and decided to restrict the 'bands' for whom it will provide services. For example:

> Mr B. was assessed as having 'moderate' needs and a care package was put in place to address these. In the meantime, his local authority has had to make cutbacks. It has decided no longer to provide services to those with moderate needs but to restrict its help to those in the 'substantial' and 'critical' categories. Even though Mr B's situation has not improved, he is no longer eligible for services.

It will be apparent that the possible consequence in both of these scenarios is that the older people's situations will deteriorate once services are withdrawn. However, in assessing and reassessing need, the practitioner has to consider the risks to independence if the service is not provided (see Chapter 3); in other words, the likely future situation has to be considered, as well as present circumstances. In the examples given above, this could lead to Mrs A's needs being assessed as still in the 'substantial' category or to Mr B's needs being reassessed as in the 'substantial' category and, therefore, to both still being eligible to receive services. As clarified in the *Gloucestershire judgment* and highlighted in Activity 4.2 (see page 104), there should be no reduction or withdrawal of services without a reassessment of the individual's needs. In addition, when services are withdrawn, the older person should be informed in writing of the reasons for this and be informed about the complaints procedure (Department of Health 2002b).

ACTIVITY 4.5: A NEEDS-LED SERVICE?

Care management was promoted as being 'needs-led' rather than service-led (see previous chapter). Can local authorities take account of their resources in deciding:

- Whether to carry out an assessment?
- Who should be given help?
- What services to provide?
- Whether to continue providing services after a period of time?
- Whether to accept responsibility for providing residential care?

This chapter and the previous chapter have focused on four key stages in working with older people – assessment, care planning and the provision of services, monitoring and review – and particular attention has been given to clarifying the legal framework so that social workers are aware of where their responsibilities lie and where there is room for manoeuvre in seeking to maximise the rights and well-being of older people. This has highlighted some of the fundamental conflicts and dilemmas inherent within community care policy and practice. Attempting to practise in empowering ways with service users, attending to issues of quality of life and well-being and respecting and responding appropriately to diversity, has been juxtaposed with the realities of resource constraints, stringent eligibility criteria and restrictive organisational policies and processes. In this climate, it may seem easier for social workers simply to focus on the detail of the tasks and processes that preoccupy their organisations, for example the organisational mechanics of the implementation of the *Single Assessment Process*, making decisions about eligibility in terms of *Fair Access to Care Services* or achieving government targets for the start and completion times for assessment (McDonald and Taylor 2006). This is certainly a more straightforward option than grappling with problematic and seemingly irresolvable values issues (Braye and Preston-Shoot 1995; Jones, C. 2001).

In examining social workers' dual and conflicting responsibilities to advance service users' interests, on the one hand, and to be accountable to their organisations, on the other, Beckett and Maynard (2005) conclude that social workers have a duty to advocate for their service users *and* a duty to contribute to their agency's agenda of using resources as fairly, efficiently and effectively as possible. They argue that social workers have 'a duty of realism' (ibid.: 97), by which they mean a duty to take account of what is achievable. Given that resources are finite, this involves weighing up the relative benefits of different ways of deploying resources. However, they point out that a duty of realism does not imply accepting the status quo: 'Part of the duty of realism is to publicly state when resources are inadequate to the task, being clear about the duties that are not being discharged and the risks that are being taken' (ibid.: 104). This means that social workers should challenge the breaching of statutory duties, the disregarding of central policy directives and the interpretation of the law in ways that have negative implications for older people's well-being, rather than accepting them with resignation as the inevitable realities of practice. There are a number of prerequisites for social workers to be able to do this: a detailed working knowledge of legislation and policy, a commitment to retaining a values focus at the forefront of their work and critical reflection on all aspects of their practice. Another vital dimension that can make a crucial difference to older people's experiences of both the outcomes and processes of intervention is the range and level of skill that social workers deploy in their practice. This is the focus of the next chapter.

KEY POINTS

- ☐ Requirements for planning and providing care are set out in *Fair Access to Care Services* and the *Single Assessment Process* guidance.

- ☐ There are a number of pieces of legislation concerned with the provision of care services. The Chronically Sick and Disabled Persons Act (1970) contains 'strong' duties to individuals.

- ☐ Local authorities have a duty to provide services to meet need assessed as 'eligible'.

- ☐ Despite the emphasis in policy on promoting well-being, in practice services remain targeted on those with high levels of need.

☐   Although central objectives of the community care reforms are being realised, there is evidence that this has not always resulted in positive outcomes for older people.

KEY READING

Clements, L. (2004, 3rd edn) *Community Care and the Law*, London: Legal Action Group.
McDonald, A. and Taylor, M. (2006) *Older People and the Law*, Bristol: The Policy Press.

CHAPTER 5

SKILLS IN WORKING WITH OLDER PEOPLE

OBJECTIVES

By the end of this chapter you should have an understanding of:

- the relationship between social work skills and particular methods and approaches, including care management;

- the meaning of the 'exchange' model and the obstacles encountered to its use in practice;

- the importance of general and specific communication skills;

- the relevance of 'person-centred' and 'holistic' assessment and intervention;

- positive practice in recording information.

The previous two chapters provided an overview of the legal, policy and organisational framework of assessment and care planning that leads to service provision in social work with older people. A detailed understanding of the law is important for ensuring that social workers engage in informed and lawful practice and such an understanding provides a tool for them to advocate in service users' interests. However, if the intended outcome of social work intervention with older people is that it improves their well-being (see Chapter 3), this is not just a matter of working mechanically within the legal, policy and organisational framework. Social work is an interpersonal activity, rooted in relationships between people and dealing with emotions. Social workers need skills to work sensitively and effectively with older people, those in their informal support networks and other workers and agencies, as well as skills in reflection and an ability to manage their own feelings (Gorman 2003). Chapter 6 will consider issues related to working with others. The focus of this chapter will be on skills and approaches for working effectively with older people.

SKILLS AND CARE MANAGEMENT

Chapters 2, 3 and 4 have identified the legal, policy and organisational context in which much social work with older people takes place. Many writers have highlighted the bureaucratic and managerial processes stemming from this context, associated with 'purchasing services' and 'managing care', and have regarded these processes either as having eclipsed or as threatening to eclipse the relational and therapeutic components of social work (see, for example, Harris, John 1998; Postle 2001; 2002). Others argue that it is possible and, indeed, essential that social workers develop strategies to engage in creative, flexible and empowering practice within these service contexts (see, for example, Evans and Harris, John 2004b; Lymbery 2004). It is important to bear in mind that there was not a halcyon time, before care management, of social workers deploying high levels of skill to advance the interests of older people. Rather, as noted in Chapter 2, work with older people was seen as of low status, often being delegated to unqualified staff, and bureaucratic and administrative demands were an integral part of the social work role, well before the advent of care management. Furthermore, the care management role was originally conceived as requiring interpersonal as well as management and administrative skills. Soon after the implementation of the NHS and Community Care Act (1990), the Department of Health commissioned work to: identify the 'interactional skills' required by staff carrying out assessment and care management; show how service users could be empowered to exercise choice about how their needs were met; and show how members of the wider social network could be involved so that the support provided from statutory, independent and informal sources was interwoven (Department of Health/Price Waterhouse 1991; Smale and Tuson 1993). Smale and Tuson distinguished three key skills necessary for 'joining' with people in assessment as an interpersonal collaborative endeavour:

- *Authenticity*: 'The care manager's ability to relate to others with integrity; to be aware of their own feelings and values as well as the significance of their agency role and the other roles they occupy dependent upon gender, race and cultural background' (Smale and Tuson 1993: 48).
- *Empathy*: 'A person's ability to communicate understanding; to understand what the other person is thinking and feeling, their position, their perception of the situation and what they want' (ibid.: 50).
- *Respect*: 'The care manager's ability to communicate their acceptance and valuation of people irrespective of their personal qualities and social or professional position' (ibid.: 54).

It is interesting to note the similarity between these 'joining' skills identified by Smale and Tuson and the conditions for therapeutic relationships that form the foundation of client-centred therapy or counselling (Rogers 1951). Smale and Tuson's approach to the 'joining' with people in assessment, therefore, places a central emphasis on counselling and interpersonal skills in assessment. At the later 'arranging, maintaining and rearranging' (Smale and Tuson 1993: 66) stage of care planning, more emphasis is given to the care manager's role in working with social networks and collaborating with others.

Lymbery (2005) sees the skills required by social workers working with older people as consisting of both interpersonal and administrative components. The interpersonal skills he identifies are: counselling skills; communication skills; networking, negotiation and mediation skills; and advocacy. He sees the administratively oriented skills as comprising budgeting, financial management, organisational and planning skills. These are all skills that are essential for assessment and care planning. Lymbery relates these skill requirements to three different sets of views about the role of social work identified by Payne (2005), which he sees as competing with each other in practice.

- *Reflexive-therapeutic* views are concerned with 'seeking the best possible well-being for individuals, groups and communities in society, by promoting and facilitating growth and self-fulfilment' (Payne 2005: 8). Undertaking counselling with an older person regarding particular losses or changes they have experienced is an example of 'reflexive therapeutic' work. Another example is reminiscence work, where the aim is to develop understanding of the self or situation or to bring about change in some aspects of the person's current life (Harris, John and Hopkins 1994; Bornat 2005). Whilst reflexive-therapeutic dimensions of social work can easily be overshadowed by the managerial concerns of care management, a systematic review of research evidence concludes that counselling older people is effective, especially in response to anxiety and depression, and can improve feelings of well-being (Hill and Brettle 2006). Even if social workers are not themselves well-placed to engage in reflexive-therapeutic work, they need to be alert to these issues and involve other agencies as appropriate.

- *Socialist-collectivist* views seek to support people who are socially oppressed and disadvantaged to gain greater power and control over their own lives. An example of this approach might be working with an older person to develop self-advocacy skills or linking an older person with community groups concerned with campaigning to improve local amenities. Another role for the social worker might be challenging oppressive attitudes and practices in others. Examples include combating ageist views, such as 'it's just old age', which prevent an older person from receiving appropriate medical care (Roberts *et al.* 2002), or highlighting the discrediting and depersonalising images of older people that may contribute to elder abuse (Daichman 2005).

- *Individualist-reformist* views are concerned with meeting individual needs in order that society as a whole will maintain stability and continue to function in its present form. They focus on the maintenance of society rather than change. Much care management practice can be seen as located within this perspective since it is concerned with the 'needs' of the individual that are defined by the state as problematic and a legitimate target for intervention, rather than with securing older people's social rights.

It will be readily apparent that these three dimensions are not mutually exclusive and social work with any individual older person will frequently include all three. The perspectives do, however, provide a useful framework for practitioners to plan, analyse and evaluate their practice. For example, if the planned intervention is reflexive-therapeutic, what issues might be overlooked from a socialist-collectivist perspective? If the approach has been mainly individualist-reformist, are there issues that need addressing from reflexive-therapeutic or socialist-collectivist perspectives? Even if there are issues that are not defined as a legitimate part of the social worker's role to address, the social worker can help to identity and locate other appropriate resources and services.

Lymbery argues that although certain skills may be more central to one perspective (for example, counselling skills to social work which is primarily reflexive-therapeutic), all of the skills intersect with each of the perspectives. Furthermore, he argues that effective social work with older people needs to encompass elements of each perspective:

> There will inevitably be emphasis on specific aspects of the task at different times, but it is vital to retain the sense that social work entails more than simply the linking of people to resources, important as this task is. It is this balance and combination of roles, orientation, values, tasks and skills that distinguishes a social worker from a member of another occupation.
>
> (Lymbery 2005: 150)

SKILLS IN USING SOCIAL WORK METHODS AND APPROACHES

In Chapter 1, the importance of social workers being reflective and reflexive was noted. We saw that Milner and O'Byrne suggested that the selection of theoretical 'maps' is influenced by the worker's preferred way of understanding and responding to problems and situations. While the worker's level of knowledge and skill in relation to particular approaches will inevitably influence the approaches s/he chooses, it is also important that practitioners 'avoid being like Blaug's (1995) carpenter who, possessing a hammer, tended to see every problem as a nail' (Milner and O'Byrne 2002: 79). In other words, practitioners must be open and flexible enough to consider alternative explanations and interventions and have a knowledge and skill base that allows the competent use of different methods and approaches, as pertinent to the particular situation.

As we saw in Chapter 1, social workers often experience difficulties in thinking and talking explicitly about theories in relation to their practice (Healy 2005) and this may be a particular difficulty for social workers working with older people within the framework of care management. As discussed above, care management can be seen as fitting within the 'individualist-reformist' view of social work (Payne 2005); the role may be experienced as more of an administrative one, involving the coordination of services, rather than a role in which social workers themselves are acting as an agent of change. Although it was originally envisaged that there would be different types of care management – one based on the coordination of services and another concerned with intensive care management, featuring the ongoing involvement of the care manager engaged in a broader range of activity with more vulnerable individuals (Challis and Davies 1986) – it is the co-coordinating services model of care management that has prevailed in practice (Weinberg *et al.* 2003). Situations are 'managed' by the social worker arranging for the provision of services by others rather than being 'acted on' or changed through direct interventions by the social worker. The 'management' of the situation may be accomplished in only one or two visits to the older person, after which the 'case' is passed to another team for monitoring and/or review. This is very different from the premise upon which most social work models are based, that is, of a practitioner working with a service user over a period of time, using assessment as the basis to plan and carry out a process of intervention, aimed at producing some level of change in relation to individuals and/or their situation. One study, for example, found that care managers spent only 5 per cent of their time in counselling and support activities (Weinberg *et al.* 2003). It is not surprising that in this context, in particular, social workers and social work students struggle to find relevant theoretical perspectives to inform their practice.

The 'task-centred method' is often cited by students and social workers as the method most relevant to their practice. Its structured and time-limited approach, focus on the present and the tasks associated with arranging services have at least some resonance with care management. A task-centred approach is based on working in partnership with the service user. It begins with a focus on the areas the service user regards as problematic and the service user is involved in prioritising goals and selecting tasks. However, there are a number of tensions between a task-centred approach, as originally outlined (by, for example, Reid and Epstein [1972]) and care management. First, assessment in care management tends to be focused on identifying eligible needs (see Chapters 3 and 4); needs identified by the older person which fall outside of eligibility criteria are likely to be either referred elsewhere, recorded but not dealt with, or disregarded. We saw in Chapter 3 that the *Fair Access to Care Service* guidance sees one of the purposes of assessment as being to help the service user identify options for meeting assessed need. In many care management contexts, this would not, however, involve working alongside the older person to achieve tasks that related to non-eligible needs. These might be seen as falling outside of the social worker's remit, even though a case can be made that this activity should be part and parcel of social work (Tanner 2005). Second, a task-centred approach aims to develop the ability of the service user to resolve their own difficulties; setting carefully graded and achievable tasks is a key part of the process of developing the service user's confidence and skills in problem-solving. In care management, social workers are likely to provide information and advice or refer an older person to another agency or, perhaps, complete straightforward tasks themselves. The fragmentation and separation of the care management role into assessment, intervention and review functions (Ware *et al.* 2003) mean there may not be the opportunity to engage in an ongoing process of the social worker working together on tasks identified and selected by the older person. Third, the worker's time is itself a limited resource and this, as well as the narrow construction of the care manager's role, may preclude the broader interventions traditionally associated with a task-centred approach.

The argument here is not that a task-centred approach is irrelevant to social work with older people. Indeed, in some situations and contexts it may offer a useful framework for the social worker and older person to work together on agreed difficulties. In particular, it encourages clear and explicit identification of goals and tasks and an approach that is based on working with rather than 'doing for' people. It has the potential to empower people through helping them develop the knowledge, skills and confidence necessary to address problems. However, as with any intervention, a task-centred approach needs to be informed by a clear understanding of what the method entails; not every piece of work involving a task to be accomplished means that a 'task-centred method' has been, or should be, used. It also needs to be used critically, taking account of issues that the method does not adequately address. For example, a task-centred approach may ignore issues of an emotional/psychological nature in favour of a focus on concrete goals with more easily measurable outcomes. The focus on the latter can also lead to lack of attention to wider structural or diversity issues that are less easily addressed through specific tasks.

In practice, there is likely to be a close connection between the theoretical map used in assessment and the form of intervention the assessment suggests is appropriate. The different maps outlined by Milner and O'Byrne (2002 – see Chapter 1, page 26) each have their distinct approach to assessment in terms of the information that is obtained and the processes and techniques used to gather it. For example, a solution-focused approach to assessment would focus on the anticipated situation when the problem is no longer there; it would not gather detailed information about the onset and nature of problems that would provide the foundation for intervention from psychodynamic or behavioural perspectives. The initial stage of assessment needs to consider the situation from as many different perspectives as possible, trying out different theoretical maps in order to determine an appropriate standpoint(s) for the assessment. In relation to the *Single Assessment Process*, discussed in the previous chapter, the overview assessment can be used to establish ideas and hypotheses about the nature of the problem or difficulties experienced by the older person. At the stage of undertaking a comprehensive assessment, the social worker can gather more detailed information according to the theoretical premises, processes and techniques of the method selected.

A PROCESS OF 'EXCHANGE'?

The 'theoretical maps' summarised by Milner and O'Byrne refer to approaches that may be used in any area of social work practice. As already noted, social workers in care management contexts, such as those working with older people, may find it difficult to relate these 'maps' to their practice. Smale and Tuson's (1993) work, referred to earlier, was concerned specifically with the skills required within the context of care management. They identified three models for assessment, the exchange, procedural and questioning models. These models are closely connected to values and principles of anti-oppressive practice since the models concern dynamics of power and the role of the worker vis-à-vis the service user, as indicated by Smale *et al.* in their reprise of the models:

> A worker can either take the role of an expert who, from the outside, understands the service user, the user's problems and what might be the best option; or s/he can work alongside the person and other significant people to arrive at a mutual understanding of the problem and negotiate who might do what to help, or who might best influence behaviour seen as undesirable or self-damaging. Both approaches may end up with the person getting what

they want, or not, depending on whether resources are available or change is possible. The difference is in how power is used and its impact on the service user. Only the latter allows the citizen to be a fully involved partner in a process of negotiating the nature of his or her problem and possible resolutions.

(Smale *et al.* 2000: 132)

Smale and Tuson (1993) call the model based on mutual understanding the 'exchange' model. They compare this with the 'questioning' model, in which the worker's role is that of the professional expert, and the 'procedural' model, which is governed by the needs of the care management 'system'. Key differences between the three models are as follows.

Exchange model

- The worker's role is to act as facilitator, generating an exchange of information between the people involved.
- The work depends on establishing respect and trust.
- Understanding is negotiated between the parties, rather than information being passed in linear fashion from one person to another.
- The worker draws on wider information about the social situation in order to enhance understanding.
- 'People are, and always will be, the experts on themselves: their situation, their relationships, what they want and need' (Smale *et al.* 2000: 137).
- 'An essential part of the worker's responsibility is to contribute to, not take over from, people exercising their own social problem solving skills' (ibid.: 138).

Questioning model

- The worker's role is diagnostic; the worker takes responsibility for making an accurate assessment and taking appropriate action.
- The model assumes the worker is the expert about people and their needs.
- The worker's role is to ask questions that reflect the worker's view of the nature of the problem/situation and what should be done.
- The model assumes the assessor's judgement and actions are objective.
- The model is relatively quick and straightforward compared with the exchange model.

Procedural model

- The worker's role is to act as guide through the system, gathering information to see if the person meets the criteria that would make them eligible for services.
- The information regarded as relevant is determined by organisational policy.
- The organisation remains central to how problems are defined and the range of solutions available for dealing with them.

- The model tends to focus on dependency needs and difficulties, rather than strengths and coping strategies.
- The model is simple and quick.
- The model tends to lead to standard packages rather than innovative or individually-tailored responses: 'the explicit or implicit agenda of organisation-focused assessments cannot match the infinite variety of ways in which different people from very different backgrounds with very different expectations see their problems and the potential solutions' (Smale *et al.* 2000: 142–3).

Government guidance on the *Single Assessment Process* (see Chapters 3 and 4) appears consistent with the 'exchange' model of assessment in emphasising the central role of the service user in assessment:

> Older people are the most important participants in the *Single Assessment Process*. There are two reasons for this. First, the assessment is about and for them. Second, of all the experts in the care of older people, the greatest experts are older people themselves. They will know when they are having difficulties, the nature of those difficulties, and what might be done to resolve them.
>
> (Department of Health 2002c: 1)

In addition to highlighting that the service user is the expert about their own situation and should be treated as such, Smale and Tuson (1993) also emphasise the social, as opposed to individual, focus of assessment:

> Social services and social work intervention are a response to the nature of a person's social relationships . . . It follows that the social situation is the appropriate unit of assessment. It includes local and cultural expectations about 'normal' patterns of care and support; the 'clients', the 'carers' and other significant people's perceptions of their needs and available resources; the judgements of other professionals; and the nature and quality of the care relationships that exist. All are an integral part of any future 'package of care' which can be drawn from a combination of people's personal networks and the available voluntary and professional services.
>
> (Smale and Tuson 1993: 26)

The tendency of social workers to understand social problems in terms of individual factors (the 'psychologising' of social problems) is a point highlighted by Milner and O'Byrne (2002: 10) who, like Smale and Tuson, argue the need for practitioners to recognise the interaction between psychological and social factors. Whilst at one level this may seem an obvious point, the way need and risk are constructed in individual terms in legislation and policy (see Chapters 3 and 4) sometimes obstructs recognition of the significance of social factors in assessment and intervention.

Although the 'exchange model' is often cited as a model for good assessment practice, like all theories and models it needs to be understood in relation to the context in which it was developed. Chapter 2 identified that the objectives of care management included separating out assessment of need from considerations about service provision and reconfiguring 'clients' of social services as 'consumers' who, once their needs had been assessed in partnership with the worker, could exercise choice in the 'care market' about how their needs were to be met. Smale and Tuson's publication was intended to provide guidance about the skills and values required by workers to achieve these objectives. What is missing from their description of models and skills is any sense of the economic, political or organisational context in which care management is carried out. In particular, the conflict between empowering service users and containing public resources, which has been so central to the way that assessment and care management have developed in practice, is absent from their analysis.

ACTIVITY 5.1: IDENTIFYING AND ADDRESSING BARRIERS TO CARRYING OUT AN ASSESSMENT AS AN 'EXCHANGE'

First read the following:

Ranjana is a 72-year-old Asian woman. She is blind and has severe osteo-arthritis in her hands and legs. She has lived with her son, Ali, and daughter-in-law, Meena, and their family for the last 15 years, since her husband died. However, Meena was admitted to hospital with depression a week ago and is likely to take some time to recover. Ali has taken time off work to look after their two children and his mother but now has to go back to work. The youngest child has learning difficulties. Ali is exhausted and his doctor has told him that he too will end up in hospital unless he gets some help. There is no family support nearby. The GP, who makes the referral, says that Ranjana is 'difficult' and 'likes things her own way'. She will not accept help from anyone outside of the family. The GP says that he has discussed the situation with Ali who has reluctantly agreed that his mother should go into a home. The GP thinks that this is likely to be permanent as he believes the stress of looking after Ranjana has played a large part in Meena's depression. Ali has not been able to discuss the situation with his mother as he is too ashamed about not being able to care for her. Ranjana understands English reasonably well but can only speak a few words of it. Her first language is Punjabi.

As a social worker in a team for older people you are asked to follow up this referral. Your team is short-staffed and you know there is pressure on you to complete assessments quickly to meet targets on the waiting times for assessment. You have another four visits during the day as well as several hours of admin-istration to catch up with, completing forms and putting information on to the computer. Your team manager has just briefed the team about the need to interpret the eligibility criteria strictly in view of the council's projected high overspend. All care plans involving more than 15 hours of services a week have to be presented to a Resource Allocation Panel for approval. You are also aware of local pressures on services. Bed shortages mean that most homes in the area (except those with poor reputations) have waiting lists. The local home care services are also under pressure at peak times of the day; it is very difficult to get help before 10 o'clock in the morning or after 6.30 in the evening.

- List all of the factors that might present barriers to the assessment being a genuine exchange between you, Ranjana and other members of the family.
- What steps could you take to address these?

The situation described in Activity 5.1 illustrates some of the complexities involved in working with older people according to an 'exchange' model of practice, whereby the service user takes a lead role in the assessment and intervention process. These include the following factors.

Organisational barriers

There are likely to be a number of organisational barriers to a genuine exchange model being realised in practice. These include constraints on the time that is available to undertake a 'person-led' assessment and the barriers that may be presented by the requirements of the organisation in terms of particular information that has to be gathered (for example, financial details) or the forms that have to be completed. A study carried out between 1996 and 1997 (Postle 2002), based on observation and interviews with 20 care managers working with older people and their line managers, identified conflicts between professional and managerial imperatives. The high throughput of work was seen as conflicting with the need to conduct thorough assessments and to contribute to care managers' perceptions of reduced opportunities for relationship-based work and use of the self. These interpersonal aspects of the social work task are described elsewhere as having to be undertaken as 'undercover work' (Postle 2001). Postle's research (2002) highlighted tension between the emphasis on the professional skills required for assessment and the restricted and often computer-driven mechanisms for recording these assessments. Another tension was between the professional requirement to focus on the person and the bureaucratic dictate to focus on the detail of financial assessments.

Policy barriers

The normative definition of need operated by the agency may conflict with the expressed need of the older person, as discussed in Chapter 3. The social worker may, with great skill and sensitivity, elicit the older person's understanding of the nature of the problem and the assistance required but policy and resource obstacles may prevent this from being provided.

Service barriers

Even if an older person's expressed needs are assessed as 'eligible needs', appropriate services that are responsive to his or her needs may not be available. The social worker's knowledge of these restrictions may intrude on the assessment process since it is difficult in practice to free a 'needs-led' assessment from service considerations (Parry-Jones and Soulsby 2001).

Professional barriers

The social work role often involves conflicting duties and obligations. Social workers have a duty to 'support individuals to represent their needs, views and circumstances', but in fulfilling this role, they also have to 'assess and manage risks to individuals' (General Social Care Council 2002). Sometimes there will be a professional and legal obligation to act in ways that conflict with an individual's expressed needs and wishes.

Communication barriers

There may be communication barriers operating between the social worker and the older person that impede an 'exchange' of information and understanding. These may include language barriers or cultural differences or the impact of sensory impairments or confusion.

Environmental barriers

A free exchange of communication may also be restricted by environmental obstacles, for example, the lack of a quiet, private and safe physical space for the older person to tell her or his story.

Network barriers

The interests of other people within the care network may have to be counterbalanced with those of the older person. Sometimes needs and interests of the different parties will be in conflict and the social worker will have to negotiate with the individuals concerned and try to reach a resolution that involves balance and compromise.

Personal barriers

Because of their personal biographies, experiences and attitudes, older people may not want or feel able to take a lead role in the assessment process. As discussed in Chapter 1, ageist attitudes may be internalised by older people, leading to low expectations of services and entitlements (Wilson 1995); as a result, older people may adopt passive roles in the process, grateful for whatever help they are offered. One study found that care managers operated with a belief that service users were not interested in being involved, and took this at face value, using this to justify the failure to involve them in key processes (Baldwin 2000). The social worker may have to work with an older person to prepare her or him for assuming an active role in the assessment and care management process; simply offering opportunities for involvement may be insufficient. (Constraints on older people's involvement in assessment and care management processes are considered further in Chapter 7.)

Situational barriers

The nature of an older person's current situation – perhaps a time of acute crisis – may also act as a barrier to their involvement. For example, Richards (2000) described older people who were receiving an assessment as either 'decided' about the nature of their difficulties and the help they wanted, 'undecided', needing help to clarify the issues, or 'overwhelmed'. For older people in the last category, a period where the social worker takes charge may be necessary before the older person is ready to assume a more active role in the process.

Social work has to work within and around the obstacles and constraints raised by such barriers. This highlights further the importance of social work skills and values in working towards positive practice in difficult and complex situations.

COMMUNICATION SKILLS

Skills in communicating effectively with others are fundamental to effective social work practice, as identified by service users themselves (Department of Health 2002a). 'Communication' is a broad term that covers multiple skill components. To cite a few examples, effective communication in social work requires skills in: observing, active listening, questioning, reflecting, using silence, facilitating, explaining, informing, advising, advocating, summarising, challenging, negotiating, mediating, and recording. (There is not space within this book to explore every aspect of communication skills but there are other texts that deal with this subject [see, for example, Lishman 1994; Koprowska 2005; Trevithick 2005].) While many communication skills are generic across all areas of social work practice, there are particular dimensions of skills that are pertinent to working with different service users, for example, play techniques needed to work with young children. This section provides two examples of skills that may be particularly relevant to social work with older people: skills in working with people with sensory impairments and skills in working with people with dementia.

Sensory impairments

Particular thought may need to be given to communication when working with older people with a sensory impairment. Age is the most significant risk factor for all forms of sensory impairment, with hearing loss one of the most prevalent chronic health conditions in later life (Margrain and Boulton 2005). Older people who have become hard of hearing or deaf in later life are unlikely to use British Sign Language (BSL), even if the social worker working with them happens to have this skill. Communication techniques may be as straightforward as speaking more slowly, articulating words clearly, facing the person and not covering one's mouth (Koprowska 2005). As with other areas of social work practice, understanding, empathy and sensitivity are as significant in the encounter as particular skills. For example, many deaf or hard of hearing people find communicating difficult in group settings and where there is background noise (Heine et al. 2002); thus, carrying out assessments in settings such as a day centre or hospital ward, or in the home when a number of people are present, may be problematic. While it may be tempting to deal with these situations simply by speaking with a raised voice, this will not suffice for some people and, in any case, can raise issues of confidentiality. If it is not possible to find a quiet room, using written, rather than verbal, communication for sensitive issues such as financial matters may be one option, though clearly not for people who also have visual impairments. Research on older people's experiences of sensory loss can raise awareness of factors that social workers need to consider. For example, sensory impairment may cause embarrassment, loss of confidence, depression and avoidance of social contact; more specifically, conversation may demand a high level of concentration from the older person and be very tiring (Heine and Browning 2004). Perhaps the most important message from such research is to find out about what helps and hinders communication for the older person concerned and then work to, respectively, maximise and minimise these factors, both in the assessment process and the wider intervention.

Dementia

Skills and values for communicating effectively with people with dementia are also important for social workers working with older people. Although people in younger age groups can experience dementia, age is generally held to be the most significant risk factor for developing dementia, with approximately 5 per cent of people over 65 experiencing dementia and 20 per cent of those over the age of 80 (Woods 2005). Kitwood (1997) was an influential figure in highlighting the essential *personhood* of someone with dementia, that is, 'a standing or status that is bestowed upon one human being, by others, in the context of relationship and social being. It implies recognition, respect and trust' (ibid.: 8). Although Kitwood analyses personhood in relation to people with dementia, the basic principle of providing support and care in ways that recognise and affirm each individual's personhood is pertinent across all areas of social work practice.

Kitwood identified both negative and positive types of interactions with people with dementia. He refers to features of negative communication as 'malignant social psychology'. Examples include:

- *Treachery*: using forms of deception in order to distract or manipulate.
- *Disempowerment*: not allowing a person to use the abilities that they do have; failing to help them to complete actions that they have initiated.
- *Infantilisation*: treating a person in a patronising way.
- *Intimidation*: inducing fear through the use of threats of physical power.
- *Labelling*: using a category such as dementia as the main basis of interacting with someone or explaining their behaviour.
- *Stigmatisation*: treating someone as a diseased object or outcast.
- *Outpacing*: providing information, presenting choices, etc., at a rate too fast for the person to understand; putting them under pressure to do things more rapidly than they can manage.
- *Invalidation*: failing to acknowledge the subjective reality of a person's experience.
- *Banishment*: sending a person away or excluding them – physically or psychologically.

- *Objectification*: treating a person as if they were an object with no feelings.
- *Ignoring*: behaving as though the person were not there.
- *Imposition*: forcing a person to do something or denying them the possibility of choice.
- *Withholding*: refusing to give attention or meet an evident need.
- *Accusation*: blaming a person for actions or failures of action that arise from lack of ability or misunderstanding.
- *Disruption*: intruding suddenly or disturbingly upon a person's action or reflection.
- *Mockery*: making fun of a person's 'strange' actions or remarks.
- *Disparagement*: telling a person that s/he is incompetent, useless, worthless etc., giving messages that are damaging to her/his self-esteem.

In contrast, Kitwood identifies positive ways of communicating with people with dementia that recognise and affirm personhood. These types of interactions contribute to what he calls 'positive person work'. The positive communications he identifies are:

- *Recognition*: acknowledging someone as a person, by name, affirming his or her own uniqueness.
- *Negotiation*: consulting people about their preferences and needs in a way that gives them some degree of power and control.
- *Collaboration*: working on a shared task, using a process that involves people's own initiative and abilities – not 'doing to' someone or casting them in a passive role.
- *Play*: activities with no goal but opportunities for spontaneity and self-expression.
- *Timalation*: sensuous or sensual experiences, for example aromatherapy or massage, that do not make cognitive demands.
- *Celebration*: experiencing life as joyful.
- *Relaxation*: may be in solitude but may well be with others.
- *Validation*: accepting the reality and power of someone's experience and hence its 'subjective truth'.
- *Holding*: providing a safe psychological space where vulnerabilities (for example, grief, rage) can be exposed.
- *Facilitation*: enabling a person to do what otherwise they would be unable to do.
- *Creation*: creating or allowing opportunities for the person to offer something to the social setting.
- *Giving*: enabling the person to give to others, for example, by showing concern, affection or gratitude.

Kitwood's message is that communication has a central role in sustaining personhood. This is echoed in other work on dementia:

> If . . . the quality we call personhood is made through relationships with others, then this is clearly where the crucial issues in the care of people with dementia lie. Further, central to the business of relationships is communication. We cannot be truly in relationship with others if we are not in communication with them.
>
> (Killick and Allan 2001: 18)

As a consequence, Killick and Allan argue that people with dementia must be helped to maintain communication and relationships with others. They discuss the skill, patience, sensitivity, creativity and critical self-awareness involved in interpreting the communications of people with dementia and suggest strategies and approaches, based on experience, to enhance practice in this area. It may be helpful to consider communication with someone with dementia using imagery from a game of tennis (Harris, Joy 2005). The 'ball' is the message that is being passed between the parties but the role of the worker or carer is that of coach, rather than competitor:

> They need to put the 'ball' where the other can reach; and it is easier to coach some people than others. Consideration needs to be given to 'pre-match preparation' such as minimizing background noise and other distractions; consciously relaxing; remembering it may feel like a first for the other person; and gaining the person's full attention first – by touch, greeting, etc.
> Strategies to help people 'return a serve':

> - say what you think the other is *feeling*;
> - offer what you think the other wants to say;
> - don't correct mistakes, and avoid confrontation;
> - don't shy away from tears and laughter;
> - little and often is often better.

> Strategies for 'reaching their serve':

> - identify the emotion;
> - be open to a range of possibilities, for example, when they say x they mean y (or z or t);
> - put present and past together to understand the other's reality.
> (Harris, Joy 2005: 125)

The Social Care Institute for Excellence (SCIE) has produced a research briefing on communicating with people with dementia (Social Care Institute for Excellence 2004). It highlights key points: communication is a basic need and a human right; all behaviour should be seen as communication; behaviour needs to be interpreted and this is a skilled task. The briefing provides helpful links to other resources relevant to this aspect of practice. SCIE has also produced a practice guide for practitioners involved in assessing the social care needs of older people with mental health needs (not just people with dementia) and again this provides an accessible source of information and guidance for busy practitioners (Social Care Institute for Excellence 2006a).

ACTIVITY 5.2: ENGAGING IN POSITIVE COMMUNICATION

Read the following extract (Craig 2004: 186), describing an experience of a student art therapist on placement in a hospital ward for people with dementia.

Jack, who has been an athlete, known throughout the county for his prowess and who has represented his region at sport, lies in a sterile bed bay. This place that has been his home for the last 10, 15 years bears not a single object, possession or photograph that would indicate anything of who he is, what is important to him, where he has travelled. There is not a single clue to indicate who his family are or to provide an introduction to his vast circle of friends. The room is stripped of all identity with its white walls, white linen and a single bedside cabinet. Only his name and the name of his consultant, handwritten on a wipeable board above his bed, provide an indication of who this gentleman is. Jack's physical needs make it difficult for him to mobilise. He doesn't verbally communicate so it is impossible to let the steady stream of bank staff and temporary carers know anything about him. Many have read the notes, which speak of medication, of the regularity of his bowel movements, of the importance of turning him every few hours to prevent the development of pressure sores. There isn't a mention in these notes of what he holds as being important, about his wife, his interests, his love of jazz music, his enjoyment of being with and of seeing his grandchildren.

I watch the temporary care staff working with him and observe them speaking over this gentleman as they turn and move him in bed. Their conversation focuses on what they have been doing the evening before, what to wear tonight and the latest gossip on 'Coronation Street'. Not a single attempt is made to speak to Jack, to address him directly. He has become a body to be moved, fed and toileted. I speak with the staff afterwards and they tell me that they literally don't know what to say to him. How could they, when they don't know who he is? All they see is a person who lies in bed day after day not moving, not speaking . . .

I spend time with Jack and his family. His wife is thrilled when I ask her to bring in precious photographs of their wedding day, of their first child's christening, of a family get together with Jack sat at the head of the table. I make high quality copies of the images and discover that Jack is able to express preferences through eye pointing. We work together and he chooses images to frame. We spend time sitting, listening to jazz music as I build the frames. At times he lies with his eyes closed, moving to the music; at others he is very much involved in the decoration of the frames, in the sponging of the paint. The images are mounted and placed where he can see them. Other staff comment and I hear them speaking to Jack, talking about the images, what they can see. Conversation. The recognition of the person behind the label of the illness.

Refer back to the 'malignant social psychology' and types of positive interaction identified by Kitwood (1997). Which negative and positive features are demonstrated in the situation of Jack, described above?

One of the crucial aspects involved in recognising the person behind the dementia that emerges in relation to Jack is the way in which the student art therapist surfaced Jack's past. Social work should have a similar concern:

> Social work uses what belongs to the person – their past . . . The careful, specific, skilled use of the past seeks to promote or at least sustain for as long as possible, the person's independence . . . By sensitively using the past, the encroaching private worlds inhabited by people with dementia can be shared with others to a much greater degree than is otherwise possible . . . This work requires good basic interpersonal skills of observation, reading verbal and non-verbal cues, attending, careful listening, responding and empathising . . . Social workers . . . must take the time to find ways of talking and ways of listening . . . In understanding the past, the present may be managed better . . .
>
> (Gibson 1993: 58–60)

This is one aspect of person-centred practice.

PERSON-CENTRED PRACTICE

As discussed earlier in the chapter, policy concerning the assessment of older people endorses an 'exchange' or 'person-centred' approach that puts the older person at the centre of assessment. Thus, the *Single Assessment Process* guidance states:

> Agencies should encourage older people to contribute fully to their assessment with due regard to their individual circumstances . . . At the commencement of an overview assessment (where not already ascertained through a contact assessment), the older person should be asked to describe their needs and expectations, and the strengths and abilities they can bring to addressing their needs, in their own words and on their own terms. This person-centred beginning should set the tone for the rest of the assessment and subsequent care planning, and due account of the user's perspective should remain to the fore throughout.
>
> At overview, specialist and comprehensive assessment, where appropriate and possible, professionals should encourage the older person to provide relevant biographical information including needs they have faced in the past, key life events, relationships, motivations and beliefs. Biographies are crucial where contact with agencies and service providers is likely to be intense or prolonged.
>
> (Department of Health 2002c: Annex E, 19)

However, studies have found that social work assessment is dominated by attention to functional abilities and self-care, whilst areas such as life history, relationships and social networks are neglected (Caldock and Nolan 1994; Caldock 1996; Stanley 1999). Assessment tends to be perceived and practised in terms of its managerial function, as a means of accessing resources (see Chapter 3), rather than in its professional sense of reaching an understanding of an individual in her or his social context. A report of the Chief Inspector of Social Services noted:

> A core skill of assessment as an analytical and an evaluative tool is being lost or undervalued. We see much information gathering but not much analysis and risk assessment . . . It is very difficult to get a holistic view of the person and their unique personality from the case file. This begs the question of whether the worker has really got to grips with the reality of the person in the context of their daily life, the problems they face, their strengths, their weaknesses, their aspirations for themselves and their fears for the future. Without this understanding it is difficult to see how social work intervention can be effective.
>
> (Department of Health 1999b: paras. 1.21–1.22)

In a study mentioned earlier in the chapter, Richards (2000) explored how the assessment process with older people was carried out in two social services teams. She observed that while the use of assessment frameworks served to provide a focus and purpose to the interview as far as assessors were concerned, these frameworks led to a tendency for assessors to become 'trapped in a restricted view' (ibid.: 3): 'Structuring the interview around an assessment schedule pre-determined the areas of investigation, perhaps sidestepping the older person's concerns or failing to capture the subtlety and complexity of the situation' (ibid.: 42). Assessors tended to focus on problems rather than identifying, and building on, older people's strengths and coping strategies. Richards distinguished between the agency agenda and service user agenda for assessment and concluded that the latter needs to occupy a central place in the assessment process, rather than being subsumed by bureaucratic concerns and requirements. Listening carefully to older people's stories will, she argues, identify their views of their needs and situations and enable intervention to be planned around the problem-solving mechanisms that they have developed over their life courses. Moreover, she argues that according significance to the older person's perspective will reduce power inequalities between the social worker and the service user.

Another study based on interviews with older people compared the language and constructs used by older people when describing their situations to those used by professionals (Baldock and Hadlow 2002). It was found that the nature of 'self-talk' by the older people, centring around their feelings, family and friends, was significantly different from the professional 'needs-talk' of disabilities and risks that dominated assessment processes and procedures. The researchers concluded, 'The qualitative gulf between the realities that users and service providers inhabit is so profound that it may always be to an extent unbridgeable' (ibid.: 48). However, the categories for defining professional talk in this study were derived from written assessment criteria rather than the actual talk of professionals in assessment interviews. This did not, therefore, allow for the 'translation work' of practitioners that one would hope to find in positive assessment practice (Morrison 2001; Fook 2002).

Other research also highlights potential differences in meaning between professionals and older people. This becomes apparent when careful attention is paid to the emotional content of older people's stories about themselves. Grenier's (2004; 2006) interviews with older women in Quebec highlighted the importance of their 'inside stories', that is, the way they understand events in relation to themselves. Grenier's analysis distinguishes between 'being frail', an identity based on physical frailty that the older women rejected, and their acknowledgement of 'feeling frail' at times, which was related to particular social, personal and emotional experiences. She argues that health and social care professionals need to move beyond a concern with physical functioning to exploring the personal meanings that physical and functional impairments have for an older person's sense of self. She argues that engaging with these emotional issues will lead to a better quality of care. It will enable us to address feelings and experiences that contribute to an older person 'feeling frail', whether or not they 'are' frail in physical terms.

If older people are not given the space to tell their stories, or if these are only 'heard' through the limited ears of narrow managerially defined criteria that ignore broader social, psychological and emotional dimensions of experience, issues that are crucial to the older person's well-being will be overlooked or misinterpreted. Our sense of self 'evolves with the sense of time passing, and our life story is an essential part of our sense of self' (Rowe 1994, quoted in Hepworth 2000: 119). Consistent with life course theories of ageing (see Chapter 1), a biographical approach facilitates understanding of the individual in the context of her/his past life experiences, as well as their current situation (Bornat 1999). This is compatible with the 'person-centred' focus advocated in the *Single Assessment Process*. Gearing and Coleman (1996) developed a biographical interview schedule that they suggest can be used flexibly and adapted to specific situations. It provides 'a route map' that explores the chronology of an individual's life, from childhood, through subsequent life stages and significant events, up to the present time. They argue that the approach has a number of benefits: it leads to a better understanding of and respect for the individual's unique situation and characteristics and an appreciation of issues of diversity; it contributes to a relationship of trust and generates feelings of value and self-worth in the older person; and it has a direct influence on decisions about appropriate service provision. However, as will be apparent from the earlier discussion of barriers to an 'exchange' model of assessment, and as acknowledged by the authors themselves, there are difficulties in applying the biographical approach in practice. In particular, it is very time-consuming and costly of staff resources and it may be necessary to meet acute needs before or alongside the biographical assessment.

Engaging with individual biographies as part of the assessment process is an approach that is not just relevant for older people with good linguistic skills. The skill of the assessor lies in finding different ways of eliciting stories, making sense of them and using them to promote 'person-centred' practice. This may be more difficult in some situations, for example, when working with people with dementia (see above), but it is still possible. Important skills include: careful attention to narratives – their style and structure, as well as content; observing and responding to non-verbal communication; and respecting the value of silence. It is also possible to establish connections between the past and the present, and within personal networks, through information provided by significant others in the older person's life, though caution is needed, as information is likely to be incomplete, distorted or based on previous patterns of behaviour (Killick and Allan 2001). An extract from an autobiographical exploration of the role of memory in constructing individual and family identity illustrates the importance of finding connections with biographies in order to engage with people on their terms (Grant 1999). A central thread within the account is the memory loss suffered by the author's mother, Rose Grant, as a result of multi-infarct dementia. In spite of Rose's memory loss, she retained her life-long enjoyment of shopping until a very advanced stage in her illness and this provided a means of connection, both with her daughter and with her past life.

> And now we're in the department store, our idea of a second home. My mother has never been much of a nature lover, an outdoor girl. We used to leave the city once, years ago, when we motored out of town in the Humber Hawk, parked in a lay-by, ate cold roast chicken from silver foil then drove home early so my father could watch the racing and my mother refold her clothes. By the sixties we considered a day out to be a drive to the new service station on the M6 where we enjoyed a cup of tea as the cars sped along to London below. My mother has never got her hands dirty in wellingtons, bending down among the flowerbeds to plant her summer perennials. Or put her hands to the oars of a boat or trampled across a ploughed field in the morning frost or breasted any icy waves. She shrinks in fear from sloppy-mouthed dogs and fawning kittens. But show her new improved tights with Lycra! 'They never had that in my day,' she says admiringly on an excursion to Sainsbury's looking at dose-ball washing liquid.
>
> And no outing can offer more escape from the nightmare of her present reality than shopping for clothes, the easiest means we know of becoming our fantasies and generally cheering ourselves up all round. Who needs the psychiatrist's couch when you have shopping? Who needs Prozac? . . .
>
> Up the escalators to the first floor where the land of dreams lies all around us, suits and dresses and coats and skirts and jackets. And where to begin? How to start? But my mother has started already.
>
> (Grant 1999: 2–3)

As with the example of Jack, presented in Activity 5.2 earlier in the chapter, this extract shows that the key requisite for person-centred intervention – finding points of connection with the older person's 'self' – does not depend on her/his being able to relay her/his stories verbally. Work with older people with learning disabilities (Johnson, K. 2005) shows that people do not need to have sophisticated linguistic skills for us to be able to learn from their stories. A number of important points emerge. First, the narratives of people who are not able to tell their stories in conventional ways tend to be excluded and some voices go unheard. This is about our failure to listen and find ways to understand. Second, the person hearing the narrative needs to reflect on the influence of her/his own 'self' and social position on the story that is told and how this is interpreted. This reinforces the points made in Chapter 1 and earlier in this chapter about the need for reflexivity on the part of social workers. Third, professional training can blinker our understanding, leading us to perceive and understand situations in limited ways. Listening to narratives may open up alternative ways of making sense of situations. Fourth, we need to understand the influence of people's experiences across the life course in shaping their stories. With regard to older people with learning disabilities, Johnson points out that they may have histories of institutionalisation and experiences of loss and other painful events earlier in their lives. These events will have shaped their view of themselves and others. Finally, the hopes and opportunities of later life must be recognised. Johnson's research suggests that later life may represent 'a late picking', offering new opportunities and hopes for the future. We need to recognise the importance of older people's hopes and dreams.

Narrative approaches such as those discussed are one of the theoretical 'maps' for assessment discussed by Milner and O'Byrne (2002 – see Chapter 1). They are concerned with the broader social meanings of the stories that people tell about themselves and others. Drawing on the postmodernist emphasis on the role of language and discourse, narrative approaches focus on the accounts (or 'narratives') that individuals use to construct meaning (White and Epston 1990). A narrative can be defined as 'a story which performs social functions' (Fook 2002: 132). People tell their own 'stories' based on their particular versions of 'reality'. These are likely to change in different contexts, at different times and with different audiences. Narrative approaches are used not only to understand people's perspectives for the purpose of assessment, but also as a method of intervention. They are based on the notion that people can be helped to construct more helpful 'stories' about their situations and that this can lead to change. In particular, the emphasis is on the creation of more positive narratives, built on strengths and successes rather than problems and deficits:

> The concept of narrative is important in both the fields of practice and research, in that an analysis of narratives is a key avenue towards identifying and understanding how people construct their 'realities' and how they might then be changed for therapeutic purposes.
>
> (Fook 2002: 67)

A simple example of narrative reconstruction is provided by the experience of an older person who participated in a research study on 'unmet need' (Tanner 2005). Harriet Manders (pseudonym) had to give up driving because of health problems. Driving had always been central to her sense of independence and she was devastated at the dependency that she saw as inevitable now that she would have to rely on other people for lifts. She talked of feeling a nuisance and a burden and envisaged that she might have to relinquish some of her social activities. Harriet Manders was interviewed five times over a three-year period, and in the final interview her narrative about this issue had changed and this had impacted on her sense of identity and self-esteem. She was now receiving lifts from various friends but rather than interpreting this as a symptom of dependence, she had reconstructed it as a measure of the reciprocity and mutual support within her social network – 'we all help each other' – and as repayment for her historical role as 'giver' to others. While the study from which this example is taken shows that older people are resourceful in adapting their stories, as well as dealing with the practical contingencies of their lives as circumstances change, social workers also have a role in helping in the process of narrative reconstruction. This may involve, for example, challenging narratives that reflect internalised ageism and helping to replace them with a narrative based on social rights and entitlements. In Chapter 3, it was argued that assessment should be seen as a process of potential value to service users, regardless of whether or not it leads to the provision of services. Attending to narratives in assessment – highlighting unhelpful narratives and uncovering and validating more helpful ones – is an example of how assessment can in itself lead to constructive change.

ACTIVITY 5.3: USING NARRATIVES IN ASSESSMENT

- How might listening to an older person's narrative help a social worker carrying out a community care assessment?
- From your experience of community care assessments, or from what you have read, to what extent do they allow scope for individuals to tell their stories?
- What could you do as a worker to increase the opportunities for older people to tell their stories?
- How might this improve their experience of the assessment process and its outcomes?

HOLISTIC ASSESSMENT

'Holistic' forms of assessment seek to understand older people within the context of their whole lives – past, present and future – rather than through a narrow lens that sees them only as 'users' of social care (and perhaps other) services. Taking a 'holistic' approach also means recognising the relationship between the individual and wider social systems:

> Holism is not concerned solely with the whole person, it is concerned with whole systems and *wholeness*, in both persons and systems and the interactions between them. The simultaneous engagement with individuals, families, organisations and social structures is what should mark out social work as a profession. A holistic approach to the assessment and meeting of the needs of individuals requires a focus on the social structures which shape their lives and the mechanisms which impact upon their experiences of services.
>
> (Lloyd, M. 2002: 166)

This has implications for how older people are constructed in policy and practice; a holistic approach will treat older people as citizens with rights, rather than as dependent people in need of services (Joseph Rowntree Foundation 2004). Recognising older people's status as citizens means addressing the barriers that prevent their full participation in the society of which they are members. It also means acknowledging older people's contributions as resources for, as well as recipients of, welfare (ibid.). This holistic view of older people's requirements as citizens is presented in the Social Exclusion Unit report, *A Sure Start to Later Life*, discussed in Chapter 2. However, as we saw in Chapters 3 and 4, these principles are still far from realised in practice.

Whilst it is crucially important that social work assessment and intervention address social, environmental and economic inequalities that obstruct older people's participation, the emotional, psychological and spiritual dimensions of older people's well-being are also part of a concern with 'wholeness'. One dimension of a 'holistic' assessment, which is often neglected in practice but may have particular significance for some older people in the later stages of their lives, concerns spirituality (see, for example, Coleman, P. *et al*. 2002; Marcoen 2005). Spirituality is not to be defined narrowly in terms of particular 'named' religious beliefs. Moss (2005) defines it in terms of how an individual gives expression to their chosen worldview. Sadler and Biggs (2006) point out that an older person may express their spirituality through music, the arts or communing with nature as well as through religious practices. Spirituality may enhance older people's well-being by contributing to a sense of meaning and purpose in life and also help them adjust to losses and change (Moss 2005; Sadler and Biggs 2006). However, religion and spirituality have tended to be either ignored as irrelevant or shunned as dangerous or pathological by practitioners (Moss 2005). Moss argues that engaging with spirituality should be part of assessment as it is a dimension of building or supporting strength and resilience:

> The definition being offered – spirituality is what we do to give expression to our chosen worldview – allows the helping professional to explore with people how they see the world, and what their chosen world-view looks like. Specifically, they can tease out the ways in which such world-views enable the people who hold them to offer a (perhaps moderately) satisfying attempt to make sense of what is happening to them and to others; the extent to which their chosen world-view provides strength and resilience to deal with adversity; and the framework it offers to them about how to regard and deal with other people.
>
> (Moss 2005: 83)

Moss argues that practitioners should not be deterred from exploring religious or spiritual issues because of the lack of a shared faith. They do not need to be an 'expert' in different faiths but to have the sensitivity, willingness and confidence to explore with people the implications of their chosen 'worldview'.

SKILLS IN RECORDING

A particular aspect of social work that plays a central role in relation to all of the issues we have discussed is that of the recording of assessments, care plans and reviews. In statutory agencies, recording is likely to take the form of inputting information in a standardised form on a computerised system, which then generates reports in a prescribed format. These systems are designed primarily to meet the managerial demands of the organisation and to enable the monitoring and extraction of data required by centrally driven inspection and performance management systems (Harris, John 2003: 68–74, 93–5; Coleman, N. and Harris, John forthcoming; White and Harris, John 2007). However, at the same time social workers are required to share copies of assessments and care plans with service users and carers (see Chapters 3 and 4). There are a number of tensions between what social work agencies require from records for managerial purposes and service users' and carers' requirements. Service users and carers are likely to value records that are presented in a clear and easily accessible format and written in straightforward language. Computer generated reports that aim to convey information seen as necessary by the organisation and, in the case of the *Single Assessment Process*, other professionals, may bear little relationship to how the older person perceives their own situation. As we saw in the research by Richards (2000) and Baldock and Hadlow (2002), discussed earlier in the chapter, there may be a gulf in understanding and language between professionals and service users. Our professional socialisation means that we can forget that core social work terms – such as 'need', 'assessment' and 'eligibility' – may be alien concepts to service users. Even basic information about services, such as names of providers and days and times of contacts, may be presented in a way that makes the information difficult to extract or comprehend. Although policy requires that a named contact person is given in the care plan (see Chapter 4), responsibility for monitoring and reviewing the care plan may be allocated to a team or organisation, rather than a named person, leaving the older person uncertain about who should be contacted if there are difficulties. Given the points made earlier in the chapter about the role of narratives in constructing and reinforcing people's reality, it is also important that the written record is positive in tone and emphasises strengths. However, the need to demonstrate that difficulties are 'eligible needs' can lead to practitioners emphasising problems, which in turn can discredit and demoralise service users (Ray and Phillips 2002). Whilst the practice of giving copies of reports to service users may be seen as 'empowering' in principle, fundamental questions have to be asked about how the receiving of reports is experienced by service users in practice. Morrison (2001) reports on efforts by one team to make its recording practice more user-friendly. Two key dimensions were the need to improve the clarity of recording and the need to ensure it conveyed strengths, as well as difficulties.

ACTIVITY 5.4: POSITIVE PRACTICE IN RECORDING

Identify alternative ways of writing the following phrases so that:

- you describe the behaviour, rather than using labels;
- you use positive, rather than negative language, building on strengths, rather than emphasising difficulties;
- your language is easy to understand, unambiguous and avoids jargon.

Negative phrases	More positive phrases
Mrs Brown is incontinent.	
Mr Green is immobile.	
Ms Purple has early stage dementia.	
Mr Grey is unable to perform any personal care tasks for himself.	
Mrs White is housebound and socially isolated.	

(Adapted from Morrison 2001)

You may have experienced some concerns as a result of considering the issues raised by this activity. First, as mentioned already, there is the concern that emphasising strengths will mean that the difficulties inherent in the person's situation will be concealed. Managers may not accept that the person is 'eligible' to receive services and service providers may not understand the nature of the problems with which the person requires help. However, writing in a way that is both clear and incorporates strengths does not mean that difficulties cannot be detailed as well. You may note from your experience of completing Activity 5.4 that it requires you to describe in some detail what someone can and cannot do, rather than just using a label, such as 'immobile' or 'incontinent'. Second, trying to write simply could be interpreted as patronising towards service users. We would argue that the ability to write in a clear and straightforward way is a skill of value to all audiences, not just service users. In any case, as discussed in Chapter 1, social work has to cater for diversity in service users' needs and situations; older people will come from different backgrounds and have different needs and preferences regarding communication that can be accommodated if the starting point is attempting to write clearly and simply. In terms of judging the language with which service users are comfortable, a useful gauge is the language used by older people themselves. For example, in Activity 5.4, Mrs Brown might have said that she has 'trouble with her waterworks' and the social worker could check with Mrs Brown whether that is how she would like her account to be used in the written record. This could be followed by some detail about what 'having trouble with her waterworks' means in the context of how Mrs Brown lives and would like to live her life. Third, there may be concerns that social workers will lack credibility with other professionals if they use 'simple' language, rather than 'professional terminology'. However, the value-base of social workers requires us to challenge all working practices that are oppressive to service users and to encourage more inclusive ways of working. Professional language can provide an easy shorthand for professionals, but act as a barrier to a full 'exchange' with service users (see the previous discussion in this chapter). As Fook (2002) argues, one of the tasks of social workers is to act as 'translator' between professional and service user cultures. If it is felt to be necessary to use particular vocabulary to communicate with other professionals, these terms or concepts should at least be explained to service users so that language is not used in ways that disempower and exclude people.

Much of what has been said about skills in this chapter applies to social work generally, not just working with older people. When considering whether special skills are required for professional practice with older people, Hughes (1995) concludes that the answer is both 'no' and 'yes'. She argues that, on the one hand, it must be recognised that work with older people requires the same level of skill and expertise as other areas of practice. On the other hand, older people have an increased likelihood of experiencing certain health or social difficulties that have consequences for the skills a social worker needs to utilise. While the worker should be alert to the heightened possibility of particular conditions, such as sensory impairment and dementia, being experienced by older people, and be equipped with the skills to respond appropriately, it is vital that no assumptions are made about what is required. This echoes key points made in Chapter 1 about the need to recognise uniqueness and diversity within a broader framework of understanding about older people's needs and situations.

The range of skills necessary to provide 'person-centred' and 'holistic' social work when working with older people have been highlighted in this chapter. The focus has been on the skills involved in directly engaging with older people. The next chapter explores the interface between social workers and others in older people's service and support networks.

KEY POINTS

☐   Social work with older people requires a range of skills.

☐   Different theoretical 'maps' and approaches can point assessment and intervention in particular directions.

☐   There are barriers to the realisation of the exchange model in practice; social workers can attempt to work within and around the obstacles and constraints raised by such barriers.

☐   'Person-centred' practice entails understanding older people's biographies and listening to their stories.

☐   'Holistic' assessment and intervention require that social workers recognise and respond to the 'whole' person within the context of the 'whole' social system.

☐   The ways in which information is recorded and shared with older people can influence the extent to which they are empowered/disempowered within the social work process.

KEY READING

Kitwood, T. (1997) *Dementia Reconsidered: The Person Comes First*, Buckingham: Open University Press.

Lymbery, M. (2004) 'Managerialism and care management practice with older people', in M. Lymbery and S. Butler (eds) *Social Work Ideals and Practice Realities*, Basingstoke: Palgrave Macmillan.

Smale, G., Tuson, G. and Statham, D. (2000) *Social Work and Social Problems: Working Towards Social Inclusion and Social Change*, Basingstoke: Macmillan.

CHAPTER 6

WORKING IN PARTNERSHIP

OBJECTIVES

By the end of this chapter you should have an understanding of:

- the nature of effective partnership working in planning and delivering services for older people;

- key issues concerning the relationship between social work and health services in providing services for older people;

- the significance of housing support for older people;

- the role of the voluntary sector in providing services for older people;

- the legal framework for working with carers and the needs of carers, especially older carers.

The previous chapter explored the skills needed by social workers in working directly with older people. This chapter considers issues related to social work's broader role in working with older people's social networks and collaborating with other professionals and agencies. The chapter will begin by considering general issues related to effective partnership working. It will then focus on four areas, working with: health professionals, housing agencies, the voluntary sector and carers.

PARTNERSHIP WORKING

Buchanan and Carnwell (2005) identify three factors that have been significant in the move towards partnership working. First, society has become increasingly complex and multi-agency responses are required to address multi-dimensional needs. Second, changes have occurred in the structures, roles and functions of statutory agencies and these have made them more fluid, flexible and better able to work in cooperation with other agencies. Third, political drivers within policy require agencies to work in 'joined up' ways to deliver 'seamless services' (see Chapter 2). As we have seen, partnership working is promoted heavily in policy but there is little consensus about what 'partnership' or related terms such as 'joint working' and 'collaboration' actually mean (Glasby and Littlechild 2004). From their review of how these terms are used, Glasby and Littlechild conclude that the common components are:

- a desire to achieve benefits that could not be attained by a single agency working by itself;
- a recognition that some services are interdependent and that action in one part of the system will have a 'knock-on effect' somewhere else;
- some sort of shared purpose or shared vision of the way forward.

(Glasby and Littlechild 2004: 7)

As they argue, the key test concerning partnership is whether service users and carers experience services as coordinated and coherent, rather than haphazard and fragmented (ibid.: 7).

When considering how different agencies and individuals involved in providing support to an older person work together, a useful reference point is Hudson *et al.*'s (1998) continuum of collaboration (see Table 6.1).

Such a continuum can not only help organisations to evaluate their current relationships with other agencies but also assist in clarifying the level of collaboration

TABLE 6.1 Hudson *et al.*'s continuum of collaboration

Level	Features
Isolation	No contact or communication between agencies; inter-professional rivalry and stereotyping; goals and interests perceived differently.
Encounter	Some contact between agencies but no meaningful interaction.
Communication	More frequent contact between agencies results in the exchange of information; some formal arrangements for liaison and some commitment to joint training.
Collaboration	Information exchanged between agencies is acted on; there is engagement in joint working; general objectives are shared.
Integration	Collaboration throughout the organisation, at strategic and operational levels; very high levels of trust and respect.

Source: Hudson *et al.* 1997: 19

WORKING IN PARTNERSHIP 151

that is necessary for them to achieve their objectives. While agencies working in isolation are unlikely to lead to 'consistent and coordinated packages' for users and carers, at the other end of the continuum, integration will not necessarily be the most appropriate level of collaboration either. The key question is what level of collaboration is appropriate for the agency to be most effective in achieving its goals (Glasby and Littlechild 2004).

As has been indicated, levels of collaboration are highly influenced by policy and political objectives. Current policy requires that agencies work together (see Chapter 2). Indeed, it has been argued that partnership has been one of the key strategies of the New Labour Government in its development of public services (Parrott 2005). Given the influence of, and changes in, policy, concepts of partnership and collaboration are not static and recent changes represent shifts from the concept of 'inter-agency working', based on notions of communication and coordination, to 'partnership', based on collaboration or integration (Parrott 2005). For example, the White Paper, *Our Health, Our Care, Our Say: A New Direction for Community Services* (Department of Health 2006b) sets out the need for the commissioning of primary care and social care to be integrated:

> One fundamental change will be better integration between those working in the NHS and those working in social care. A better-integrated workforce – designed around the needs of people who use services and supported by common education frameworks, information systems, career frameworks and rewards – can deliver more personalised care, more effectively.
>
> (Department of Health 2006b: para. 8.35)

The current significance of partnership for service delivery can be summed up as follows:

> The concept can be seen in the enabling of new forms of service delivery in which management of the process is left to the partners while the service outcomes are set and quality controlled by the state. Professionals within these partnerships are enjoined to work in new ways, to change what may be considered unhelpful working practices and cultures and to reconstruct their professional and practical relationships with one another . . . The accepted faith of partnership is one of synergy in which previously separate players whether state, private or voluntary agencies can become more than the sum of their parts by joining in partnership to create collaborative advantage, i.e. in achieving what they could not have done if they had acted separately.
>
> (Parrott 2005: 29)

Although partnership working has increasingly become a focus of policy and a requirement of initiatives such as *Partnerships for Older People Projects* (Department of Health 2006d – see Chapter 2, Box 2.2), there are a number of barriers to effective collaboration being achieved in practice. These are:

- *structural*, for example, fragmented responsibilities for services both between different agencies and within them;

- *procedural*, for example, differences in planning and budget cycles;
- *financial*, for example, differences in funding mechanisms and the way service costs are paid by users of services;
- *professional*, for example, differences in ideologies, values and professional interests. A prime example is the conflicting beliefs and values underpinning the 'medical' and 'social' models of disability (see, for example, Priestley 1999); another is different professional perspectives on what constitutes acceptable risk and risk-taking (this is discussed further in Chapter 7);
- *defensiveness* in response to perceived threats to professional status, autonomy and legitimacy.

(Glasby and Littlechild 2004)

Sharing information

One area of difficulty that arises from structural, procedural and professional barriers is the sharing of information between different agencies. This is particularly relevant to implementation of the *Single Assessment Process* (see Chapter 3). There are a number of legal imperatives concerning the protection of confidentiality. Article 8 of the Human Rights Act (1998) states that 'everyone has the right to respect for his private and family life'. The Data Protection Act (1998) imposes requirements concerning the processing, sharing and security of sensitive personal data. Like NHS organisations, local authorities are required to appoint a 'Caldicott Guardian' to safeguard confidentiality: 'Acting as the "conscience" of an organisation, the Guardian should actively support work to facilitate and enable information sharing and advise on options for lawful and ethical processing of information as required' (Department of Health 2006f: 5).

However, these legal and policy mandates relating to confidentiality have to be set against policy and practice requirements to collaborate closely with other agencies and professionals. The *Code of Practice for Social Care Workers* (General Social Care Council 2002) states that social care workers must respect confidentiality (para. 2.3), but also work openly and cooperatively with colleagues (para. 6.5) and ensure that they are informed about the implications and outcomes of risk assessments (para. 4.4). Richardson and Asthana (2006) identify four possible models of information sharing that strike differing balances between protecting confidentiality, on the one hand, and openly sharing information with other professionals and agencies, on the other. These models are as follows:

- *ideal*: information is shared appropriately but only when necessary;
- *over-open*: information is shared when this is not always necessary or appropriate. This model is likely to breach confidentiality but unlikely to lead to important information being withheld;
- *over-cautious*: information is withheld when it is necessary or appropriate to share it. This creates a high risk of failure to communicate necessary information but a low risk of breaching confidentiality;
- *chaotic*: the sharing and withholding of information is indiscriminate, leading to high risks of both not communicating important information and breaching confidentiality.

Although there is limited evidence concerning the influence of professional culture on information sharing, it is suggested that health professionals, influenced by the medical model, may be more inclined to adopt an 'over-cautious' model, prioritising the protection of confidentiality over the need to communicate with other professionals, while the police may adopt an 'over-open' approach, when communicating with health and social care agencies (Richardson and Asthana 2006). As well as professional values and culture, the level of trust between professionals is also likely to bear directly on willingness to share information (ibid.). These are key areas to be addressed between all parties involved in local implementation of the *Single Assessment Process* (see Chapters 3 and 4) and more widely in professional and inter-professional training. Even when professional protocols regarding information sharing are agreed, there remain practical difficulties in terms of the need for shared recording and information systems, not least in relation to strategic planning.

Strategic planning

Chapter 4 pointed out that care planning can be undertaken at the level of planning support for individuals and at the level of planning services for a geographical area. While Chapter 4 discussed issues concerning care planning for individuals, here we look briefly at strategic planning.

There are a number of legal provisions requiring local authorities to identify and plan appropriate services to address the needs of their areas. Under the National Assistance Act (1948, Section 29), local authorities are required to maintain a register of disabled people, using the definition of disability set out in Section 29 (see Chapter 2). Individuals can choose whether or not they wish to be registered and the provision of services does not depend upon registration (Clements 2004). The Chronically Sick and Disabled Persons Act (1970, Section 1), gives local authorities a more proactive role to 'inform themselves' of the numbers of disabled people in their areas, that is, independently of people's requests to be registered. The National Health Service and Community Care Act (1990) developed the responsibility more explicitly from that of identifying need to planning appropriate provision. Under Section 46, local authorities had a duty to consult relevant health, housing and voluntary agencies, including organisations representing service users and carers, and to publish annual community care plans that set out how their services would address local need. However, the requirement to produce community care plans was removed in England in April 2002, in the light of subsequent new obligations regarding planning and the greater emphasis on joint working between health and social services (see Chapter 2; and Clements 2004). Community care planning at the strategic level now takes place primarily through Joint Investment Plans, which are produced by health trusts and local authorities. Joint Investment Plans were introduced in a government circular in 1997 (Department of Health 1997b), and reinforced in the 1997 White Paper, *The New NHS* (Department of Health 1997c). Health trusts and local authorities are required to jointly analyse their current provision in the light of the needs of their local population, identify gaps in services and agree priorities for the current and future commissioning of services (Glasby and Littlechild 2004).

As far as older people are concerned, the *National Service Framework* (NSF) for older people, discussed in Chapter 2 (see Box 2.1) sets out national standards, key interventions and milestones to be achieved so this also represents a strategic framework for NHS organisations and local authorities. However, a review of progress in achieving the NSF standards, *Living Well in Later Life* (see Chapter 3), notes the lack of a shared sense of direction in services for older people in the areas inspected (Healthcare Commission *et al.* 2006). This is seen as having led to inconsistent and uncoordinated services, ineffective use of resources and a lack of incentive to change. The report advocates developing a shared vision and strategy that are rooted in the views of older people:

> When older people are asked about the priorities that would most improve their lives, these often relate to issues beyond health and social care services, such as having a neighbourhood that is safe, access to transport, an adequate income and opportunities to meet with others. Therefore visions and strategies for older people must reflect these needs.
>
> (Healthcare Commission *et al.* 2006: 15)

The report recommends that local strategic partnerships involving all organisations that commission and provide services for older people, including those in the independent sector, are strengthened to achieve a joint strategy and coordinated approach.

Achieving effective partnerships

If partnerships are to be effective, action is required at a number of levels: structural, institutional and individual (Glasby and Littlechild 2004). Glasby and Littlechild argue that while central government has long exhorted closer working between agencies, this cannot be achieved comprehensively unless structural barriers to partnership working are addressed. The need for a new governance framework that develops partnership at and between all levels – Whitehall, government offices, local authorities/local strategic partnerships, neighbourhoods and individuals and families – is highlighted in a Local Government Association report:

> Although successes in joint working between the NHS and local government can be readily identified, much of the evidence relates to improved processes rather than better outcomes for individuals or communities. Moreover, the division between locally elected and centrally managed governance systems has remained a fundamental obstacle. The resulting differences in culture, structure and systems have substantially withstood three decades of organisational tinkering. The forces sustaining two separate systems have, on the whole, proved too powerful in the face of limited initiatives to bridge their boundaries. More radical approaches which align and integrate decision-making, resource allocation and accountability in the organisational mainstream rather than at its margins are now required.
>
> (Wistow 2006: 2)

Wistow proposes a comprehensive and integrated local governance system, bringing together social care, health and other local agencies, all sharing a strategic focus on the well-being agenda. He suggests that the framework should be based on a democratic local government model and he highlights the contribution of social care services in addressing issues of comprehensive well-being, social inclusion and community capacity building. While these proposals concern major structural and institutional changes, there are steps that can be taken by practitioners and managers at organisational and individual levels to improve partnership working in their localities. Buchanan and Carnwell outline key principles for effective partnership working (see Box 6.1).

BOX 6.1   PRINCIPLES FOR EFFECTIVE PARTNERSHIP WORKING

- Make time to create, nurture and maintain partnerships. This is often best achieved through face-to-face contact.
- Develop a mutual understanding and respect between the agency partners. This demands time and commitment.
- Do not try to force partnership but allow time for it to develop organically and in response to local needs and conditions.
- Guard against lapsing into 'multi-agency inertia', where ideas are discussed but never implemented.
- Maintain a shared focus on service delivery and the needs of service users.
- Develop a commitment to partnership at both strategic and operational levels.
- Establish the basis and boundaries of the partnership, for example, the basis on which agencies can withdraw from the partnership and the scope for agencies to act independently outside of the partnership.
- Consider the need for agencies to maintain their own identity and difference.
- At the same time, promote the partnership's corporate identity, for example, through an independent chair.
- Concentrate on process and the quality of experiences of service users, not just practices and procedures.
- Involve service users actively in the partnership and listen to their views.
- Guard against exploitation and power imbalances, for example, larger agencies dominating the partnership.
- Clarify the boundaries of confidentiality and expectations regarding the sharing of information across the partnership.
- Evaluate the success of the partnership.

(Buchanan and Carnwell 2005: 272–7)

It is important to evaluate partnerships in terms of outcomes, rather than assuming that partnership is in itself 'a good thing'. Partnership working may be ineffective but, more than this, it may have deleterious consequences. Heywood *et al.* (2002) highlight some of the dangers of joint working. First, a focus on joint working can be used to conceal inadequate funding for services. With regard to the nature and extent of support someone receives, 'ultimately, it may be that it is resources rather than partnership that really matter' (Cornes and Manthorpe 2004: 24). Second, joint working can easily come to be seen as an end in itself rather than as a means to the delivery of services that are responsive to service users' needs. Third, 'joint working can be used to stifle dissent' (Heywood *et al.* 2002: 146), particularly in terms of silencing the voices of small voluntary sector agencies. Hence the importance of Buchanan and Carnwell's (2005) principle of guarding against power imbalances (see Box 6.1).

ACTIVITY 6.1: EXPERIENCES OF PARTNERSHIP WORKING

- Identify people/other agencies with whom you are working or have worked previously (this does not necessarily have to be in a social work/social care capacity).
- What attributes of partnership and collaboration have you found in these relationships?
- What benefits of partnership and collaboration have you observed?
- What barriers to partnership and collaboration have you noticed?
- How were/could these be addressed at structural, institutional and individual levels?

(Adapted from Carnwell and Carson, A. 2005: 19)

Having reviewed general issues concerning partnership, the next section considers particular issues arising in supporting older people at the interface between social work and health services.

HEALTH SERVICES

As people age, they become more likely to experience ill health and disability. Whereas just over a quarter of men and women aged 50–64 in Great Britain reported a long-term illness or disability in 2001, for people aged 85 and over this figure increased to two-thirds of men and three-quarters of women (Office for National Statistics 2004). Although women have a longer life expectancy than men, they are more likely to live longer in poor health. The most frequently reported health problems for people over the age of 65 are heart and circulatory diseases and musculoskeletal ailments. For those over the age of 75, women are more likely than men to have arthritis and rheumatism, while men are more likely to suffer respiratory diseases, such as bronchitis and emphysema (ibid.).

There is a close interrelationship between physical health and social and emotional well-being. Social and economic conditions create and perpetuate health problems, while access to social and economic resources can help to mitigate the consequences of disability and ill health (McLeod and Bywaters 2000). Moreover, there is no direct relationship between objective measures of physical health and an individual's subjective evaluation of how 'healthy' they are. A key factor for older people in defining themselves as 'healthy' appears to be whether they are able to continue doing the things that are important to them (Reed *et al.* 2004). This indicates an important role for social workers, working alongside health colleagues. This role encompasses: helping to prevent and alleviate circumstances that contribute to poor health (for example, addressing issues such as poverty, which contributes to inadequate nutrition and heating); improving access to appropriate health care services; and helping people to manage health-related problems in ways that enable them to maintain valued roles and activities.

However, despite the interrelationship of physical, social and emotional dimensions of well-being, the separation of 'health' from 'social' care in policy and practice has obstructed the delivery of coherent and holistic support for older people. As mentioned in Chapter 2, the post-war Welfare State was founded on the notion that the health needs of sick people would be met by the National Health Service and the social care needs of frail people would be met by families or local authorities. However, this distinction has become increasingly blurred, with local authorities assuming increasing responsibilities for older people who are sick as well as frail (Glasby and Littlechild 2004). As noted in Chapter 2, improved working relationships between key organisations involved in supporting older people, including the facility for integrated health and social care teams through the establishment of care trusts, has been a key strand of New Labour policy. This section will focus on two key areas that relate to the interface between health and social work services: the distinction between personal care, nursing care and continuing health care; and intermediate care and delayed discharge.

Personal care, nursing care and continuing health care

The professional assessment of whether an older person has personal care needs, nursing care needs or continuing health care needs is significant as it determines who bears financial responsibility for meeting the need. The funding of care is complex and the different arrangements that may apply are set out in Figure 6.1.

In England, personal care is regarded as a 'social' need, and therefore individuals are subject to a means-test to determine the charge they should pay for services arranged to meet these needs (see Chapter 4). 'Health' needs, on the other hand, are met by the NHS, free at the point of delivery. Personal care has increasingly come to be defined as 'social care', even though it involves care of the body through touch, which has traditionally been the remit of health care (Twigg 2000). A Royal Commission, set up to look at ways to fund the long-term care of older people, was critical of the way in which people with personal care needs are penalised by having to pay for care, in contrast to those with physical health needs, whose care is provided free of charge by the National Health Service (Royal Commission 1999). The Commission recommended separating out a person's living costs (that is, everyday expenses such as food, heating, etc.), their housing costs (such as their rent and council tax) and their personal care costs. It proposed that personal care costs should be met through the taxation system, with services such as domiciliary care and equipment to aid daily living being provided free of charge to those with assessed personal care needs. (In Scotland, personal care is provided free of charge, under the Community Care and Health [Scotland] Act [2002],

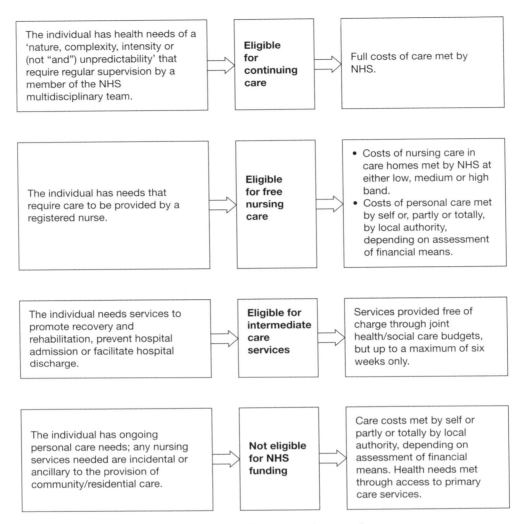

FIGURE 6.1 Funding arrangements for meeting different types of care needs

and this has fuelled the debate about how to fund long-term care for older people [Philpot 2004].)

In its response to the Royal Commission (Department of Health 2000), the government rejected the proposal for free personal care but introduced free nursing care under the Health and Social Care Act (2001, Section 49). While the local authority remains responsible for the accommodation, board and personal care of those who meet the conditions set out in Section 21 of National Assistance Act (1948), any 'nursing care' required is the responsibility of the NHS and is provided free of charge to the resident. Free nursing care in care homes applies, regardless of a person's financial circumstances. This means that even where a resident is paying their own care home fees, that part of the care that is 'registered nursing care' will be provided free of charge, paid for by the NHS. Registered nursing care is defined as care provided by a registered nurse. This includes care that is planned, supervised or delegated by a registered nurse.

The NHS may make one of three different levels of contribution to care costs (high, medium or low), depending on the level of the person's assessed nursing need. All residents who may be eligible for free nursing care have to have an assessment of their physical and mental health needs, carried out by a nurse following specific guidelines (Department of Health 2001c). The assessment tool is called the *Registered Nursing Care Contribution* (Clements 2004).

As recommended by the Royal Commission, there is a view that the state should accept responsibility for meeting personal care needs, as well as nursing care needs. A discussion paper, based on the work of the Joseph Rowntree Foundation's Long-term Care Advisory Group, proposes ways forward to develop a clearer, fairer and more coherent system for funding long-term care. These fall within three broad areas: devising more coherent systems for allocating resources to those in need of long-term care; acknowledging the need to devote more public resources to this area; and developing mechanisms for private resources to complement public funding (Hirsch 2005).

A further dimension of responsibility (see Figure 6.1) relates to people who are assessed as having continuing health care needs. Continuing care refers to people who need NHS care because their health needs are extensive and complex. In these situations, the NHS assumes responsibility for paying the full care costs, not just a nursing care component. A number of ombudsman investigations in the 1990s highlighted various restrictive practices of health authorities that prevented people who should have been receiving continuing care from accessing it. A significant Court of Appeal ruling in 1999, the *Coughlan judgment*, based on the case of a disabled woman, Pamela Coughlan, held that the NHS should accept responsibility for funding nursing home care if it is primarily the person's health need that gives rise to the need for care. It held that local authorities can only legally accept responsibility for nursing care where this is 'merely incidental or ancillary to the provision of accommodation'. This is determined by considering the type and level of nursing care needed. Despite the 'Coughlan test' for determining when continuing care should be provided and the issuing of various sets of guidance and directions, clear eligibility criteria for the provision of continuing care did not materialise and there was wide geographical variation in the criteria used. Guidance issued by Department of Health (2001d) outlines 'key issues' that the NHS should 'bear in mind' (note the weak wording) when making decisions about continuing care:

- The limits of local authority responsibilities. Following the *Coughlan judgment*, the eligibility criteria for continuing care operated by strategic health authorities should not require local authorities to provide services beyond those that fall within the duty to provide residential accommodation under the National Assistance Act (1948, Section 21). Nursing services can only be provided by councils if these are 'incidental or ancillary' to the provision of residential accommodation.

- If the 'nature, complexity, intensity *or* [not "*and*"] unpredictability' of the individual's health needs requires regular supervision by a member of the NHS multidisciplinary team, this should indicate eligibility for continuing care. Supervision does not, therefore, have to be required from a consultant but can come from a member of the multidisciplinary team. Similarly, ombudsman investigations indicate that the word 'regular' should not be interpreted too narrowly.

- The need for the use of specialist health care equipment, under the supervision of NHS staff, is also an indicator of the need for continuing care. An example might be gastric feeding tubes for someone unable to swallow.
- The person's medical, physical or mental health condition is 'rapidly deteriorating or unstable' and requires regular supervision by a member of the NHS multi-disciplinary team.
- The person is in the final stages of a terminal illness and is expected to die in the near future. Guidance indicates that it is inappropriate to apply very short timescales in respect of life expectancy.

The remaining two 'key issues' highlight factors that do *not*, in themselves, indicate eligibility for continuing care:

- The need for care or supervision from a GP or registered nurse does not on its own provide sufficient grounds to receive continuing care.
- Continuing care can be provided in hospital, a nursing home, hospice or the person's own home so the location of care does not on its own determine eligibility for continuing care. Eligibility for continuing care is also not affected by who is providing the care. Someone may be receiving a care package within their own home, including social care components, and be entitled to full funding of the care by NHS if the continuing care criteria are met.

(See Mandelstam 2005: 360)

Since the introduction of free nursing care bandings, or the Registered Nurse Care Contribution, referred to earlier, there has been concern that assessment at the high band is being used when individuals meet continuing care criteria and should be having the total costs of care met by the NHS. This issue was tested in the Grogan case in 2006, which challenged the refusal of continuing care by Bexley Care Trust. The High Court found that the Coughlan Test had not been used and that the Trust had unlaw-fully refused continuing care on the basis that nursing costs could be met through the Registered Nurse Care Contribution banding. The Grogan ruling has, therefore, reaffirmed the need to consider, on the basis of the totality of someone's needs, whether there is a primary need for health care. Advice for older people, their families and professionals on these complex issues has been issued by a collaborative grouping of organisations, including a suggested letter for challenging decisions that have been made about continuing care (Age Concern England *et al.* 2006).

This section has illustrated some key points about social work's interface with health at the level of practice. It has highlighted: the blurred and shifting bound-aries between the definition of 'personal/social care' needs versus 'health/nursing' care needs; the scope for both contestation and collaboration between health and social care agencies in determining their respective responsibilities; and the potentially significant financial implications for older people and their families according to the ways in which these issues are resolved.

Avoiding unnecessary hospital admissions and ensuring timely discharge

Standard 3 of the *National Service Framework for Older People* (see Box 2.1, page 54) sets out its aim, 'to provide integrated services to promote faster recovery from illness, prevent unnecessary acute hospital admissions, support timely discharge and maximise independent living' (Department of Health 2001a: 41). This is to be achieved primarily through intermediate care services. The provision of intermediate care, as outlined in the NSF, aims to:

- prevent people from being admitted to hospital where this can be avoided;
- help people to be discharged swiftly from hospital care;
- prevent early admission to residential and nursing care.

It involves services that:

(a) are targeted at people who would otherwise face unnecessarily prolonged hospital stays or inappropriate admission to acute in-patient care, long-term residential care, or continuing NHS in-patient care;

(b) are provided on the basis of a comprehensive assessment, resulting in a structured individual care plan that involves active therapy, treatment or opportunity for recovery;

(c) have a planned outcome of maximising independence and typically enabling patient/users to resume living at home;

(d) are time-limited, normally no longer than six weeks and frequently as little as 1–2 weeks or less; and

(e) involve cross-professional working, with a single assessment framework, single professional records and shared protocols.

(Department of Health 2001e: 6)

Intermediate care is, therefore, targeted at older people with high levels of need who are at risk of requiring or continuing to be in either hospital or residential care. The NSF cites figures that suggest that 20 per cent of the days during which older people occupied acute hospital beds were inappropriate and resulted from the lack of available alternative services. The need to tackle unnecessary or prolonged hospital or care home admissions arises largely because of concerns about the costs of institutional care but it is also justified on the basis of the negative outcomes for older people, such as disruption of their social networks, disorientation and the risks of acquiring infections (ibid.). While many older people will share the concern to return home from hospital as soon as possible or to avoid being admitted to hospital or a care home, intermediate care has been seen as motivated primarily by cost, rather than quality of life, considerations (Nolan 2000).

Intermediate care can operate at a number of junctures and in different forms. It can provide intensive support in the home setting, for example through rapid response teams, preventing the need for hospital admission; it can be provided immediately following discharge from hospital, for example through 'hospital at home' schemes, thus enabling people to be discharged from hospital more quickly; and it can be offered on a day or residential basis between hospital care and discharge home, offering a period of rehabilitation for people who might otherwise need admission to residential or nursing care. The planning and provision of intermediate care requires partnership working across professional and organisational boundaries; it is likely to involve collaboration between, for example, doctors, nurses, physiotherapists, occupational therapists, social workers and social care workers, drawing on provision from the voluntary and private sectors as well as the statutory sector. As yet there is a lack of sound research evidence on the effectiveness of intermediate care services, including only limited evidence about older people's own experiences of this form of provision (Petch 2003). Evaluation is hampered by wide variation in the nature, purpose, target service user group and organisational arrangements of different services provided under its remit. Concern has been expressed that some services have been designated as intermediate care when this amounts simply to the renaming of existing services, rather than a new form of provision. The focus of intermediate care on a short intensive period of rehabilitation also seems to have largely excluded older people with dementia, who are seen as having a progressive disease that is not amenable to intervention (Read 2005), despite contrary arguments that proactive and positive interactions to help people to function better can play a role at all stages of dementia care (Marshall 2005: 15).

While intermediate care, as stated above, may operate at different junctures, between home and hospital, home and care home and hospital and care home, the delayed discharge policy is specifically concerned with accelerating the discharge from acute medical care of people who are assessed as medically fit for discharge. Implemented in January 2004, the Community Care (Delayed Discharges) Act (2003) introduced a 'reimbursement policy' whereby social services may be obliged to reimburse the NHS for the costs incurred through 'blocked beds'. These are 'blockages' in the system when the patient has been medically assessed as fit for discharge but discharge is delayed and the bed is 'blocked' because the necessary social care services are not in place. Although this policy is not exclusive to older people, it is older people, often targeted as 'bed-blockers', who are primarily affected by the policy. This is in itself ageist in deeming older people's needs for careful discharge planning and proper rehabilitation as being less significant than those of younger people. In effect it places the blame on older people for the systemic failure to provide appropriate and timely services.

Under the policy, if a patient is thought likely to need social care services upon discharge from hospital, the NHS issues a 'Section 2' notice of the need for assessment to the local authority (an 'Assessment Notification'). This must be given at least two days prior to the proposed discharge date. The patient and any carers should be consulted prior to the notice being issued. The local authority, on receiving the notice, must assess the person's needs for community care services and decide on the services that should be provided. It may also need to carry out an assessment of carers' needs. However, the focus of the assessment is the services that are needed to enable the person to move on from their occupancy of the acute bed; further assessment may be required to put in place more comprehensive or long-term care arrangements. Under Section 5 of the Act, the NHS must notify social services of the proposed date of discharge (a 'Discharge Notification') at least one day in advance of the day itself, excluding weekends and public holidays. Social services will be charged for each day, commencing the day following the given discharge date, that the patient remains in hospital solely as a result of either the assessment not being carried out or the services planned, either for the service user or the carer, not being made available (Mandelstam

2005). If the delay is in any way caused by factors that are the responsibility or part responsibility of the NHS, rather than solely social services (for example, if the delay is caused by a jointly commissioned service not being available), then the reimbursement charge cannot be levied (Clements 2004).

Additional funding (£300 million over two years) was made available to local authorities to support the reimbursement policy. This funding was to be used to develop services to support discharge, rather than just to pay fines. Early evaluation of the impact of reimbursement indicated that delays in hospital discharge had decreased since the policy's introduction (Commission for Social Care Inspection 2004c). However, later figures, published in 2006, show a dramatic increase in 'bed-blocking' (Gainsbury 2006). The increase, linked to announcements of deficits in the NHS, is attributed to insufficient funding, budget cuts in primary care trusts and hospitals' efforts to fast-track patients through the system. Hospitals receive payments for individual patients, regardless of the amount of time they occupy a bed, so this increases the incentive for hospitals to increase their rates of admission, which, in turn, necessitates speedier discharges (ibid.). This is an example of the interlinked and shifting boundaries between health and social care, discussed in Chapter 2. Accelerated discharges have direct consequences on the demand for social care services. Given that, as we have seen, reimbursement fines may be levied on local authorities who are not able to arrange appropriate services within the required timescales, some of the deficits within NHS Trusts' budgets can be offset by fines imposed on social services, even though a prime reason for delayed discharges may be changes in policies and practices in the NHS that increase demands on social services resources.

While concerns with targets and budgets have led to a focus on the speed of discharge, 'timeliness of discharge alone will not deliver quality outcomes' (Commission for Social Care Inspection 2005b: 50). In terms of outcomes for older people, the 2004 research by CSCI only examined short-term outcomes, a few days or weeks after the older person had been discharged (Commission for Social Care Inspection 2004c). A subsequent report revisited the older people to find out about longer-term outcomes (Commission for Social Care Inspection 2005b). Lessons highlighted by this later research are shown in Box 6.2.

BOX 6.2   LEARNING FROM EXPERIENCES OF HOSPITAL DISCHARGE

In 2004, the Commission for Social Care Inspection (CSCI) interviewed over 70 older people who needed social services support on discharge from hospital across seven locations in England. Interviews were carried out a few days or weeks after their discharge. The report concluded that the reimbursement policy had speeded up hospital discharge and, in parts of the country where there was access to good community support services, older people were recovering well. However, where community services were unavailable or inadequate, older people's recovery was undermined. It appeared that some older people were propelled into making hasty decisions to enter institutional care while there was some evidence that others were

continued

being readmitted to hospital as a result of premature discharge or inadequate post-discharge support (Commission for Social Care Inspection 2004c).

In 2005, the CSCI revisited the same sample of older people to explore longer-term outcomes of the reimbursement policy. The report of the follow-up research presents a number of learning points.

- Continuity in terms of a named person with responsibility for monitoring and reviewing care is important to older people: 'People moving frequently between hospital and home particularly benefited from there being one person who had a longer-term relationship with them and knowledge of their needs and preferences' (p. 46).
- 'Good, ambitious care management' (p. 46) is important in achieving positive outcomes. The failure of care managers to offer older people the opportunity to use direct payments was particularly noted.
- Many hospital readmissions could potentially be avoided with improved risk assessment and forward planning to prevent and respond to crises.
- An orientation towards rehabilitation can result in long-term improvements in people's lives: 'Positive outcomes for people were more common in places where rehabilitation was seen as a principle underpinning all services rather than as a specialist service, organised in a building, with a limited intake' (p. 47).
- Ongoing coordination of community health and social services is vital to successful outcomes for older people with multiple needs. Effective multi-disciplinary working was more common at acute stages than in longer-term management and support.
- A focus on preventive services has been eclipsed by the concern to reduce pressures on hospital resources. Coordination of a wide range of services across all local authority services is needed to address quality of life issues for older people.
- More effort is needed to ensure a consistently high quality of home care. At present, this is very variable.
- Care homes need to play a more flexible role in supporting independence, alongside other community services, for example, by offering shared care.
- Hospital or care home admissions that arise through breakdowns in the caring network can be prevented by the provision of more practical and flexible support for carers.
- Improvements are needed in meeting individuals' cultural needs and preferences.
- Strategic partnership between health and social services are vital and these are being strengthened over time. Reimbursement grant money was increasingly being invested in services, rather than used to pay hospital trusts for delayed discharge.

(Commission for Social Care Inspection 2005b)

A key point is that the level and quality of post-discharge support services is crucial to achieving positive outcomes for older people's lives. The report notes that while detailed monitoring takes place of the frequency of and reasons for delayed discharges, much greater attention needs to be directed at monitoring the outcomes for older people.

Whilst research has explored the nature and extent of joint working between the NHS and social services, less attention has been given to working relationships with the voluntary sector (Cornes and Manthorpe 2004: 19). Yet the voluntary sector plays a significant and increasing role in delivering services that would once have been provided by statutory agencies. Voluntary sector organisations, such as Age Concern, may be contracted to provide services such as hospital aftercare, either under the remit of intermediate care or with a more preventive focus, such as social rehabilitation (Le Mesurier 2003). An evaluation of five voluntary sector pilot hospital aftercare social rehabilitation projects found that the safe transition of older people from hospital to home was jeopardised by premature discharge, lack of available services and poor coordination of health and social care services (McLeod *et al.* forthcoming). In this study the voluntary sector service functioned as a significant source of support for older people discharged from hospital in a number of respects: providing help with practical domestic tasks, such as shopping and cleaning; undertaking an advocacy role to help the older person gain access to particular resources, such as welfare benefit advice; and providing 'educational' help which enabled the older person to develop or regain skills necessary for their independence, for example restoring confidence in using public transport or using a telephone following a stroke. However, it was noted that in providing support post-discharge, the voluntary sector may be drawn into substituting for the statutory sector, which may mean less help is available for the 'lower level' support that was originally the remit of the project (ibid.). Similarly, in research on Help the Aged's intermediate care programme for older people, it was noted that volunteer coordinators often played a significant part in the provision of care, having to 'step up' their role to compensate for the fact that social workers were not employed as part of the intermediate care team. Thus, 'the reality for many older people was that the volunteers and their co-coordinators were effectively the "jam and sponge" as well as the "icing" on the top of the cake' (Cornes and Manthorpe 2004: 22).

A synthesis of qualitative research findings on older people's views of hospital discharge was undertaken by the Social Care Institute for Excellence (2006b). Although primarily concerned with methodological issues, the synthesis highlights some significant findings in terms of experiences and outcomes of hospital discharge processes for older people. Older people were noted as having a low level of participation in their own discharge planning and to experience considerable anxiety and apprehension about discharge. Factors unrelated to whether the patient was ready to be discharged, such as the pressure on beds, influenced the decision-making, which was primarily in the hands of doctors:

> it was the role of the doctor to decide on discharge. The role of social workers was to respond quickly to demands/pressure to discharge, leaving them with limited time to see the person; indeed it was found that an older person could be discharged to residential care without seeing the social worker who was making the arrangements.
>
> (Social Care Institute for Excellence 2006b: 39)

Of particular significance for health and social care professionals involved in discharge planning is the need to understand and respond to older people's management of the process within a life-planning framework:

> older people view discharge as simply an integral part of the process of coming to terms with the impact of illness on life planning. Experiencing illness, being treated in hospital and leaving hospital is therefore a major event or process that threatens self-sufficiency and control over one's life,

particularly if complete physical recovery is not expected in the longer term
. . . The synthesis shows that, in older people's eyes, coming to terms was
not a passive process of acceptance but an active process of working out
how to manage, and how to preserve control over the most important things,
while accepting what must be given up.

(Social Care Institute for Excellence 2006b: 47–8)

If there are increased pressures on social workers to effect the swift discharge
of older people from hospital, the consequences for older people may be that they are
discharged directly to care homes without the benefit of a period of rehabilitation that
might have enabled them to recover sufficiently to return home. Alternatively, they
may be discharged home before they are ready, creating physical, psychological and
emotional risks, the prospect of early readmission and imposition of additional pressure on informal carers. These circumstances run directly counter to supporting older
people's control over life planning processes.

The examples of intermediate care and hospital discharge illustrate the interdependence of health, social work and social care services and the potential consequences
for older people when 'joined up' care is not delivered in practice. While policies are
directing professionals to collaborate in providing timely support to address objectives that concur with what older people want – remaining or returning home – these
same polices can also jeopardise both partnership working and person-centred care.
The central focus for practitioners can easily become managerial-driven processes
and requirements pertinent to their particular organisation, such as reaching targets and
avoiding fines, rather than achieving user-centred outcomes related to well-being.

A particular threat to partnership working and person-centred care is the climate
of retrenchment in both health and social care, which leads to both needing to make
cuts and restrict services. As already indicated in relation to delayed discharge, there
is evidence that cuts within NHS services are having an impact on social care. A telephone survey of local authorities situated in areas where there were NHS Trust deficits
revealed that 67 per cent of the 55 authorities that responded felt that their councils
had been adversely affected by the NHS deficit. 40 per cent reported an increase in
the number of referrals where there appeared to be an NHS responsibility, while 35 per
cent stated that the NHS had withdrawn funding from agreed or jointly funded services
(Local Government Association 2006). NHS financing, priorities and provision have
a direct impact on social work and 'cost-shunting' is likely to increase inter-agency
conflict about boundaries and responsibilities (Carson, G. 2006). Different organisational audit and performance systems may also lead to conflicting priorities, as each
organisation is working to achieve different targets and meet different performance
measures, the achievement and meeting of which are likely to be affected, and possibly
compromised, by the policies and practices of other organisations. The voluntary sector
may be pushed into the position of compensating for deficits in the statutory system,
which in turn may generate pressure on its own resources and undermine its goals.
These factors all threaten to undermine partnership working, fostering blame and
antagonism, rather than collaborative goodwill, between agencies.

For intermediate care and hospital discharge services to be effective in terms of both
conserving costly resources and promoting independence, an integrated, whole-system
approach is needed. Unless these services are supported by adequate and appropriate
provision at other stages in the service pathway, including preventive and longer-term

rehabilitative support, there is a danger that problems will simply shift from one part of the system to another. A comprehensive and coherent strategy to achieve both cost-effectiveness and well-being objectives needs to be underpinned by fundamental principles, throughout all levels and types of provision. Thus, it is argued that key principles underpinning intermediate care – person-centred care, multi-agency working and an enablement approach – should be integral throughout mainstream services, rather than being confined to a specialised, targeted and time-limited intervention (Young and Stevenson 2006: 340).

ACTIVITY 6.2: DISCHARGE PLANNING

You are a hospital social worker with responsibility for ensuring effective discharge planning for older people referred to you by the ward staff. Identify the different expectations that the following parties may have of your role, bringing out the possible tensions and conflicts:

- hospital managers;
- ward staff;
- community support services;
- your line manager/budget holder;
- your social work profession/colleagues;
- the older person;
- carer(s)/family members.

This section's consideration of issues involved in partnership between health and social care services has illustrated the significance placed on working together in current policy and practice. It has become clear that partnership depends on effective systems of inter-professional collaboration. However, Lymbery (2006) argues that the literature on the sociology of the professions and on inter-professional working suggests that such collaboration is difficult to achieve, not least because of the vast differences in power between the occupational groupings involved and the competition for territory between them. He argues that unless these issues are understood and addressed, rhetorical calls for more partnership will be ineffective.

HOUSING AND HOME

Housing issues are a legitimate focus for social work's attention because of the connections that housing has with health, physical and social functioning and psychological well-being; housing-related provision can be central to supporting older people in the community. Issues related to housing and home for older people have to be located within the broader policy context of a reduced stock of council housing, growth in owner-occupation, a decline in the provision of places in residential care homes and emphasis on supporting people to live independently in the community (Heywood *et al.* 2002; Kellaher *et al.* 2004). Older people are particularly likely to live in sub-standard housing. Age Concern England present figures that show that about 32 per cent of pensioner households live in housing classified as non-decent, with inadequate heating being a common deficiency. Amongst home owners, those most likely to live in non-decent housing are people over the age of 60 who live alone (Age Concern 2006d). The likelihood of living in poor housing increases with advancing age, with older women over 80 who are living alone being the most likely to live in inadequate housing (Adams 2003). Older people are not only more likely to live in poor housing but also potentially less likely to be able to take action to improve their housing conditions as a consequence of interlinked difficulties such as frailty, disability, isolation and poverty (ibid.). Internalised ageism, discussed in Chapter 1, may also leave older people with little sense of their right to improved conditions.

The experience of poor housing conditions earlier in the life course lays 'a sure path to more ill-health and social need' in later life (Heywood *et al.* 2002: 156). Demonstrating a direct causal relationship between poor housing and ill-health is problematic because of the difficulty of disentangling related variables, such as poverty, poor nutrition and inadequate heating. However, policy (Acheson Report 1998) and research (for example, Marsh *et al.* 2000) have highlighted health problems that are related to living in poor housing. The physical and mental health problems associated with particular housing conditions are shown in Box 6.3.

BOX 6.3   SUMMARY OF COMMON HOUSING FAULTS AND THEIR IMPACT ON HEALTH

Damp, condensation and mould growth:

- asthma;
- bronchitis;
- other respiratory problems;
- arthritis and rheumatism;
- mental health problems such as depression.

Cold homes:

- respiratory illness;
- cardiovascular conditions;
- hypothermia;
- increased risk of accidents and falls;
- impaired mental function;
- mental health problems including depression and isolation;
- rheumatism and arthritis.

Defective and inadequate electrical wiring:

- risk of injury caused by electric shocks or house fires;

- risk of accident or injury if circuits fuse or trip frequently and if sockets and switches are inadequate or poorly located;
- trip hazards caused by trailing wires and extension cables;
- mental health problems – worry about fire risk.

Defective gas appliances, or coal fire:

- carbon monoxide poisoning;
- risk of explosion in case of gas;
- fire hazard from blocked chimneys or flues.

(Care and Repair England 2006)

Living conditions within the home, such as the accessibility of front entrances, toilets, showers, stairs and kitchen equipment, have a significant impact on physical and social functioning. Parkinson and Pierpoint (2000) explored the role of housing in preventive services for older people, looking at particular examples of good practice. Their conclusions highlight the role of the environment, rather than impairments, in determining disability, thus supporting a social model of disability:

> There was frequently little correlation between levels of disability and dependency, if the physical environment was right. Well-designed or adapted kitchens and bathrooms allow clients to retain independence, reduce the need for hands on care and support prompt discharge from hospital.
>
> (Parkinson and Pierpoint 2000: 9)

The report concludes that housing is not just about bricks and mortar, but about much wider forms of support that people need to maintain quality of life within their home environments.

Despite the relationship between housing and health and well-being, housing and home have been largely neglected within community care policy (Heywood *et al.* 2002). Analysis of community care plans and Director of Public Health reports in three health regions noted the lack of attention given to older people's housing needs in health, housing and community care planning processes (Harrison and Heywood 2000). Heywood *et al.* (2002) argue that one reason for this neglect is that housing is experienced as a private, rather than a social and political, issue. Approximately 90 per cent of older people live in ordinary housing in the community, while 5 per cent live in some form of sheltered or supported housing and 5 per cent live in residential care (Department of Health/Office of the Deputy Prime Minister 2000). However, literature on the housing needs of older people has tended to ignore the majority of older people who are living in ordinary housing (Appleton 2002). A Task Group that was convened by the Joseph Rowntree Foundation to look at the role of housing and care in meeting the needs and preferences of older people took the position that housing for older people should be considered in relation to all older people, not just the minority who require specialist forms of housing (Joseph Rowntree Foundation Task Group 2004). Key requirements identified were:

- housing that is designed in ways that support people's independence, including access to assistive technology and adaptations that enable people to 'age in place';
- flexible forms of help to support home living;
- housing, health and care services that are 'joined up' in integrated teams within communities.

The concept of 'ageing in place' refers to enabling older people to continue living in their preferred home environment for as long as possible:

> It means coordinated effort is required to adapt the physical and social environment to the person by providing flexible supports as needs change rather than moving the person to a new environment where the required level of support is already in place – adapting the environment to the person rather than moving the person to a new environment.
>
> (Bigby 2004: 159)

Various forms of support are available to facilitate 'ageing in place'. As part of their preventive provision, many areas operate 'handyperson' schemes, run by charitable organisations such as Age Concern, home improvement agencies or Help the Aged. These schemes have been shown to be crucial in enabling older people, especially those who are owner-occupiers but living on low incomes, to remain living in their own homes for longer and to retain their quality of life (Adams 2006). However, despite the growth in the number of handyperson schemes in recent years, they are not part of the mainstream of services and suffer from not being clearly the responsibility of any one organisation, given their interface with housing, health and social care provision (ibid.).

Home improvement agencies (HIAs) are not-for-profit organisations that usually receive some financial support from central government (specifically the Department for Communities and Local Government) and local authorities. They carry out home improvements and adaptations to enable older people to 'stay put' in their own homes for longer. This may include major adaptations, such as fitting a downstairs bathroom, as well as small repairs, such as fitting door and window locks. HIAs also provide advice and guidance about housing repair issues, financial advice, for example about applying for local authority grants or equity release, and technical help, for example overseeing repairs and ensuring work is completed satisfactorily. 'Foundations' is the national co-ordinating body for home improvement agencies in England (see www.foundations.uk.com). According to the Foundations website, there are currently HIAs operating in over 300 local authority areas. They are usually known as 'care and repair' agencies or 'staying put' schemes. The relationship between health and housing is recognised through a growing number of joint initiatives between HIAs and primary care trusts. Schemes include those where HIAs carry out work to reduce the risk of falls within people's homes, for example by fixing rails, securing carpets and fitting brighter lights, and those that undertake repairs and adaptations necessary for safe discharge from hospital (Easterbrook, 2002; Adams 2003). Research into the role of HIAs by Smart and Means (1997) highlighted the complexities involved in determining the cost-effectiveness of HIAs. However, based on detailed case analyses, they concluded that the cost of HIA intervention is low compared with other forms of domiciliary support.

An alternative to the reactive approach of delivering services to help older people address problems is to work proactively in planning and designing the environment to promote independence and well-being. Coleman refers to this as moving 'beyond a problem orientation' to inclusive design that has benefits for everyone, not just older people (Coleman, R. 2000). Older people can continue to live in 'ordinary' housing, even when very frail, if the environment is supportive. The development of technology has created numerous possibilities. The Joseph Rowntree Foundation has developed two demonstration 'smart homes' characterised by small computers, positioned around the house, which enable systems and devices to communicate with each other. For example, it is possible to dial into the house from outside so that lights and heating can be turned on in advance of returning home; smoke detectors can automatically trigger a call to the fire brigade; a motion detector can automatically turn on lights for someone who gets up in the night; in the morning, a single switch can turn on lights, draw back curtains and run the bath (Joseph Rowntree Foundation 2006).

ACTIVITY 6.3: THE ROLE OF TELECARE

Read the following extract:

> The role of technology in supporting people to live at home ('telecare') is increasingly recognised. The Preventative Technology Grant, announced in July 2004, consists of £80m in grant finance allocated over two years commencing in April 2006. Local authorities are allocated the funding but are expected to work in partnership with housing, health, voluntary and independent sector agencies and with service users and carers in planning and delivering telecare. Telecare equipment and services include: community alarm systems that act as an emergency response mechanism; sensors in the home to detect and monitor movement; devices to detect falls, fire or gas and trigger a warning at a response centre; lifestyle monitoring systems that provide warning of a change or deterioration in an individual's normal pattern of behaviour; telemedicine that monitors vital signs such as blood pressure and transmits the information to a response centre. Thus telecare is seen as having the potential to:
>
> - reduce the need for residential and nursing care;
> - reduce acute hospital admissions;
> - reduce accidents and falls that occur in the home;
> - act as an adjunct to hospital discharge and intermediate care services;
> - contribute to preventive services;
> - provide support to people who wish to die at home;
> - increase service users' independence and choice;
> - give more relief and freedom to carers.
>
> (Department of Health 2005c)

Consider the potential advantages and disadvantages of telecare from the perspectives of:

- older people themselves;
- those who form part of their informal caring networks;
- service commissioners/funders;
- service provider agencies.

So far we have considered housing need in terms of its physical dimensions. Yet 'home' also has particular significance for positive emotional well-being:

> Home is existential and experiential. It is where domestic lives are played out. Home is a myriad of things: a set of relationships with others, a statement about self-image and identity, a place of privacy, a set of memories, and a social and psychological space.
>
> (Oldman 2002: 330)

Thus, supporting older people to 'age in place' may enable them to retain integral components of their identity as autonomous and independent individuals (Oldman 2002; Twigg 2002). Later life may be a time of loss and change and in this context home and environment can be a significant source of stability and continuity and a site of self-determination (Peace 1998; Percival 2002; Kellaher *et al.* 2004). A study carried out as part of the Economic and Social Research Council's *Growing Older* programme revealed the significance of secure domestic spaces for constructing and maintaining identity and for providing an anchor from which older people could feel confident to engage in their neighbourhoods and communities (Peace *et al.* 2006). However, it cannot be assumed that this will be the case for all older people. Indeed, older people may have a sense of greater autonomy and independence in a residential setting if key dimensions of choice and control have been lost within the sphere of the private home (Peace 1998). Similarly, if social contact with others is highly valued, this may be more easily achieved within a residential care setting than in the home environment (Richardson and Pearson 1995).

Retirement communities or retirement villages, like 'smart homes', are a form of housing that combines some elements of 'ordinary housing' with specialist provision. Retirement communities are seen as having four defining characteristics:

- residents are retired from full-time employment;
- there is a community element in terms of people within a certain age cohort living in a geographically defined area;
- there are elements of collective living, with some sharing of activities and facilities;
- there is a sense of autonomy alongside security.

(Kingston *et al.* 2001)

When comparing the health and social status of members of a residential community with a community sample, Kingston *et al.* reported a 'feelgood factor' and optimistic outlook in the residential community samples. The main reasons for deciding to move to a retirement community were the greater sense of security and a desire to relieve pressure on families. Community security was a significant concern identified by the community sample and one of the features most highly valued by the residential community sample, along with friendship and peer support:

> Positive aspects of life in the residential community revolve around a general sense of optimism, and a tangible pioneering spirit that this does indeed represent a new beginning for many residents. This spirit perhaps recaptures the sense of community, neighbourliness and security they feel was lacking before they entered a new community.
>
> (Kingston *et al.* 2001: 233–4)

A review of existing literature on retirement communities and data from ongoing evaluations notes a number of advantages of this form of housing provision for older people. Because retirement communities consist of more than 100 dwellings, it is possible to provide facilities that are both more cost-effective and more flexible. While facilities such as fitness centres and cafés are not focused on providing 'care', they address aspects of social, recreational and educational need, with associated benefits to health and social well-being. There is some evidence of benefits to local health and social care services. For example, resources are saved by being able to deliver services (such as GP visits and health promotion activities) to older people living in one place and there is some evidence that access to on-site care and support reduces the need for hospital admission and facilitates early discharge from hospital (Croucher 2006). The Joseph Rowntree Foundation Task Group (2004) summarises the potential benefits of these forms of housing in terms of: their function as an alternative to residential care; the extension of choice and the potential to meet diverse needs and preferences; the support opportunities for people with dementia; the role of such schemes in community regeneration and support. However, places in retirement communities are not readily available and affordable. Also, as noted by the Task Group, these forms of specialist provision should not be promoted at the expense of support to enable older people to live in ordinary housing, when this is their choice.

This section has discussed some examples of forms of housing support that may need to be considered in planning services for older people. A key barrier to older people accessing such help is lack of information, both about sources of support to maintain their homes and alternative housing options (Office of the Deputy Prime Minister 2006). A social worker who is well-informed about the various types of housing support available locally will be able to help older people address housing-related needs by proving information and/or involving relevant housing agencies in care planning.

Although there is not space here to explore in detail the issue of homelessness, it is important to note that some older people may not have a settled home at all. Sometimes homelessness is an outcome of wider difficulties, such as rent arrears, financial problems and bereavement, and some of these contributory factors to homelessness may be preventable. Proactive measures, coordinated between different agencies, such as offering help and advice to older people who have rent arrears, who are struggling financially or who are depressed, may be effective in preventing homelessness (Crane *et al.* 2006). This is an example of the need for holistic responses, as discussed in Chapter 5, that recognise the interacting physical, social and emotional dimensions of individual situations.

VOLUNTARY SECTOR AGENCIES

As we have already seen in relation to hospital aftercare and housing support services, voluntary sector agencies often play a significant and central, rather than subsidiary, role in providing support services to older people. Moreover, their practices and values may be more closely attuned to the needs of service users than those within the statutory sector. For minority ethnic groups in particular, the voluntary sector may act as an important 'bridge' to other agencies, providing information and advice in accessible and acceptable forms, especially to people whose first language is not English (Butt and Moriarty 2004). Black and minority ethnic organisations have often developed in response to their awareness of communication barriers and the lack of cultural awareness and competence within mainstream services. In this sense, voluntary sector organisations act not just as a bridge to mainstream providers but also as an alternative source of support (Policy Research Institute on Ageing and Ethnicity 2005).

The culture and values enshrined in a voluntary organisation's practice may render the process of receiving help acceptable and also personally validating. For example, a study that looked at what older people valued about different schemes operated by Help the Aged highlighted the 'whole person' orientation of the schemes and promotion of positive attitudes and approaches, rather than a focus on deficit (Reed *et al.* 2004). Chapter 2 discussed the promotion of the 'mixed economy' that occurred as part of the community care reforms of the 1990s, whereby the provision of services was increasingly contracted out to the independent sector. As a consequence, many services provided by the voluntary sector are commissioned by statutory agencies, which, in effect, delegate their statutory functions to the voluntary (or private) sector through commissioning and contracting processes. The danger for voluntary sector providers is that the business culture required to engage effectively in contracting can conflict with and eclipse the key values and practices that most endear their services to service users (Harris, John 2003: ch. 8). Research by Patmore and McNulty (2005) reveals the influence of the values of service commissioners on the nature of the service provided by voluntary sector agencies (this study is discussed further in Chapter 7). The work of a voluntary agency may also be restricted by specific indicators and outcomes required by commissioners, leading it to be driven by responsiveness to commissioners, rather than to service users. For example, voluntary sector providers may be required to set access or eligibility criteria for their services, prescribed by their external funders (Cornes and Manthorpe 2004). Some services provided by the voluntary sector may fall outside of the remit of the statutory sector. For example, 'low level' help with shopping, cleaning and gardening may be left entirely to the voluntary sector. Despite the increased emphasis on prevention in policy (Department of Health 2006b; 2006d), the statutory imperative to meet eligible need, discussed in Chapters 3 and 4, is likely to mean that in times of resource shortfall, these lower level forms of support are accorded low priority (Cornes and Manthorpe 2004). For the voluntary sector this means that statutory funding for this type of provision, if provided in the first instance, may be reduced or cut. While this may allow the agency greater autonomy, the lack of statutory support can create financial insecurity for the service, hinder planning and development and consume precious staff resources in the search for alternative sources of funding. The nature of its relationship with the statutory sector therefore poses some dilemmas for the voluntary sector:

the process of contracting and collaboration needs careful thought . . . strategies have to be developed that will establish relationships between the formal and informal sectors in ways which do not compromise the independence and flexibility of the informal sector and which offer some stability of funding and support.

(Reed *et al*. 2004)

Having considered the roles of formal services, statutory and voluntary, in a range of settings and services, we now turn to carers, often described in accounts of the 'mixed economy' as 'the informal sector'.

CARERS

It is estimated that around 11 per cent of the UK population provides unpaid care (Carers UK 2005). The bulk of caring has always been undertaken by unpaid members of informal support networks. As the Seebohm Committee (1968) noted:

> we must emphasise that any comprehensive plan to meet the needs of the elderly . . . must pay great attention to the contribution to the care of old people which is, or could be, made by relatives, friends and the wider community. The care which a family gives to its older members is of prime importance and nothing is quite an adequate substitute. Therefore, the social services . . . should make every effort to support and assist the family which is caring for an older member.
>
> (Seebohm Report 1968: para. 294)

Despite the central contribution to older people's lives made by such informal support, it is only in recent years that 'carers' have been socially constructed as an identity category (Bytheway and Johnson 1998). The voice of carers, through national organisations such as Carers UK and local carers' groups, has been increasingly influential in bringing to public attention the often undervalued work of carers and the substantial saving in public revenue that their input represents (Carers UK 2002). This has led to a campaign by carers' organisations for the title of carer to be used exclusively in connection with unpaid caring (Lloyd, L. 2006b).

As outlined in Chapter 2, one of the objectives underpinning the community care reforms of the 1990s was to provide support to carers (Department of Health 1989). Throughout policy since that time there have been numerous injunctions to involve and support service users *and carers*, as well as specific pieces of policy and legislation concerned with assessing and responding to carers' needs. The implications for older people of the way 'care' and 'carers' are constructed in policy and practice will be explored further in Chapter 7. This section will outline the legal framework for working with carers, before proceeding to highlight particular issues relevant to social work's role in relation to carers.

The law relating to carers

In line with the objective of providing support for carers set out in the *Caring for People* White Paper (Department of Health 1989 – see Chapter 2), the first piece of legislation specifically aimed at carers was introduced in 1995. The Carers (Recognition and Services) Act (1995) defines a carer as 'someone who provides or intends to provide a substantial amount of care on a regular basis'. The Act gives carers a right to request an assessment of their ability to provide and continue to provide care. The duty to assess depends on a request by the carer. The results of the assessment have to be taken into account in the assessment of needs, carried out under Section 47 of the NHS and Community Care Act (1990), of the person for whom the carer is providing care. However, 'taking the assessed needs of carers into account' does not impose any obligation to provide services. The Act did not bring any additional funding for supporting carers, although limited new resources were pledged in *A National Strategy for Carers* (Department of Health 1999c).

The Carers and Disabled Children Act (2000) extends the rights of carers but does not repeal the 1995 Act. It removes the connection between an assessment of need of a 'cared for' person under Section 47 of NHS and Community Care Act and the assessment of a carer's needs. It gives carers a right to an assessment even if the 'cared for' person has refused a community care assessment. However, the 'cared for' person must be someone for whom the local authority may provide or arrange for provision of services. The term 'carer', as in the previous legislation, refers to someone who provides 'substantial and regular' care. Guidance states that in determining the meaning of 'substantial and regular', the whole caring situation should be considered, not simply the number of hours per week someone is involved in caring (Department of Health 2001f). The local authority has a duty, on request by the carer, to assess the carer's needs but there is only a power, not a duty, to provide services to meet any needs revealed by the assessment. Following the assessment of the carer's needs, the local authority decides: whether the carer has needs in relation to the care s/he is providing; whether the local authority could meet those needs; and if so, whether services should be provided. These 'services' are described under Section 2(2) of the Act as: 'any services which the local authority sees fit to provide and will in the local authority's view help the carer care for the person cared for'. This leaves the local authority with potentially wide discretion about the services that could be provided (Brammer 2003). Examples of services provided under this section include taxi fares for a carer to attend a carers' support group, funding for a carer to attend a leisure/exercise class, funding of a holiday for a carer and payment for driving lessons (Macgregor and Hill 2003). Carers receive any such services that the local authority decides should be provided independently of the 'cared for' person. However, the 'cared for' person must agree to any services that are delivered directly to her or him. Local authorities also have powers to issue vouchers to enable carers to have respite from caring and carers can receive a direct payment in lieu of services assessed as necessary to support them. As the Act distinguishes between services provided to support carers and those for the 'cared for' person, it provides for carers to be charged in their own right for services they receive. However, the local authority should take account of costs that the carer bears in relation to caring before deciding what to charge.

Whereas assessment under the 1995 and 2000 Acts depends upon a request for assessment by the carer, Section 1 of the Carers (Equal Opportunities) Act

(2004) imposes a duty on local authorities to inform carers of their right to an assessment. This means that there is now a duty to be proactive in informing carers of their right to an assessment, not merely to be reactive in responding to requests for assessment (Department of Health 2005d). Section 2 of the Act also imposes a duty on local authorities to take into account a carer's wishes in relation to outside interests, including work, study, and leisure, when undertaking a carer's assessment. Section 3 places a duty on local authorities to promote better joint working with health and other agencies in relation to the provision of services relevant to carers. The Social Care Institute for Excellence has produced an online practice guide, *Implementing the Carers (Equal Opportunities) Act (2004)* (Social Care Institute for Excellence 2005). The guide identifies steps that need to be taken at a strategic level within local authorities to implement the Act. These include involving carers in all aspects of local arrangements, producing clear eligibility criteria for service entitlement, developing a multi-agency strategy and arranging jointly commissioned and funded projects.

ACTIVITY 6.4: THE IMPACT OF CARERS' LEGISLATION

First, read these research findings:

> Between May and September 2002, Carers UK carried out a postal survey with carers to find out about the role carers' assessments had played in identifying and addressing carers' needs. 1,695 responses to the questionnaire were received. In addition, telephone interviews were carried out with 30 respondents. 35 per cent of the carers who responded to the postal survey were aged 65 or over and 53 per cent of the people 'cared for' were categorised as older people. Survey respondents were located at the 'heavy end' of caring. 95 per cent were providing care of more than 20 hours per week and 46 per cent of respondents had been caring for more than 10 years. Despite this, only 32 per cent of respondents had received a carer's assessment. Of these, only 37 per cent had received any increase in services following the assessment. Two-thirds of respondents reported that they did not receive all of the help they needed. The barriers included:
>
> * the service they wanted was not available locally (39 per cent);
> * they were put off from receiving services by their poor quality (32 per cent);
> * they were put off from receiving services by charging policies (29 per cent);
> * they were on a waiting list to receive services (28 per cent);
> * the person they cared for did not want help provided by anyone else (13 per cent).
>
> (Macgregor and Hill 2003)

Why do you think only 32 per cent of carers in the study had received an assessment following implementation of the Carers and Disabled Children Act (2000)?

What action could be taken to:

- increase the number of carers receiving an assessment;
- help more carers receive the services they need following assessment?

The needs of carers

When they are devising care packages, social workers may relate to carers primarily as 'resources', identifying the needs that carers will meet and the tasks they will undertake. However, Twigg and Atkin (1994) identified other models of the relationship between carers and services/professionals in addition to the 'carer as resource' model. Rather than being seen as resources for the professional to draw on, carers may be seen as 'co-workers', working in partnership with professionals in planning and delivering appropriate support for an older person. Clearly this model depends on trust, openness and some equalising of power between carers and professionals. It is important to acknowledge the potential of the 'co-worker' model to disempower the older person and the need for the older person to be included as far as possible as part of the co-working relationships. Carers may also be 'co-clients', eligible for services in their own right as service users, as well as in their role as carer to another service user. This may be the case for some older carers, discussed in the following section. The final type of carer/worker relationship identified by Twigg and Atkin is that of 'superseded carer', where the aim is to change or replace the carer's role, for example for the sake of the carer's health or that of the older person, perhaps in a situation of abuse. These four models may be useful as tools to help social workers to reflect on how they perceive and respond to carers, though a mix of models is likely to apply in practice. The appropriate model(s) in any situation will need to be determined by how the carer perceives and aspires to carry out their role, allied with how this meshes with the wishes of the older person. There may, of course, be a conflict of interest, for example, if the older person and professional want the carer to be a 'resource' but the carer wants to be 'superseded'. (The potentially differing needs and wishes of carers and older people will be considered further in Chapter 7.)

There are a number of publications concerned with the needs of carers in general terms (for example, Nolan *et al.* 1996; Heron 1998; Stalker 2003) and some that are specifically concerned with the needs of carers of older people (Qureshi and Walker 1989; Phillips *et al.* 2002; Yeandle and Buckner 2005). It is vital that every caring situation is treated as unique and that full consideration is given in every case to the individual needs and preferences of those involved in caring, the needs and preferences of the older person, and the nature and dynamics of the caring relationship. However, there are some key general messages emanating from the above and other literature on caring that provide a useful backcloth to social workers' engagement with carers. First, support provided informally for an older person may be seen as an intrinsic part of a close relationship, rather than in terms of a role as a 'carer'. This means that people providing informal support may be unaware of their entitlements as 'carers' and the services available to them and may need information and advice. Second, there are a number of services that research identifies as particularly valued by carers. These include: services that provide respite from caring; help with practical tasks, such as cleaning, laundry and shopping; access to emergency care; welfare benefits advice; access to health services to address carers' own health needs; and workplace support to enable carers to continue in employment, such as flexible working practices and special leave provisions. Third, emotional and psychological support emerges as of paramount importance to carers. They need to feel that they are valued and that they have access to someone who cares and is prepared to listen. Fourth, carers want a choice about whether to provide care 'for' someone (as opposed to caring 'about' them) and choice about the level and nature of the support they provide.

Older carers

Earlier work on the needs of carers emphasised gender inequalities in caring and the impact of community care policy on the 'burden' of caring borne by women (Finch and Groves 1980; Graham 1983). Subsequent critiques have developed a more sophisticated understanding, highlighting the significance of other social divisions, such as disability (Morris 1997) and ethnicity (Gunaratnam 1997), for 'caring' and how this is experienced. Another social division impacting on caring is that of age itself. Alarmist pronouncements on the future drain on economic and social resources that will be posed by the growing number of older people in the population neglect the fact that many older people are themselves carers. Based on 2001 Census information, Yeandle and Buckner (2005) state that there are over 1.5 million people over the age of 60 providing unpaid care. Older women carers slightly outnumber men in the 60–74 age group, but over the age of 75 there are more male carers than women. A significant finding is that, with advancing age, there is a corresponding increase in the amount of care that carers give. Two-thirds of men and a half of women carers aged 60–64 provide care for up to 20 hours a week. However, for carers over the age of 85, over half of men and almost half of women provide 50 or more hours of care per week (ibid.).

Older carers may face multiple and overlapping inequalities. Health problems are more likely to be experienced by those providing high amounts of care and older carers tend to be most concentrated in areas of social and economic deprivation. Moreover, evidence suggests that substantial numbers of older carers are missing out on Pension Credit and Carer's Addition (Carers UK 2005).[1] Carers from Black and minority ethnic communities appear more likely to experience financial hardship (ibid.). Research by Merrell et al. with Bangladeshi carers (not specifically on older carers) in South Wales found that information about support services was often poor and that even where carers were aware of available services, access may be prevented by feelings that services are insensitive to cultural and religious needs. Older women carers may be particularly affected by language barriers and this study suggests that there is rarely access to professional interpreting services (Merrell et al. 2006).

Yeandle and Buckner (2005) identify the types of support required by older carers. Many of these echo the findings on carers' needs more generally. Older carers want: comprehensive information about caring; flexible services that enable them to remain in employment; flexible employment policies and practices; specific advice regarding major financial decisions, such as early retirement; effective age discrimination legislation; an adequate income; services that help to prevent deterioration in health; opportunities and support to participate in educational and leisure activities; recognition from professionals of the care they provide and their expertise as carers; a valued status; and specifically targeted support for carers in Black and minority ethnic communities (ibid.).

There are a number of implications for the role of social workers that emerge from these research messages. Social workers can make a difference by simply listening to carers and valuing what they do. They can offer emotional support and validation of the carer's role and contribution, recognising the expertise of the carer and harnessing this in the planning and monitoring of support arrangements (Nolan *et al.* 1996). They also need to act as a resource bank, linking carers to sources of information, advice and support that are pertinent to their specific needs. Carers need to be made aware of and encouraged to utilise services that will support their own health and well-being. In line with the Carers (Equal Opportunities) Act 2005, this includes educational, leisure and employment opportunities. Often carer support services will be provided by local charitable carers' organisations that may receive funding from local authorities. National charitable organisations, such as Carers UK and the Princess Royal Trust for Carers, may also be valuable sources of information and support for carers.

ACTIVITY 6.5: ENGAGING WITH CARERS' NEEDS

Joe Hunt is aged 82. He was born in Jamaica. His mother died in childbirth and he was never given any information about his father. He was brought up by his grandmother and an aunt. After his grandmother died in the early 1950s, Joe came to England and settled in London. He had a seven-year relationship with a white British woman and they had a daughter, Sonia, but after the relationship broke up Joe moved away from London and lost contact with Sonia. Joe had trouble finding long-term employment and developed an alcohol problem. He lived an itinerant life style and spent some years sleeping rough. In his early 70s, following a series of hospital admissions for emphysema, he was housed in a one-bedroom flat. Five years ago, his daughter, Sonia traced him and made contact with him. Her mother had recently died and she was keen to resume a relationship with her father as he was her only known living relative. She began to visit Joe regularly. Two years ago, Joe's health deteriorated following a stroke. He is now partially paralysed on the right side of his body and can only walk short distances using a walking aid. He also has speech impairment. Sonia insisted on Joe moving in with her and her partner. They have no children and Sonia, who is a trained nurse, was happy to give up her part-time job to look after Joe. The living room is being used as ground floor bedroom for him and they have converted the garage into a bathroom. Over the last six months, Joe's behaviour has become increasingly difficult to manage. He insists on Sonia buying him alcohol and on some days he drinks heavily. This can lead to additional mobility problems and, at times, continence problems. He has days when he is tearful and talks constantly of wanting to go 'home'; on other days he can be aggressive, throwing things at Sonia, pinching her when she is helping him dress or swearing at her. Sonia is determined to continue to look after her father but her partner is saying that he will no longer put up with the disruption Joe is causing in the household or the stress that his behaviour is causing to Sonia.

- Make a list of the possible needs Sonia may experience in this situation.
- What support services could you suggest that might be helpful to her? (You may want to get ideas by finding out about services provided for carers in your locality or by looking on websites of national carers' organisations, like Carers UK and Princess Royal Trust for Carers.)
- How would you make sure that Joe's needs and wishes are also considered?

This chapter has focused on the interface between social work and other individuals and organisations that may be involved in supporting older people. It has discussed general issues regarding partnership working and looked at specific issues concerning health services, housing support services, voluntary sector agencies and carers. As noted in Chapter 4, social workers are likely to be involved in situations where older people have complex needs and where many agencies and individuals are involved. These situations will feature different, and perhaps conflicting, views about the nature of difficulties and what should be done about them. Drawing on skills discussed in the previous chapter, social workers may be particularly well-equipped for the role of facilitating partnership working between the parties involved. They can use their skills in eliciting different viewpoints, recognising and valuing each person's contribution and negotiating a pathway through complex, and perhaps conflict-ridden, networks of relationships and resources. They can play a lead role in formulating a 'whole person' response that retains the older person at the centre of planning services and delivering support. In inter-professional contexts, social workers can pose constructive challenges to negative attitudes and poor practice and seek to educate by example. The next chapter is concerned with further dimensions of social work's complexity: value constraints, dilemmas and conflicts that may arise in practice.

KEY POINTS

☐   There is a continuum of different approaches to partnership working.

☐   Partnership is an increasingly significant aspect of policy. It faces a number of barriers to its implementation but there are principles that can form the basis for effective partnership, given the right conditions.

☐   The separation of 'health' from 'social' care in policy and practice has obstructed the delivery of coherent and holistic support for older people.

☐   Housing issues are a legitimate focus for social work's attention. In addition to the importance of physical standards of housing for older people, 'home' has a particular significance for positive emotional well-being.

☐   Voluntary sector agencies often play a significant and central role in providing support services to older people.

☐   It is only in recent years that 'carers' have been identified as an official category in policy, although the bulk of caring has always been undertaken by them. Their needs should be considered when social workers are working with older people.

KEY READING

Glasby, J. and Littlechild, R. (2004) *The Health and Social Care Divide: The Experiences of Older People*, Bristol: The Policy Press.

Heywood, F., Oldman, C. and Means, R. (2002) *Housing and Home in Later Life*, Buckingham: Open University Press.

Yeandle, S. and Buckner, L. (2005) *Older Carers in the UK*, London: Carers UK/Sheffield Hallam University.

CHAPTER 7

VALUES-BASED PRACTICE

OBJECTIVES

By the end of this chapter you should have an understanding of:

- values and value conflicts in social work with older people;

- the importance of working in partnership with older people and limitations encountered in practice;

- dilemmas in dealing with issues of risk and protection;

- the need to work with different and conflicting perspectives;

- the components of high quality care and support for older people.

Social work is complex, contested and contradictory (Thompson 2005), increasingly so, in recent years, because of what has been termed its 'institutional destabilisation' (McDonald 2006: 32–8). As we have seen in earlier chapters, the assumption underpinning the post-war Welfare State – of collective responsibility for citizens – has been increasingly challenged and largely discredited in mainstream politics (see, especially, Chapter 2). As a consequence, social work is caught up in, and destabilised by, a sometimes bewildering barrage of ideas about policies and organisational forms and what they mean for working with older people. Earlier in the book, it became clear that there is an uncomfortable fit between political injunctions to social workers to 'empower' people to become self-determining citizens, whilst they are required to implement policies that maintain forms of social injustice and restrict the use of resources to improve people's lives (see, especially, Chapters 3 and 4). This more recent contradiction in the practice of social work co-exists with a much older tension; social workers are exhorted to be 'person-centred' (or 'client-centred', as it would have been put in the past) but, as well as focusing on the older person, they have to take account of the interests and potentially conflicting needs of carers, other members of informal networks, other professionals and agencies, their employing organisations, social work's professional values and codes and the interests of 'society' (Thompson 2005). This recent contradiction and older tension result in value dilemmas for social workers, as different responsibilities and concerns come into conflict.

Banks (2001) outlines different sources of value conflict for social workers. The conflict may be between two competing social work values, for example, self-determination and protection from harm. It may involve competing interests between different individuals in a situation; for example, promoting the autonomy of one individual may infringe the needs and interests of another. Conflict may arise when the rights and freedom of one individual are in opposition with the 'greater good of society as a whole'; for example, an older person may choose to live with very low standards of cleanliness within their home but this may have environmental health consequences for those living in adjacent properties. The conflict may be between personal values and professional social work values; for example, a particular social worker might have a personal value that sons and daughters should look after their parents in later life, but social work values include being non-judgemental and respecting the wishes and values of others. The conflict may entail a clash between personal and/or professional values and organisational values and practices; for example, personal and professional values may support the position that society should promote the well-being of the older population but this may be undermined by policies and practices related to the application of stringent eligibility criteria (see Chapters 3 and 4). In their practice, social workers have to find ways of negotiating and managing these conflicts and dilemmas. Thus Dominelli refers to the 'negotiated realities' of social work practice:

> social workers are constantly negotiating within a context of ambiguity and uncertainty, involving the rationing of resources in the face of need, not being available when vulnerable clients require their services most, and having to adhere to policies that may be at odds with their own personal beliefs.
>
> (Dominelli 2002: 182)

Many of the 'negotiated realities' involved in social work with older people have been touched on in earlier chapters. This chapter aims to provide more in-depth discussion of practice issues that involve particular value complexities or conflicts for social workers. There are inevitably no 'right answers' to present. However, as argued in Chapter 1, an important tool for social workers working in complex, changing and conflict-ridden situations is that of critical reflection and reflexivity. The discussion in this chapter aims to facilitate processes of critical reflection on some of the key areas of value tension and conflict in social work with older people.

WORKING IN PARTNERSHIP WITH OLDER PEOPLE

The book began with a discussion of service user involvement and the need to base practice on engagement with the direct experiences and perspectives of older people. This has been a central theme throughout the book and it is appropriate that it is also a key focus of this final chapter. As mentioned in Chapter 1, the requirement to involve service users derives from legislation and policy, professional responsibilities and values and from the demands and actions of service users themselves (Braye 2000). In terms of policy mandates, a central thrust within current policy, as discussed in Chapter 2, is on 'active ageing', supporting and enabling older people to play an active role in their own self-care, in service planning and provision and as citizens in their local communities. For example, the national ageing strategy, *Opportunity Age* (see Chapter 2), states: 'Our vision is of a society where later life is as active and fulfilling as the earlier years, with older people participating in their families and communities' (Department for Work and Pensions 2005: para. 23). The document goes on to say, 'The primary responsibility for keeping active and participating in communities lies with older people themselves. Central government and local authorities need to work with them to remove the barriers which prevent them from contributing to their full potential' (ibid.: para. 24).

Alongside this policy direction, professional drivers for service user involvement and working in partnership can be found in traditional social work values such as self-determination, which involve supporting individuals to make their own choices and decisions and to act as far as possible on their own behalf (Banks 2001). More 'radical' social work values recognise the limits to self-determination that may be imposed by social and economic conditions. This brings the additional obligation for social workers to work to challenge and address barriers to older people's participation (Braye and Preston-Shoot 1995; Dominelli 2002). The *Code of Practice for Social Care Workers* (General Social Care Council 2002) states that a worker's responsibilities include 'supporting service users' rights to control their lives and make informed choices about the services they receive' (para. 1.3) and 'promoting the independence of service users and assisting them to understand and exercise their rights' (para. 3.1). In addition, the *National Occupational Standards for Social Workers: Values and Ethics Performance Criteria* state that social workers must involve and empower individuals, families, carers, groups and communities in decisions that affect them (Training Organisation for the Personal Social Services 2002). Service users themselves have been increasingly vocal in asserting their right to equality and inclusion. This encompasses demands for involvement as consumers of services and also challenges to power structures that shape their experience of 'personal' problems (Braye 2000; Turner, M. and Beresford 2005).

Whilst there is this range of strong drivers to involve service users, reflective practitioners need to adopt a critical and questioning approach towards notions of 'involvement', 'partnership' and 'empowerment' in their practice. Mandates to 'involve' older people are not necessarily the same as 'working in partnership', which implies some rebalancing of power in the relationship between the 'partners'. Involving an older person at a very basic level might mean meeting with them following a discharge planning meeting to tell them what had been discussed and decided; working in partnership might involve discussing fully with them before the meeting the nature, process and purpose of the meeting, discussing and rehearsing their contribution, helping them to clarify and express their views and preferences and ensuring that full account is taken of these in the decision-making. As with Hudson *et al.*'s (1998) continuum of collaboration (see Chapter 6), there is a continuum of involvement, from a very minimal level of giving information to service users to a maximum level where service users are in control of decisions and resources. Heywood *et al.* (2002: 139 – based on work by D'Aboville 1994), present these different 'levels' of involving older people as follows:

- providing information to help older people understand how to access services;
- consulting older people individually to enable them to identify their own needs and their preferred options for meeting them;
- consulting older people in groups about their service requirements;
- involving older people in developing services, for example in writing service specifications or deciding on quality standards;
- delegating control to older people for decision-making or service provision.

However, while we have talked about partnership implying some degree of equality in the distribution of power, it has to be remembered that social workers, as (usually) agents of the state, are invested with massive amounts of power compared with users of social work services, who are likely to be drawn from oppressed and marginalised social groups. In this sense, 'partnership working' with service users can never be based on an equal distribution of power (Beckett and Maynard 2005). Similarly, there are significant constraints on 'patient empowerment', in terms of the exercise of power and control by people in receipt of health care (Descombes 2004), perhaps particularly when they are older. However, whilst recognising its limits, social workers can nevertheless endeavour to maximise partnership in their work with older people (see Chapter 5, Activity 5.1).

As well as different levels of involvement, ranging from information giving to service user control, there are also different levels or tiers of change at which involvement may be directed. The focus of older people's involvement may be:

- *Individual*: working with the social worker in planning and managing their own care services.
- *Service*: working with other older people, and perhaps other service users, in planning, delivering and evaluating service provision more generally. This will often be at a local level, for example, through local Older People's Partnership Boards. Partnerships for Older People Projects (see Chapter 2) provide another example of the involvement of older people in local service development.
- *Institutional*: the involvement of older people in representation and campaigning on issues affecting older people, for example, through political parties or voluntary organisations representing older people's interests. Research has demonstrated that older people face barriers to involvement in traditional political activity and that they are disillusioned and disaffected with these forms of involvement (Postle *et al.* 2005). However, it indicates that older people, along with other service user 'groups', may be carving out other channels for political activity – for example, through local forums and support groups – that enable them to make their voices

heard and effect change (Harris, John 2001). Postle *et al.* argue that workers need to support older people's participation in these forms of activity in order to promote social inclusion and citizenship.

All three levels are important but we focus here on the individual level of involving older people in assessment and care planning, since this is the level most likely to concern social workers in their work with older people. As we have seen earlier in the book, in carrying out assessments and planning services (see, especially, Chapters 3 and 4) there can be a tendency for social workers to focus on arranging services that are known to be available, either from their own or other organisations. This can lead to a 'doing for' approach with older people, rather an approach reflecting the 'exchange model', discussed in Chapter 5, which treats older people as experts on their own situation and seeks to elicit and support their own coping strategies. Research with older people in Leeds and Hartlepool noted:

> formal service support is only a part, in many cases a small part, of the resources used by older people to meet . . . needs. Even the frailest older people invested significant time and energy in taking responsibility for and looking after themselves, while a substantial input of help from family, friends and neighbours on a day-to-day basis was evident for many. Older people were frustrated when formal services appeared neither to understand their contribution to, or value their expertise about, meeting their own needs.
>
> (Godfrey *et al.* 2004: 208)

The starting point for assessment and care planning is with the older person's own views about their strengths, difficulties and how these can be addressed. This will incorporate exploring with the older person their past and current strategies for managing difficulties, what they have found to be effective and ineffective, and how their own preferred coping strategies can be supported. A comprehensive, person-centred assessment will provide a solid foundation for care planning since key information about the older person's biography, preferred life style, values, preferences, and so on, will already have been obtained and a relationship of trust established. (This will require the skills discussed in Chapter 5.)

However, not all older people will be already equipped to participate actively in their own assessment and care planning. As mentioned in Chapter 5, maximising their participation in decision-making may require more than simply offering opportunities for involvement. Research by Baldock and Ungerson (1994) with people recovering from strokes found that their degree of participation in the 'care market' was influenced by their 'habits of the heart', that is, particular values and attitudes about their role in relation to the state and the market. Those whose attitudes featured 'clientelism' tended to adopt passive and dependent roles. As discussed in Chapter 1, older people may have internalised ageist attitudes and may have low expectations about the level of involvement possible (Minichiello *et al.* 2000). Working in a meaningful partnership may involve challenging and changing particular discourses in order to increase older people's understanding of systems and processes and develop the skills they need to participate meaningfully in them.

Consumerist notions of service user 'involvement', and some current policy constructions of 'independence' and 'enablement', are predicated on the ability and willingness of service users to express preferences, exercise choice and be actively engaged in taking action on their own behalf (Harris, John 2003: ch. 7). However, for many older people in poor states of physical and mental health and unfavourable social and economic conditions these assumptions are erroneous:

> often social workers' decisions about how best to assess and respond to need are taken at a time when an older person's capacity to engage in decision making is compromised by shattering events such as bereavement, moving house, serious illness and loss of mobility. At such times, it is difficult to see how the rational exercise of choice and control is viable or desirable ... Assumptions about older people's readiness to assume a position in a process of rational decision making can be counterproductive. In such circumstances, care is required, which acknowledges the effect of shattering events and allows the older person time to recover.
>
> (Lloyd 2006a: 1180)

The resourcefulness of older people and sense of responsibility for their own situations is not inconsistent with them being at times unable to take an active role in the assessment and care planning process. As noted in Chapter 5, Richards's (2000) study found that during assessment some older people were 'overwhelmed' by their situations and needed the social worker to take more of a leadership role. Working in partnership with older people entails exploring with them not only what *services* will be helpful to them but also what *processes*. This should be reviewed over time. Older people in a state of crisis or beset by practical difficulties may welcome the social worker taking charge but then may gradually be able to assume more responsibility as their situation becomes easier. Other older people, perhaps following a lifetime of hardship and/or experiences as passive 'clients' of services, may need help and encouragement to contribute to decision-making. A key point is that the social worker should not begin with a fixed view about how and at what level an older person 'should' be involved. A focus on outcomes will help here. If the desired outcome is the enhancement of older people's well-being, what this means and how it is achieved has to be negotiated with them on their own terms. Without this, notions of 'empowerment' and 'partnership' are professionally defined and controlled, reinforcing, rather than challenging, oppression and marginalisation.

Referring back to the professional mandates for service user involvement, effective partnership with older people, at whatever level, has to be founded on central social work values. Godfrey *et al.*'s (2004) research with older people, referred to earlier in this chapter, highlighted the importance attached by older people to being treated with dignity and respect. This is echoed in the research on older people's positive experiences of schemes run by Help the Aged (see Chapter 6); it was particular qualities of the services that were valued and the personal meanings that these conveyed to the older person:

> First among the personal meanings was a strong sense of being valued as an individual and a person. Common themes that emerged from the

data included: not being patronised, being respected as an older person in ways not always present in other organisations, and being treated as an individual. Their involvement enhanced a sense of mutuality, ownership and commitment.

(Reed *et al.* 2004: 179)

Within a broad framework of values such as respect, dignity and citizenship, social workers need to attend to specific manifestations of inequality. For example, particular attention needs to be given to addressing issues of powerlessness in work with people with dementia (see Chapter 5). Research with older women with dementia noted their experiences of powerlessness in relation to their gender, age and social class, as well as their cognitive impairment (Proctor 2001). They felt that they had not been involved in key decisions about the services they received. The researcher points out that although this may be related to loss of memory about communications that had taken place, the outcomes are, nevertheless, experiences of marginalisation and powerlessness. This demands specific strategies, such as providing information in a way that can be more easily understood and remembered, and devoting plenty of time to listening to concerns and validating emotions, rather than using dementia as a reason for not involving people.

Similarly, Bigby discusses the discrimination often faced by older people with learning disabilities (see Chapter 5), for example, the low expectations held by service providers and others, and the lack of support and options made available. The value base of social work accords social workers particular responsibilities for identifying and challenging discriminatory attitudes and practices. One way of exercising these responsibilities is by countering negative stereotypes in processes of assessment and care planning and ensuring that older people with learning disabilities are recognised as individuals of worth and significance (Bigby 2004: 54).

ACTIVITY 7.1: PROMOTING INVOLVEMENT

Fryderyk Gorski is an 87-year-old white Polish man. When he was in his 50s, both of his legs were amputated below the knee following an industrial accident. He has used a wheelchair since this time. He has become frailer with age and now needs considerable help transferring from the wheelchair. He has shown increasing signs of confusion over the last couple of years and he becomes easily agitated and disorientated. Although he normally reads and speaks English well, he reverts to Polish at times of stress. His daughter, Julia, lives with him and meets most of his support needs, with some help from day care provision and a carer respite service. However, Julia has suffered a stroke and been admitted to hospital. It is not yet known how seriously Julia has been affected and whether or when she will be able to return home. You are asked to carry out an urgent review of Fryderyk's needs with a view to drawing up a new care plan in the light of the disruption in the informal care arrangements.

- In what ways might Fryderyk exercise power/lack power in this situation?
- In what ways do you as the social worker exercise power/lack power in this situation?

- How would you try to promote Fryderyk's involvement in the process of reassessing his needs and devising a new care plan?

RISK AND PROTECTION

We do not focus specifically on safeguarding vulnerable adults since this is the subject of another book in this series (Parker and Penhale 2007). Rather, we discuss issues of risk and protection as they relate to social work with older people more generally. As with service user involvement, identifying and responding to risk can place social workers in the midst of conflicting values and responsibilities. The *Code of Practice for Social Care Workers* (General Social Care Council 2002) states that workers must 'promote the independence of service users while protecting them as far as possible from danger or harm' (para. 3) and 'respect the rights of service users while seeking to ensure that their behaviour does not harm themselves or other people' (para. 4). These dual responsibilities – on the one hand, to promote independence and rights and on the other hand to protect people (both service users and others) from harm – relate to the points made at the beginning of the chapter. Social work is concerned with the welfare of individuals as well as the 'wider good of society', endowed with both 'care' and 'control' functions. Policy has indicated a commitment to shifting health and social care services away from paternalism and more in the direction of promoting rights. In line with its emphasis on increasing independence and choice, the White Paper, *Our Health, Our Care, Our Say* (Department of Health 2006b) has stated its intention of developing a national approach to the management of risk that would put individuals at the centre of the decision-making process. The role of practitioners would be to support individuals in making and carrying out their own decisions.

Supporting individuals to make their own choices and decisions accords with the traditional social work value of self-determination, mentioned at the beginning of the chapter. However, as Preston-Shoot (2002) argues, self-determination as a guiding principle on its own is problematic for a number of reasons. First, everyone's choices are limited by the extent to which they impact on other people's choices: 'one person's autonomy might compromise another person's self-determination' (ibid.: 196). Second, self-determination implies choice but choice is only a relevant concept when there are different options available. For example, an older person's refusal of the offer of assistance may be taken at face value as the exercise of self-determination. However, if the older person does not realise that there are viable sources of help available, or her/his response is influenced by intimidation from someone else, then this cannot be seen as self-determination. Third, while anyone may make 'bad' or irrational choices, sometimes this may be the result of not having access to the necessary information to make a reasoned decision. Finally, people may need help to consider longer-term outcomes, since a 'self-determining' decision may be based on a restricted and short-term view. These arguments indicate that social workers need to be critical in their approach to self-determination. In particular, leaving individuals to be 'self-determining' should not be an excuse for inaction. Preston-Shoot distinguishes between:

- *negative freedom*: leaving individuals to do as they choose when, in reality, there are constraints on their choice;

- *positive freedom*: intervening in ways that enable individuals to exercise greater self-determination. This would include working to remove barriers to their exercise of choice, for example, by providing information, offering alternative perspectives or making available other options.

A key concept at the intersection between individual rights and protection is that of risk. Identifying and managing risk has gained an increased profile in social work practice in recent years. Contributory factors include the drive for improved 'evidence' and 'certainty' as the basis of practice and the culture of 'blame' that leads to practitioners 'covering their backs', rather than taking risks for which they will be held accountable (Parton 1996). The significance of risk in contemporary social work practice can also be related to wider political and policy developments (see Chapter 2). As we noted at the beginning of this chapter, whereas the 'welfare state' was premised on the provision of universal services to meet collective need, much of this responsibility has now devolved to individual citizens. Older people are encouraged to age 'well' and 'successfully' by working for as long as possible, volunteering, being responsible members of their communities and careful guardians of their own health and well-being. The state has a residual role, targeting intervention at particular individuals who have failed to discharge effectively their personal responsibility for managing risk (Kemshall 2002). Thus, in adult services, defining 'eligible needs' in terms of those needs that represent critical or substantial risks to independence (see Chapter 3) means that in practice much assessment work with older people, at least in the statutory sector, is centrally concerned with risk. However, a social model of disability would question discourses that construct risk as a personal issue and would highlight the risks that result from society's failure to address older people's needs (Stevenson 1999). One example is the way that fear of crime and feelings of threat and insecurity can lead to older people withdrawing into their homes (Reed *et al.* 2004). This can inhibit access to social activities and relationships and make meeting more basic needs, such as shopping for food, problematic. This is likely to have a detrimental effect on quality of life more generally, as well as increasing the risk of isolation and depression (Godfrey and Denby 2004).

As well as its individual focus, another facet of risk that can be detrimental to older people's well-being is its overwhelmingly negative connotations as far as older people are concerned. Age and gender stereotypes lead to inconsistencies in social attitudes (Orme 2001); society is prepared to condone or even extol risk-taking when it involves young men, but finds it hard to accept risk-taking by older women (Braye and Preston-Shoot 1995). The construction of older people, and especially older women, as vulnerable, dependent and powerless leads to physical risk being seen as something to be avoided at all costs. However, this can create social and psychological risks for older people. Ballinger and Payne examined ways in which risk was managed in a day care setting for older people. They found that staff were primarily concerned with physical risks, such as the possibility of older people having falls, while the older people themselves were concerned with the risks to their personal and social identities, for example increased dependence and loss of dignity. Measures introduced by staff to reduce physical risk could increase the social and psychological risks:

the service response to the signs of physical risk in the day hospital resulted in an environment in which people were dissuaded from independent activity

. . . The focus on physical activity and risk, and the staff's role in limiting 'inappropriate' patient behaviour, reinforced passivity among the service users, and also meant that the potential for psychosocial interventions, for example, to promote self-esteem or confidence, was not recognised and under-utilised.

(Ballinger and Payne 2002: 319)

Older people's internalisation of ageist views may contribute to feelings of passivity and dependency and it is important that professionals are aware of their own power to influence service user decision-making about risk. A report into risk-taking and older people (Wynne-Harley 1991) highlighted older people's low sense of self-worth and their tendency to allow others to make decisions for them. Older people may reduce or avoid risk in order to allay the concerns of their families, even if this runs counter to their own wishes (Tanner 2001). In such a context, older people may agree to a course of action, for example, on the basis that 'the doctor knows best' or 'I don't want to worry my family'. The social work role may entail encouraging older people to examine their own thoughts and feelings and assisting them to reach a decision that is compatible with these, rather than following unquestioningly the recommendations of others. This stance has received official support in a report, *Making Choices: Taking Risks* (Commission for Social Care Inspection 2006b). It points out that older people have had considerable experience of dealing with and adapting to risk in their lives, well before they need to call upon assistance from services. As one of the older people mentioned in the report commented: 'You should be able to make your own decisions, depending on what level you feel safe at. You spend your whole life making decisions about things – You don't want to suddenly give up that responsibility because you're older' (Commission for Social Care Inspection 2006b: 6). The report calls for robust and sensitive approaches to dealing with risk that take account of people's dignity, independence and well-being. This is easier said than done. For example, if medical representatives and carers are arguing in favour of a risk-averse option, it may be necessary to involve an advocate to help determine and represent the older person's interests. (The role of advocacy is discussed later in the chapter.)

Although risk is often seen in negative terms – the likelihood of unwanted outcomes occurring – assessing risk means weighing up potential benefits as well as potential harms or losses; taking risks involves deciding that the potential benefits of a proposed act outweigh the potential drawbacks (Carson, D. 1988: 248). As Carson argues, there are no risk-free options; an option that reduces some risks is likely to create other risks. For example, admitting older people to a care home may be seen as a 'safe' option, compared with supporting them at home. However, whilst this option may reduce some risks, such as self-neglect and loneliness, it may increase other risks, such as disorientation, depression, loss of social contacts and abuse (Pritchard 1997). The aim in any situation should not be to remove risk; indeed, 'reasonable, informed and calculated risk taking plays an important part in contributing to the quality of life for young and old; this is a matter of choice, demonstrating an individual's right to self-determination and autonomy' (Wynne-Harley 1991: 29). This point is echoed by Stevenson: 'Risk is inherent in life itself, a necessary component in the exercise of personal autonomy' (Stevenson 1999: 201). The concern, rather, has to be with identifying and managing *unacceptable* risk (ibid.). This raises a further issue: who determines what type and level of risk is unacceptable and what processes are used to do this? This highlights the close connection between risk and values (Tanner 1998). Making judgements about risk is ultimately a subjective process, since individual values influence how different outcomes are evaluated and the degree of risk that is felt to be legitimate in order to achieve a desired goal. For example, older people who place a premium value on personal privacy and autonomy may be prepared to tolerate a high level of risk to remain living in their own home.

ACTIVITY 7.2: DIFFERENT APPROACHES TO DEALING WITH RISK

Titterton (2005: 82) contrasts two models for dealing with risk, the 'safety-first' model and the 'risk-taking' model:

Safety-first model	Risk-taking model
• Physical health • Disabilities (what the person *can't* do) • Danger • Control • What the assessor thinks is right	• Physical, psychological and emotional well-being • Rights and responsibilities • Abilities and disabilities (what the person *can* achieve) • Choices and opportunities • Involvement of individual and family/carers

Refer back to Activity 3.1 at the start of Chapter 3. Consider these two models in relation to the situation of Mr A. Which dimensions of these models are evident in the two different scenarios presented?

Given that social workers are inevitably involved in decisions concerned with risk, it is important to have a comprehensive and coherent framework for assessing and managing risk. This will improve the quality of assessments and decision-making and also enable practitioners to give a clear account of their actions to others. Brearley's (1982) framework is often used as the basis for models of risk assessment. Brearley makes clear that he does not see his framework as a way of removing the uncertainty in decision-making, but as a way of structuring the knowledge, ideas and values involved in the process. Coherent and detailed risk assessment will clarify values issues, but not remove them. Brearley sees risk analysis as involving two key tasks:

- *estimation* of risk, that is, consideration of probability; how likely is it that a particular outcome will occur?
- *evaluation* of risk, that is, the value attached to the outcome; how serious are the consequences deemed to be?

Furthermore, he argues that risk assessment must take account of:

- *hazards* – the factors that increase the possibility of a negative outcome; a greater number of hazards will increase the likelihood of danger;
- *strengths* – the factors that reduce the likelihood of a negative outcome.

Brearley highlights the importance of distinguishing hazards (that is, the factors likely to increase risk) from dangers (that is, the feared outcomes themselves). For example, an older person may be said to be 'at risk of falling'. This indicates something about the feared outcome (a fall), though not its potential consequences, but nothing about the factors that will increase or reduce the likelihood of it occurring. Yet it is through enhancing strengths and reducing hazards that risks can be managed. For example, in relation to someone 'at risk of falling', greater clarity and precision would result from starting to analyse risk in the following way:

- The *dangers*: broken limbs; threats to physical health through lying unattended and being unable to summon help; death.
- The *hazards*: steep stairs; poor mobility; poor eyesight; loose rugs.
- The *strengths*: a stair rail; an alarm call in each room; a neighbour who calls in twice a day.

Each danger can be assessed in terms of the likelihood of it occurring (estimation) and, if it does happen, the likely severity of the consequences (evaluation). The assessment would take account of both the hazards and strengths present in the situation. This sort of detailed risk assessment would help in the formulation of a plan to manage the risks, which is likely to involve a combination of interventions to decrease the hazards, on the one hand, and increase the strengths, on the other. (A more detailed example of a risk assessment completed according to Brearley's model is given in Box 7.1, page 196.)

Sheppard (1990) demonstrates the conceptual clarity arising from the distinction between *estimation* and *evaluation* of risks (see Figure 7.1). In Figure 7.1, quadrant A represents a high risk of serious danger. For example, someone with severe dementia who smokes heavily and who has already had two house fires caused by lighted cigarettes might fall into this category. (This does not necessarily imply, however, that the risk cannot be managed within the home environment.)

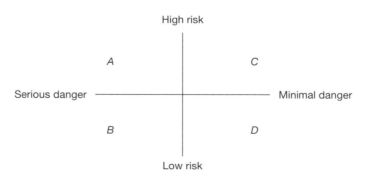

FIGURE 7.1 Assessing the seriousness and likelihood of risk

Quadrant D represents a low risk of minimal danger; for example, an older person who is no longer able to go out on her own to do her shopping but who has family nearby who are prepared to take her shopping might fit this category. However, this example highlights that it is not possible to evaluate the seriousness of risks without understanding how the potential consequences are perceived by the person concerned. It is also necessary to consider within the risk evaluation the consequences for other people in the caring network. In this example, the risks may be higher than first appears if doing shopping independently of her family is crucially important to the older person's sense of identity and well-being. Equally, the risks may be higher if helping with the shopping would adversely affect wider family members or their relationship with the older person.

In quadrant B there is a low risk of serious danger. For example, an older person may have inadvertently caused a house fire some years ago through a moment of carelessness but there could be few current factors indicating continued risk. However, some events or situations have a powerful influence because of the potential level of danger they represent. These situations may lead professionals to avoid risks because the potential consequences are very serious, even though the actual likelihood of the feared outcome occurring is quite low.

In quadrant C there is a high risk of minimal danger. For example, there is evidence that women (especially) can become demoralised when they are unable to maintain their usual household standards (Clark *et al*. 1998; Tanner 2001). As already noted, individuals will differ in their evaluation of the seriousness of a particular outcome and individual priorities will not always accord with those of organisations. Thus, household cleaning is generally regarded as an area of 'low risk' in terms of eligibility criteria, even though it has been found to be highly significant to older people's sense of well-being (Clark *et al*. 1998; Tanner 2001). Therefore, the estimation and evaluation of risk has to be undertaken with a full understanding of the biography, current circumstances, values and attitudes of the individuals concerned, along with an understanding of the meaning and significance of the risk in the context of their daily lives. An example from one of our research studies concerns Harriet Manders (pseudonym), who was mentioned in Chapter 3. She had asked for help from her local authority with cleaning; in particular, she had always kept her kitchen spotless and she was concerned that she could no longer mop the kitchen floor. The social worker who assessed her needs told her that she was not eligible for help as 'no one ever died of a dirty floor'. Harriet Manders made some important points about this: her balance was very poor and she could well die from the dirty floor if she slipped and fell badly on some spilt food or grease; she could die or seriously injure herself if she struggled to clean the floor herself (as she was likely to do in the event of not receiving help); the emotional and psychological consequences of not being able to maintain her usual standards could lead to her becoming depressed and 'giving up'.

A basic principle in managing risk is to look for the least disruptive change that will appropriately manage the risk (Brearley 1982). Titterton (2005) concurs with the point made earlier: managing risk does not mean eliminating it. Rather, he argues that risk management should aim to increase strengths or benefits in a situation as well as minimising harms. He sees risk management as a process of compromise and negotiation in which everyone involved is consulted and these views then inform a risk plan. The risk plan should detail: who has been consulted; who is responsible for putting together and implementing the plan; the steps that will be taken to minimise possible harm; the steps to be taken to increase possible benefit; agreed timescales; the points at which intervention will occur and how this will happen; the milestones for measuring success or failure of the plan; and arrangements for record keeping.

There are a number of points that can be summarised from this review of the concept of risk and its application in practice. First, 'risk' should be interpreted broadly, including risks to social and emotional dimensions of well-being, as well as physical risks. This is acknowledged in current policy. As mentioned in Chapter 3, both the *Single Assessment Process* and *Fair Access to Care Services* state that assessment of risks to independence should include 'autonomy and freedom to make choices' and 'involvement in family and wider community life', as well as 'health and safety' and 'the ability to manage personal and other daily routines' (Department of Health 2002c: Annex E, 21). Second, a thorough assessment of risk cannot be undertaken 'objectively' by identifying various risk factors in an individual's situation. It also has to engage with the values and life history of the person concerned and with their understanding of the implications and meaning of the risks and the different options for addressing them. Third, risks cannot be assessed only in relation to the older person; risk assessment has to encompass all of those in the wider network whose lives potentially will be affected by the risks and the different ways of managing them. This issue will be discussed further later in the chapter. Fourth, related to this point, decisions about risk cannot be taken by one worker in isolation but need to incorporate the perspectives of all sources of informal and formal support in an older person's social network.

Box 7.1   EXAMPLE OF A RISK ASSESSMENT USING BREARLEY'S MODEL

Ann Lee is an 85-year-old physically fit woman with Alzheimer's disease who lives alone. The main concerns highlighted at referral are Ann's propensity to wander at all hours of the day and night and her irregular and haphazard food intake.

A risk assessment following Brearley's model might comprise the following:

- The **hazards** in this situation are the wandering and the lack of an adequate and appropriate diet.
- The **strengths** are Ann's familiarity with the local environment and ability to find her way back home; the availability of a daughter who looks in twice a day; and the fact that Ann will get herself some food, even if this is at odd times and unusual combinations of food items.
- The **dangers** are the possibility of injury through road accident, mugging or hypothermia or Ann getting lost and becoming disorientated and distressed as a result of wandering; the possibility of malnutrition or food poisoning because of poor eating habits; and her daughter's mental distress as a result of continual anxiety about her mother.

Estimation of the risks might be that mugging and a road accident are unlikely as it is a quiet rural location; Ann is unlikely to get lost as she can find her way home, also she is well known in the area; the risk of hypothermia is greater as Ann sometimes goes out at night, inadequately dressed, for several hours at a time. The risk of malnutrition is low as she does eat a reasonable amount over the course of the day and her daughter ensures there is nutritious food available; there is some risk of food poisoning as Ann sometimes eats uncooked food or leftover food from previous meals. There might be quite a high likelihood of her daughter experiencing mental distress as she is known to have a history of depression and to be very anxious about her mother's welfare.

Evaluation of the risk may be that the fairly high risk of hypothermia at certain times of the year is serious and needs to be addressed in the action plan; the risk of food poisoning is of medium severity but is unlikely to have serious consequences given safeguards that can be introduced (for example, someone taking responsibility for regularly discarding out-of-date or leftover food). The consequences of further mental distress for Ann's daughter are quite serious in terms of the distress and disruption in her own life and in relation to the implications this would have for Ann's support network.

Applying the model illustrates the way in which a coherent and comprehensive risk assessment can highlight key areas for action in a care plan and also assist in weighing up potential advantages and disadvantages of different courses of action. If Ann's GP, for example, was arguing for residential care, the risk assessment could be used to demonstrate that the risks in the situation are not insurmountable and compare favourably with risks that might ensue with a residential option (for example, depression, loss of familiar environment, routine and independence).

Practitioners need recourse to a range of knowledge to inform their risk assessments; in this example, knowledge would be needed about dementia, its likely course and management strategies; knowledge of the local environment to identify potential hazards and strengths; knowledge of research about outcomes to help assess the merits of different courses of action; and crucially, knowledge of Ann's own life history, values and attitudes.

The skills to communicate effectively with Ann and to engage her daughter in contributing her expertise to the assessment and care planning process will be necessary. Professional values are also central. A clear professional value-base will assist in attaching weight to the various possible outcomes of a situation. For example, depending on what is established about Ann's wishes, upholding the value of 'empowering an individual in decisions affecting her' (Training Organisation for the Personal Social Services 2002) may lead the social worker to supporting Ann in her wish to continuing to live at home, even though this involves possible risks.

ACTIVITY 7.3: MANAGING RISKS

Based on the assessment information given in Box 7.1, outline a care plan that would address the risks identified.

What values would be important in working with Ann and her daughter to manage the risks?

Mental capacity

Returning to the question of identifying and managing unacceptable risk, a key question in judging the acceptability of risk will be the level of the individual's mental capacity. Thus, although the White Paper, *Our Health, Our Care, Our Say* is committed to supporting individuals to make choices, this is subject to their having the capacity to make these decisions. Whether or not the individual concerned is deemed to have mental capacity will be a key factor influencing the social work response to the situation. For example, if older people are living in very poor conditions but they refuse all offers of help, there is no legal authority to intervene, provided that those concerned have the mental capacity to make the decision about how they live, they are not suffering from a mental disorder that would call for intervention under Mental Health Act (1983) and they are not infringing the rights of others. However, the restrictions on self-determination, discussed earlier, would have to be borne in mind. In such situations, the social worker would try to establish whether individuals who appear to be 'at risk', whether from self-neglect, self-harm or abuse, are making a free and informed choice to live in that particular way. The social worker should: endeavour to explore the older person's understanding of the situation; provide information about possible sources of help; explain and make available alternative ways of dealing with the situation that the older person may find acceptable; address and allay concerns the older person may have about the possible consequences of intervention (for example, anxieties about financial charges that might be levied for services or fears about being placed in residential care); and leave clear information about how contact can be renewed if help is needed at any point in the future. Ultimately, though, if someone who has mental capacity and is not suffering from a mental disorder refuses help, their right to privacy and family life under Article 8 of Human Rights Act (1998) must be respected.

For older people whose mental capacity is impaired, for example because of severe dementia, the Mental Capacity Act (2005) (fully implemented in October 2007, although the provision for an Independent Mental Capacity Advocate Service was implemented in England in April 2007) establishes a new legal framework for decision-making. Prior to this Act, provisions existed for other people to manage the property and financial affairs of someone who lacked mental capacity but there was no legal framework for decision-making in respect of more general matters. The Mental Capacity Act (2005) covers decision-making in relation to welfare, health and financial affairs. It is relevant to decisions about day-to-day matters, such as the support services or dental care someone needs, as well as decisions relating to major life-changes, such as a move to residential care. Section 1 of the Act sets out five key principles:

- All adults (people over 16) are presumed to have capacity to make their own decisions unless it is proved that they lack capacity.
- Individuals should be given all possible help to make their own decisions before they are treated as though they are not able to make their own decisions.
- Making what others perceive as unwise decisions does not indicate a lack of capacity to make those decisions.
- Any action taken or decision made on behalf of someone who lacks capacity under the Act must be made in their best interests.
- Any action or decision taken on behalf of someone who lacks capacity should be the option that is the least restrictive on their basic rights and freedoms.

Section 2(1) of the Act defines what is meant by lack of capacity:

> For the purposes of this Act, a person lacks capacity in relation to a matter if at the material time he [*sic*] is unable to make a decision for himself in relation to the matter because of an impairment of, or a disturbance in the functioning of, the mind or brain.

There is, therefore, no blanket judgement about someone's level of mental capacity; this is decided in relation to specific decisions. For example, someone may have the capacity to make minor decisions, such as what they want to eat, but lack the capacity for making major decisions, such as those involved in making a will. The Act applies to those whose lack of capacity is both temporary and permanent. The test of capacity is set out in Section 2(3):

> a person is unable to make a decision for himself if he is unable:

- to understand the information relevant to the decision;
- to retain that information;
- to use or weigh that information as part of the process of making the decision; or
- to communicate his decision (whether by talking, using sign language or any other means).

The person who wishes to take a particular action or decision on behalf of the person thought to lack mental capacity must reach the view about capacity. For legal matters, this is likely to be a solicitor; for medical matters, it is likely to be a doctor; for many matters of everyday living, it is likely to be a carer or family member. Professionals, such as a doctor or psychologist, may be asked to provide an opinion on someone's level of capacity in relation to the decision in question. Those making decisions on behalf of someone who lacks capacity must work through a checklist in determining what is in the person's best interests. This includes: considering all relevant circumstances; considering whether and when the person is likely to regain capacity (and, therefore, be able to resume decision-making); encouraging the person to participate as fully as possible in decision-making; taking account of the person's past and present wishes and feelings, beliefs and values in the decision-making; and taking account of the views of carers or other interested parties, as appropriate. The test of capacity becomes more stringent with the seriousness of the decision. Anyone, including both informal and professional carers, who acts in the reasonable belief that someone lacks capacity and that they are acting in the person's best interests cannot be held legally liable, unless they can be shown to be negligent.

Under the Mental Capacity Act (2005), people can plan ahead and appoint an attorney to act on their behalf, if at some point in the future they lose capacity. This is called a Lasting Power of Attorney. (A Lasting Power of Attorney is similar to the Enduring Power of Attorney, which existed previously, but it applies to health and welfare matters as well as business and financial affairs.) People can also make advance directives regarding future medical treatment (Sections 24–26). However, an advance directive can only specify treatment that someone wishes to refuse, not treatment that they would like to have. If the directive concerns refusal of life-sustaining treatment, it must be in writing, signed and formally witnessed and include a statement that the decision stands 'even if life is at risk'. Both a Lasting Power of Attorney and an advance directive can only be made if the person has mental capacity at that time. For someone in the early stages of dementia, therefore, it will be important that the potential benefits of a Lasting Power of Attorney and/or advance directive are considered while the person still has the capacity to consent to these decisions.

The Mental Capacity Act (2005) also establishes a new Court of Protection that will have overall responsibility for the Act. The Court can make decisions and orders regarding complex issues on behalf of those who lack capacity and it can appoint court deputies to take decisions regarding property and affairs, health and welfare matters. An Office of the Public Guardian supports the Court of Protection, acting as the registering body for Lasting Powers of Attorney and deputies, overseeing the work of deputies and providing information to assist the Court of Protection in its decision-making.

For people who lack capacity but do not have family, friends or others to advocate for them, an Independent Mental Capacity Advocate can be appointed where the decisions to be made involve serious medical treatment or significant changes in accommodation. The Independent Mental Capacity Advocate acts on what can be established about the person's wishes, beliefs and feelings and this may involve challenging the person appointed to make decisions on their behalf. However, the Act gives only a limited entitlement to advocacy, rather than, as campaigners urged, a more general right to advocacy for all those who lack capacity. The legal protection of people who lack capacity is further strengthened in that the neglect or ill-treatment of someone who lacks capacity becomes a criminal offence, punishable by up to five years' imprisonment.

A detailed Code of Practice is issued alongside the Mental Capacity Act (2005) and this will be periodically reviewed and updated. A Draft Code of Practice was issued for consultation in 2006, prior to implementation of the Act (Department of Constitutional Affairs 2006). The Draft Code provides guidance in relation to the Act and practice examples (see Box 7.2). (The Code itself was issued in April 2007.)

BOX 7.2   AN EXAMPLE OF THE APPLICATION OF THE MENTAL CAPACITY ACT 2005

Mr E is 87 years old and has lived alone since his wife died three years ago. He is supported by his daughter, who visits every evening, and a home carer who comes for an hour each morning to help him get up. Mr E has little short-term memory and is often confused about the time of day, so he forgets to eat. He also neglects his personal hygiene but usually agrees to have a bath when his daughter persuades him. She would like him to move to residential care, but having discussed it with him, she feels satisfied that he understands the risks involved in staying at home and is capable of deciding to take those risks. Two months later, Mr E has a fall and breaks his leg. While being treated in hospital, he becomes more confused and depressed. Although he says he wants to go home, at this point in time his daughter feels he cannot understand the consequences or weigh up the risks of doing so. She takes steps to involve relevant professionals in assessing his capacity to make this decision.

(Department of Constitutional Affairs 2006: 35)

Social workers have a duty to have regard to the provisions of the Code and their failure to do this could be used in legal proceedings. It is vital that social workers working with older people who lack mental capacity familiarise themselves with the Code's content. The Department of Health has made additional resources available to local authorities to train staff, commission an Independent Mental Capacity Advocate service and allow for the staff time involved in carrying out assessments of capacity and best interests.

An additional complexity in the law, which may be relevant to older people, concerns those who are being treated in hospital or who are placed in a care home but who lack the capacity to consent to these decisions. As was stated earlier, it may be possible for professionals and others to cajole older people with dementia into going into hospital for assessment or treatment related to their mental health or to enter a care home but the person could not be regarded as having freely given informed consent. Compulsory detention under the Mental Health Act (1983), which brings with it certain legal safeguards, is generally used only when someone objects to detention. Where someone does not actively object but does not have the capacity to consent either, it is possible that the person could have been deprived of their right to liberty under Article 5 of the Human Rights Act (1998). This situation has become known as the 'Bournewood Gap', following the case of a man with autism who was detained in Bournewood hospital without his having consented to the detention or his being made subject to compulsory detention under the Mental Health Act (1983), with its built-in safeguards. The European Court of Human Rights has ruled that being in a hospital or care home without having consented to this does not necessarily amount to a deprivation of liberty and that whether or not a deprivation of liberty has occurred has to be decided by examining the circumstances in each individual case. 'Bournewood safeguards' are being introduced to protect those who lack capacity to make decisions about their care and who are being deprived of their liberty outside of the remit of the Mental Health Act (1983). The changes will be implemented in amendments to the Mental Capacity Act (2005) that are contained in the Mental Health Bill that is planned to amend the Mental Health Act (1983). There will be new rules that require authorisation to be obtained before depriving someone who lacks capacity of their liberty. It is anticipated that a relatively small number of people will fall within these rules but in some circumstances they may apply to people in the more advanced stages of dementia. As with the other provisions of the Mental Capacity Act (2005), an advocate will be appointed to represent people who do not have anyone to act in their interests.

These new provisions offer a clearer legal framework for decision-making that is carried out on behalf of people who lack capacity and introduce safeguards to protect their rights. However, some argue that further safeguards are needed (see, for example, the *Making Decisions Alliance* website, an alliance of older people's and disability organisations that have campaigned to improve the law in relation to capacity and decision-making: www.makingdecisions.org.uk).

Advocacy

As we have seen, the role of advocates in representing the interests of people who lack capacity is recognised in the Mental Capacity Act (2005), though in a limited way in that advocates will only be provided for people who do not have anyone to act on their behalf. Provided that there is someone who can potentially act for them, it is assumed that this will be appropriate and in line with the person's wishes. One of the criticisms of the Mental Health Bill that amends the Mental Health Act (1983) is that it contains no right to advocacy. This is different from Scotland, where people detained under the Mental Health (Care and Treatment) (Scotland) Act 2003 (implemented in 2005) have a right to independent advocacy. Advocacy is a way of helping to protect the rights of older people who, for various reasons, are unable to represent their own interests. The *Single Assessment Process* guidance recognises the role of advocacy, advising:

> Agencies should consider at the earliest opportunity whether older people might need, or benefit from, the assistance of advocates, interpreters and translators, and specific communication equipment, during the assessment process and subsequent aspects of care planning and service delivery. Where such a need exists, councils should either arrange for this support or facilitate access to it . . . The role of an advocate is a specialism in its own right, and should ideally be provided by professionals who are independent of both statutory agencies and the older person.
>
> (Department of Health 2002c: Annex: 19–20)

The values and ethics requirements of the *National Occupational Standards for Social Workers* state that social workers must be able to: lobby on behalf of service users; challenge their own organisations on behalf of service users; challenge injustice and lack of access to services; and challenge poor practice, as well as advising service users about independent advocacy (Training Organisation for the Personal Social Services 2002). However, challenging their own organisations, the lack of access to services and poor practice may be difficult for social workers because of their multiple accountabilities, as outlined at the beginning of the chapter. As employees, they have organisational roles and responsibilities that may conflict with their role of advocating in service users' interests. This is recognised implicitly in the *Single Assessment Process* guidance, quoted above. Advocacy is both a specialist role and one that is best performed by people who are otherwise independent of the assessment and support arrangements in order to avoid conflicts of interest. The importance of independent advocacy is confirmed in a review of information, advice and advocacy for older people (Dunning 2005). This study highlights the significance of information, advice and advocacy services in promoting the citizenship of older people: 'They can be essential to preparation, participation, prevention, protection and power throughout the life course. As such, they are indeed keys to continuing independence and remaining in control of one's later life' (ibid.: 67).

However, in many areas access to independent advocacy remains limited and older people often do not know about schemes or how to access them (Margiotta *et al.* 2003). Also, as independent advocacy is usually provided by the voluntary sector, some of the general issues facing this sector apply, not least, those concerning funding (see

Chapter 6). Community-based groups who undertake advocacy on behalf of members of Black and minority ethnic communities may be limited in their power to effect change because of their own marginalisation; moreover, they may reinforce, rather than challenge, barriers to accessing 'mainstream' services (Bowes and Sim 2006). A registered charity, Older People's Advocacy Alliance, was set up with a specific brief to promote independent advocacy for older people and address some of these issues. It aims to improve access to independent advocacy and enhance standards, increase the involvement of older people themselves and develop links with minority ethnic communities (Older People's Advocacy Alliance 2006).

WORKING WITH DIFFERENT NEEDS AND PERSPECTIVES

As identified at the beginning of the chapter, and an underlying theme throughout, one of the value dilemmas facing social workers occurs when there is an obligation to act on behalf of two (or more) individuals and they have competing needs and interests. In particular, this may occur when there are conflicting needs and perspectives of an older person and their carer(s). The requirement in policy documents is invariably to involve or take account of 'service users and carers', as though their interests are the same. Yet balancing older people's needs and concerns with those of significant people in their care networks is often not straightforward (Harris, John 2002). It is important that older people's needs are not conflated with those of their carers, and vice versa, and that their individual support requirements and perspectives are considered. However, the polarisation of 'older person' and 'carer' identities and needs when planning support is problematic too. In this section, we explore some of the potential differences in the perspectives of service users and carers, before proceeding to consider approaches that seek to address and balance the needs and interests of all parties.

Critical consideration of how 'care' and 'caring' are constructed in policy and practice highlights some potential tensions with the perspectives of service users. A number of points can be highlighted. First, some disability rights activists see the term 'care' and the concept of people having 'carers' as oppressive, representing service users as dependent and subordinate (Priestley 1999). 'Care' often contains overtones of monitoring, supervision and control (Johnson, J. 1998). Second, the term 'carer' implies that the relationship is one-way, whereas research attests to the reciprocity and interdependence within older people's personal and social relationships (Phillipson et al. 2001; Godfrey et al. 2004). As we have seen in the discussion of older carers in the previous chapter, older people are themselves significant resources in giving care and support to others. Third, it is argued that the focus on supporting carers fosters an uncritical acceptance of the conditions that have created the need for 'care' in the first place; attention should instead be directed at addressing the factors that contribute to people's need for 'care' (Morris 1993). For example, removing an older person's 'need' for a relative or neighbour to do her/his shopping might mean ensuring local and accessible shopping facilities and transport and removal of environmental hazards such as steps and uneven pavements. The older person might then not need 'care'. Fourth, often neither older people themselves, nor those in their informal networks who are involved in providing support, define this as 'care'; 'care' is an intrinsic part of the interpersonal relationship but not its defining characteristic (Henderson and Forbat 2002). One proposal is to replace categories that polarise and artificially restrict people's roles and identities ('carer' versus 'cared for') by concepts that reflect the complexity and fluidity of relationships, for example, 'working alliances' (Brechin 1998) or 'caring systems' (Bytheway and Johnson 1998).

However, others argue that rather than rejecting the notion of 'care' as oppressive, we need to retain it and revalue it in positive terms. Rather than viewing the receipt of care as a negative quality of those who have failed to match up to an ideal of independence, it should instead be recognised as a universal characteristic of human relationships (Lloyd, L. 2006a). Lloyd argues that social workers can play an important role in challenging the ideal of 'the independent, autonomous individual' and the assumption that dependency is something to be eliminated or managed. She points out that some types of dependency (for example, the dependency of affluent older people on paid help) are accepted; it is only certain types of dependency that are constructed negatively in policy and public discourses. Defining independence in terms of self-sufficiency is also a particular cultural construction characteristic of white western values. In other cultures, older people can receive high levels of care from family members and still retain a powerful status as head of the family; receiving care can contribute to one's status by indicating that one is of 'good family' (Grewal *et al.* 2004). Secker *et al.* (2003) make a helpful distinction between dependence, meaning reliance on others, and independence, meaning an individual's subjective sense of autonomy. In these terms it is possible, as for some of the minority ethnic older people in Grewal *et al.*'s research, to be receiving high levels of support from other people but to retain a sense of personal independence. Using this distinction, it could be argued that policy and practice objectives should focus more on fostering feelings of independence than removing dependence on services.

Returning to the question of what this all means for social workers trying to provide effective support for carers, while at the same time working in partnership with older people, Brechin (1998) argues that 'good care' must be evaluated from the perspective of both (or all) parties to the care arrangements: 'On this model, care would only be deemed to be good if the consequences were good from the point of view of both parties' (ibid.: 179). She presents this model in a diagram (see Figure 7.2).

Brechin argues that there are three key areas when evaluating the quality of care:

- The extent to which the care relationship extends the choices and opportunities available to each party. A carer, for example, might benefit from satisfaction, status or payment as a consequence of the caring role. This might provide opportunities for new relationships and mutual support mechanisms with others in similar situations, for example through membership of carers' groups.
- The nature of interpersonal processes between the parties to the relationship, that is, what takes place within the relationship between older person and 'carer' and the level of satisfaction of each party with the relationship.
- The intra-personal experience of the relationship in terms of its impact on self-esteem:

> There are important issues to do with such things as sense of personal identity, agency, empowerment, and self-confidence, which would be an

important part of judging the extent to which any care relationship and process is rewarding or damaging. The impact on the self-esteem of the person being cared for and the impact on the self-esteem of the carer seem self-evidently central to defining the success or otherwise of the relationship and process.

(Brechin 1998: 181)

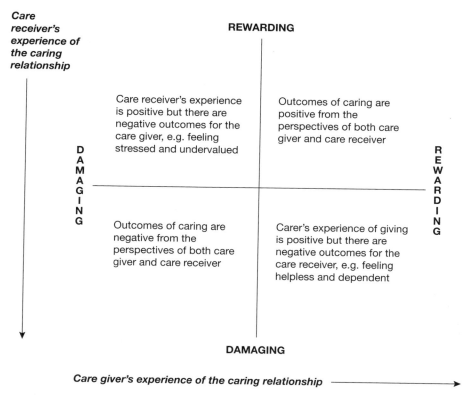

Care receiver's experience of the caring relationship

REWARDING

Care receiver's experience is positive but there are negative outcomes for the care giver, e.g. feeling stressed and undervalued

Outcomes of caring are positive from the perspectives of both care giver and care receiver

DAMAGING

REWARDING

Outcomes of caring are negative from the perspectives of both care giver and care receiver

Carer's experience of giving is positive but there are negative outcomes for the care receiver, e.g. feeling helpless and dependent

DAMAGING

Care giver's experience of the caring relationship

FIGURE 7.2 Quality of care
Source: Adapted from Brechin 1998: 179

This indicates the high level of complexity, and therefore skill requirements, for a social worker seeking to address the needs and concerns of both older people and their carers. It is not simply a case of establishing each party's practical needs, but reaching an understanding of how each party perceives and experiences the relationship and of the impact of this on her/his own sense of self.

Nolan *et al.* (2003) also recognise that all parties in caring relationships both have needs and contribute to addressing the needs of others. They propose a framework based on 'six senses', representing the shared needs of the person 'cared for', the 'carer' and formal carers/professionals. This framework provides a constructive starting point for planning support since it is premised on needs and concerns common to all, rather than assuming that one party has 'needs' while the other parties' role is to meet them. The six senses are as follows:

- *a sense of security*: feeling that you are safe;
- *a sense of belonging*: feeling that you are part of something or have a place;
- *a sense of continuity*: feeling that there are links between your past, present and future;
- *a sense of purpose*: feeling that you have a goal to aim for;
- *a sense of achievement*: feeling that you are getting somewhere;
- *a sense of significance*: feeling that you matter.

These senses are seen as interacting with each other and also as changing in their significance to individuals over time. A social worker involved in planning support for older people and carers can use the framework to: assess current needs and experiences; plan support that will help the 'senses' to be addressed; and evaluate whether and how the intervention has met the 'senses' for each party in the caring relationship. At the same time, the framework can also be applied to those in the wider caring network. It recognises that care staff have needs, for example, to experience a sense of achievement and significance in their work. It also helps social workers to reflect on their own needs and the implications for their practice of whether and how these are met.

ACTIVITY 7.4: PLANNING AND PROVIDING 'GOOD CARE'

Nora Williams is an 89-year-old white British woman who lives alone in a first floor flat that she purchased 25 years ago from the council. The flat is in a run down area of the town; there is a high crime rate and Nora is afraid to go out on her own. Over the years new residents have moved into the flats and Nora is suspicious of them. She believes there are a lot of drug users in the complex and she always keeps her doors and windows locked, fearing that they will rob her. She has angina, diabetes and high blood pressure. She is very overweight and has limited mobility. She is isolated and lonely and she relies heavily on her son, Alan, for both emotional and practical support. Alan lives five miles away and visits Nora at least once a day, also phoning her each morning and evening to check that she is all right. He does her shopping and pays her bills for her. He takes home her laundry to his partner, Sylvia, and every day brings over a meal that Sylvia has cooked for Nora to reheat. Sylvia and Nora have never got on so it is rare that Sylvia visits. Nora visits Alan and Sylvia on special occasions, such as birthdays and Christmas, but these tend to be tense occasions because of the poor relationship between Nora and Sylvia.

  Alan, aged 65, has recently retired and he and Sylvia planned to spend several months each year in a small apartment they have bought in Spain. Sylvia suffers from painful arthritis and they hope the warmer climate will help her. However, having promised Sylvia that they would spend more time in Spain once he retired, Alan now says that he cannot leave Nora. In addition to his daily visits, she has taken to phoning him several times during the day, and sometimes at night, either saying that she thinks she is having a heart attack or that she thinks someone is breaking in. Alan always has to drive over to reassure her. The situation has now reached crisis point, with Sylvia threatening to leave unless Alan 'sorts things out'. Sylvia thinks that Nora would be happier in a home as then she will have company and won't be anxious. Nora has always refused all help. She believes that Sylvia wants her 'put away' and she thinks that any professionals who have tried to help in the past are in league with Sylvia. She has refused to let them through the door.

Alan is struggling to adjust to retirement and the changed role and status this has brought. He feels helpless, caught between the demands of Nora and Sylvia. He has started drinking heavily. A few days ago he was charged with driving while under the influence of alcohol. He realises that the situation cannot continue and, on the advice of his GP, has contacted the local authority to see what help is available.

- What aspects of the relationships would you aim to address to move this situation to one of 'good care', as defined by Brechin (1998)?
- What services and approaches could be used to meet the needs of Nora, Alan and Sylvia, in terms of the 'six senses' identified by Nolan *et al.*?

DELIVERING QUALITY CARE AND SUPPORT

Working to ensure that the needs and concerns of all parties within the 'caring network' are addressed is directly related to delivering high quality care. People are more likely to provide 'good' care if their own 'senses' are met. This section develops the previous discussion, focusing on the delivery of high quality services. In defining 'quality' care, it seems that the key criterion as far as service users are concerned is the way in which they are treated by the people who work with them. Research has shown that the relationships that older people have with those on the front line of providing services are often the key factor in determining their satisfaction with services (Henwood *et al.* 1998) and that these relationships can be as important to them as the practical help they receive (Clark *et al.* 1998). As far as social workers are concerned, the service user focus groups set up by the General Social Care Council as part of the consultation regarding the reform of social work education (see Chapter 1) emphasised the importance of social workers' personal qualities. Service users wanted social workers to be: available in both physical and emotional terms; supportive and reassuring; respectful; patient and attentive; committed to promoting independence; punctual; trustworthy; reliable; friendly; honest; warm; and empathic (Department of Health 2002a: 7). When older people from minority ethnic groups (African-Caribbean, South Asian, Chinese, Vietnamese) were asked about their expectations of health and social care services, 'the highest expectations related to being treated with respect; feeling safe and comfortable; having dignity respected; and that professionals behave with integrity' (Policy Research Institute on Ageing and Ethnicity 2005: 6). In inter-professional environments, one of social work's significant contributions may be its underpinning values and principles. For example, it has already been noted that values are central to defining social work's specific contribution to work with people with dementia. This contribution is rooted in a social model of disability and practice based on principles of citizenship, partnership and equality (Manthorpe *et al.* 2004; Manthorpe and Iliffe 2005; Parsons 2005). Prime facets of a quality service relate directly to core values and to some of the skills discussed in Chapter 5.

Research commissioned by Age Concern to find out older people's priorities from health and social care services involved nine focus groups that included older people whose voices often go unheard (Age Concern 2006c). It was found that although the priorities identified by older people were in tune with policy objectives, these policy objectives were not, in the older people's experience, being realised in practice. In terms of social care, one respondent's comment was that 'social care needs to include the "social" aspect as well as the "care" aspect' (ibid.: 4). The report continues:

> As was pointed out by one older person living alone with a mobility problem, she hugely appreciated the stair rail that was installed in her home when she needed it. But what she would like more than anything else is someone to talk to. For her, social care means seeing more than one person for more than ten minutes each week. The perception among many of these respondents, especially those who have mobility problems and are very much restricted to their homes, is that they do indeed receive the basic care they need in order to survive. However, they wish for so much more. They miss conversation and activity. They would like companionship and stimulation and see these things as a vital part of staying 'young at heart' and interested in the world around them.
>
> (Age Concern 2006c: 4–5)

(These comments echo Margaret Simey's experiences, explored at the beginning of Chapter 1.)

A review of the performance of home care services for older people comments that although older people usually express general satisfaction with home care services, they raise a number of concerns when questioned in more depth (Commission for Social Care Inspection 2006a). These include: home care visits being unreliable and 'rushed'; inflexibility in the tasks that care workers are permitted to undertake; and difficulties in getting care plans reviewed. The report notes that in many areas home care services are struggling to meet demand, with difficulties in recruiting and training workers and equipping them for new ways of working. It concludes that action is needed to develop and manage the social care 'market', including strategies to develop the social care workforce. The 'cultural shift', which the report identifies as needed in the way home care is commissioned and provided, is seen as entailing service users having more control over purchasing decisions to ensure that services meet their needs and includes their having direct control of their individual budgets (see Chapter 4).

As we noted in Chapter 6, social workers are often involved in arranging support services that are commissioned from the private or voluntary sectors. As far as older people are concerned, it is the values and practices of these key personnel on the front line that will determine whether or not they experience a quality service, as illustrated in the quotation above. Research by Patmore and McNulty (2005) reveals the influence of service commissioners on the nature of the service provided by independent (private and voluntary) sector agencies. The study explored factors that promote home care services for older people that are flexible and person-centred. It comprised a literature review, telephone interviews with managers of home care provider services and in-depth case studies of agencies purchasing and providing home care (four of these providers were independent sector agencies and two were local authority providers). The research highlighted the influence of staff values on the extent to which person-centred, flexible care was provided: 'Flexible person-centred care for older people may be dependent as least as much on the staff values and the ethos promoted within an organisation as on particular assessment, service planning or review procedures' (Patmore and McNulty 2005: 9).

A key factor promoting person-centred care was the level of continuity of home care. An established and ongoing relationship between the older person and the home carer enabled the carer to become familiar with the older person's preferences and aspirations, whilst the relationship also provided motivation for staff to provide a responsive service. Another factor was the degree of flexibility carers were allowed in responding to needs and wishes identified by service users. The values and attitudes of service commissioners were significant, as these were the people determining the conditions under which home care was provided. Some purchasers permitted flexibility whilst others did not. The research distinguished two types of purchaser:

- *'customer-centred'* purchasers who were oriented to providing flexible, person-centred help;
- *'system-centred'* purchasers who were primarily concerned with restricting the costs of the service and maintaining its efficiency.

The researchers point out that the use of large block contracts increases the influence that purchasers exercise on provider practices and values. If purchasers do not encourage person-centred, flexible practices, then it is difficult for providers to deliver this within the constraints set down by the purchaser. Statutory social services providers enjoyed greater discretion than independent sector agencies, though how this was exercised depended to an extent on the values of the managers of the statutory services. Although the study set out expecting to identify particular systems and processes for promoting person-centred, flexible home care, its main conclusion is the centrality of values:

> Caring values seemed the motive force behind flexible, person-centred home care – whether at the level of the home care worker, the provider manager, or the Social Services purchaser . . . 'Caring for the whole person' seems the prime source for flexible, person-centred care. It is an outlook which seems to develop easily and naturally among many home care staff, once they get to know a customer. Among provider managers, to practise it requires either the command of staff time which is held by some Social Services provider managers or the support of like-minded purchasers. The importance of purchasers who value holistic care is a major finding from the study.
>
> (Patmore and McNulty 2005: 19–20)

So far the discussion has focused mainly on the quality of home care services but work has also been undertaken on quality of life of frail older people in care homes (Tester *et al.* 2004). The research focused on the transition to residential care, with interviews carried out with older people who had entered homes in the previous six months. The study identified both positive and negative influences on quality of life. The main interrelated components of quality of life identified were: sense of self; care environment; activities; and relationships (see Figure 7.3).

Older people's sense of self was expressed through: the sense that people made of their frailty, ill-health and strengths compared with those of others; their presentation

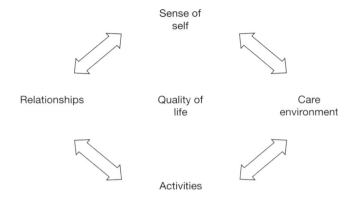

FIGURE 7.3 Components of quality of life in a care home environment

of self through appearance; and their preferences regarding personal space, with some residents favouring peace and privacy and others preferring company. A key factor in relation to the care environment was that residents were able to exercise choice over their daily living arrangements: 'Having choices, expressing preferences and opinions and making complaints were all ways in which participants might express themselves as individuals' (ibid.: 215). Relationships with other residents and with family members were important in helping residents maintain a sense of self. The study found that memories of relationships with people no longer alive were significant for older people with dementia. The main activities for most residents were those associated with daily living, for example, getting up, and going to bed and meals. Trips outside the home were rare and only one of the homes studied organised any daily leisure activities.

The factors summarised by the study as exerting a positive and negative influence on the quality of life of older people in care homes are reminiscent of the 'six senses' identified by Nolan *et al.* (2003), discussed earlier in the chapter. They include: the exercise of autonomy, choice and control; meaningful communication with others; meeting of emotional needs; experience of continuity; and a positive response to increasing frailty. Other important factors highlighted concern the wider context, in particular whether there is a positive structural, cultural and spiritual environment. The study concludes:

> quality of life can be promoted by good quality individualised care. This study demonstrates the key role that care providers and practitioners can play in enabling residents to maintain their sense of self, to communicate verbally and non-verbally, to exercise control and rights, to maintain and develop relationships, and to have meaningful activity and interaction within the contexts of institutional care settings.
>
> (Tester *et al.* 2004: 224)

However, there is worrying evidence that there is a persistence of negative cultural attitudes towards older people, reflected in poor standards of practice. In particular, a lack of respect and dignity in the way older people are treated within hospitals has been reported (Healthcare Commission *et al.* 2006). Deficiencies in the value base of services for older people have been recognised by the Department of Health in its *Dignity in Care Campaign* (Department of Health 2006g), which recognises that the 'emphasis on throughput has at times been at the expense of the quality of care provided' (Lewis, I. 2006: 1). The campaign declares the intention 'to put dignity at the heart of care' (ibid.). The 'Dignity Challenge' posed by the campaign states that high quality care services that respect people's dignity should:

- have a zero tolerance of all forms of abuse;
- support people with the same respect you would want for yourself or a member of your family;
- treat each person as an individual by offering a personalised service;
- enable people to maintain the maximum possible level of independence, choice and control;
- listen and support people to express their needs and wants;
- respect people's right to privacy;
- ensure people feel able to complain without fear of retribution;
- engage with family members and carers as care partners;
- assist people to maintain confidence and a positive self-esteem;
- act to alleviate people's loneliness and isolation.

(Lewis, I. 2006: 3)

Measures introduced to support the 'Dignity Challenge' include additional resourcing for capital investment to improve physical standards within care homes, a programme for service improvement and the publication of an online *Dignity in Care Practice Guide* (Social Care Institute for Excellence 2006c).

The value base of social workers should place them at the forefront when it comes to identifying and challenging factors that detract from quality services. Equally the skills and values of social work make it well positioned to promote and implement positive changes in cultures, attitudes and practices. Despite the conflicts and constraints that are an inevitable and intrinsic part of social work, a central tenet of this book is that there is much that social workers can do to ensure that practice upholds central social work values. Often this will be achieved through micro-level encounters in which social workers engage with older people in ways that affirm their individual worth and significance, connect with their unique perspectives and experiences and acknowledge their diverse needs and preferences. At other times, social work's role may be to question and challenge wider policies and practices that compromise social work values and to advocate or initiate ways of working that move practice in more 'person-centred' directions. The central challenge for social workers is never to lose sight of both the private troubles experienced by older people *and* the public issues that shape those experiences, as a consequence of the political, policy and organisational responses directed at them.

KEY POINTS

- ☐ Social workers need to think critically about the nature and level at which they involve older people and seek to maximise this whenever possible.

☐　Assessing and managing risk has to be based on explicit and comprehensive analysis and a full understanding of the older person's biography and values.

☐　The differing needs and perspectives of service users and carers must be recognised.

☐　All parties to 'caring networks' have needs that require acknowledging and addressing.

☐　Key components in delivering high quality care are the nature of the relationship between older people and support staff and the values that are upheld in practice.

KEY READING

Brechin, A. (1998) 'What makes for good care?' in A. Brechin, J. Walmsley, J. Katz and S. Peace (eds) *Care Matters: Concepts, Practice and Research in Health and Social Care*, London: Sage.

Lloyd, L. (2006) 'A caring profession? The ethics of care and social work with older people', *British Journal of Social Work* 36: 1171–85.

Nolan, M., Grant, G., Keady, J. and Lundh, U. (2003) 'New directions for partnerships: relationship-centred care', in M. Nolan, U. Lundh, G. Grant and J. Keady (eds) *Partnerships in Family Care*, Maidenhead: Open University Press.

Preston-Shoot, M. (2002) 'Evaluating self-determination', in B. Bytheway, V. Bacigalupo, J. Bornat, J. Johnson and S. Spurr (eds) *Understanding Care, Welfare and Community: A Reader*, London: Routledge.

CHAPTER 8

ACTIVITIES: POINTERS TO THE ISSUES

This final chapter outlines possible responses to the activities elsewhere in the book. They are 'pointers'; they do not provide complete 'answers' or definitive prescriptions for practice. They are intended simply to provide a degree of guidance on key issues that are raised by the activities.

ACTIVITY 1.1 WHAT IS IT LIKE TO BE 'AN OLDER PERSON'?

There are, of course, an infinite number of possible responses to this activity, in the same way that there would be to the questions, 'What is it like to be middle aged?', or 'What is it like to be a younger person?' Everybody's experience will be unique. However, it may be possible to discern some common themes, as well as different ways in which these are played out in the lives of older people in diverse circumstances. The bullet point questions to guide your note-taking, which are provided within the activity itself, should have already provided pointers to some issues to consider. Underpinning all of those pointers is the importance of beginning from the experiences of older people themselves and emphasising their accounts, rather than making assumptions about what their experiences might be. In reflecting on this activity, you might want to pay particular attention to anything that surprised you and consider why it did so. This may tell you something about cultural and your own personal constructions of 'old age'.

ACTIVITY 1.2 COMPARING EXPERIENCES

We cannot know what has emerged from comparing your findings with the research findings. We also cannot know what you have learned about older people's experiences and perceptions of later life and the messages you have identified for social work practice. Some of the messages that are important for us are:

- People we perceive as 'older people' may not regard themselves as old.
- Later life can be a time that provides increased opportunities for fulfilling relationships and activities.

- Factors like health and income can influence the extent to which older people are able to benefit from these opportunities.
- Older people are likely to have their own strategies for dealing with the difficulties they may face.
- Older people have views about what they want from services and about how services should be provided.
- Older people have rich life histories that have a bearing on their current situations. We need to see them as 'whole people'.
- Like all of us, older people need to have a sense of meaning and purpose in life.
- Older people need to feel that they are 'givers' as well as 'receivers' in their relationships with others.

ACTIVITY 1.3 THE SOCIAL CONSTRUCTION OF AGEISM

Some examples (you may have different ones):

- Economic structures – the emphasis on 'productivity', understood narrowly in terms of paid work. Because many older people are no longer in the workforce, they are seen as being unproductive, and therefore of limited social value.
- Political values – depicting the changes in the population structure in negative terms such as 'demographic timebomb' or 'increasing dependency ratio'. This ignores older people's positive social roles and legitimates restrictive policies.
- Cultural heritage – in mainstream (white) western culture, traditional cultural representations of older women include the benign and powerless (for example, granny knitting in the armchair) and the malevolent and repulsive (for example, old witch/ugly hag).
- Historical legacy – older people as passive and dependent, with services provided on the basis of others knowing what was best for them.
- Social attitudes – expectations of inevitable decline: 'What do you expect at your age?'

ACTIVITY 1.4 THE RELATIONSHIP BETWEEN BODY, SELF AND SOCIETY

Margaret grew up with cultural values that saw retirement as a period of rest and decline. This conflicted with her own identity, acquired over the life course, as an active person who could influence the world around her. Although Margaret was able to resist dominant expectations and continue to be active in retirement, a sudden loss of physical mobility imposed restrictions on her ability to be socially involved, purposeful and powerful, in the way she had been previously. It also changed the way that others responded to her. She was seen in one-dimensional terms in relation to her physical needs, rather than as a fully rounded individual with a life history and many components to her identity. Inside she was the same person, with the same interests and desire to be active and make a difference, but institutional and social responses to her physical needs, in the form of care services, reinforced her limitations and dependence and 'disabled' her from fulfilling her former roles. This in turn had an adverse impact on her own sense of self. She was on the receiving end of cultural and social values that left her feeling that she did not have a meaningful role. She was seen as a receiver and not as someone who had anything to give.

A social worker in contact with Margaret obviously could not change the wider social and cultural values to which she is exposed. However, s/he could seek to counter them by enabling Margaret to exercise choice and control in the social work process and in her social network more broadly. Margaret could be treated as the expert on her own situation. By learning from Margaret about her life history, her interests, strengths and aspirations, the social worker could relate to Margaret as a whole person, rather than just as someone with physical needs. The social worker could find out from Margaret about the roles and activities that give her life meaning and work with her to see what sort of support will enable her to maintain these. The social worker could also help Margaret to continue to make a contribution to the lives of others. For example, the social worker could help to remove environmental obstacles, such as lack of transport, so that Margaret can continue with her voluntary work, rather than attending a day centre. Or if environmental obstacles are insurmountable, alternative forms of voluntary work, for example based on use of the telephone, could be explored. A creative and flexible response from the social worker would allow support services to be planned around Margaret's preferences and requirements, rather than her being expected to slot into existing services.

ACTIVITY 1.5 CHALLENGING AGEISM

The ageist attitudes underpinning the comments can be challenged in a number of ways, such as:

- *Old people don't make any contribution to society* – older people have contributed in their lives up to older age and they continue to contribute through paid and voluntary work, through roles played in households, in pressure groups, political parties, etc.
- *Old people are a huge drain on taxpayers' money but are always moaning about how hard-up they are* – older people have been taxpayers themselves or are still taxpayers and have contributed or still are contributing towards provision for their own older age. Pensions have not been linked to average earnings and older people are often reluctant to claim benefits to which they are entitled. Perhaps older people are justified in 'moaning', though many don't!
- *'As a GP, I'm very busy. There's no point me going to see Mrs S. just because she's a bit confused and forgetful. She's just getting old and there's no treatment for that'* – older people who experience health problems have as much right as anyone else to expect that medical practitioners will take those problems seriously. Confusion and forgetfulness are not a symptom of old age *per se* but may indicate, for example, a vitamin deficiency or a urinary infection. For these conditions, or for early stage dementia, prompt diagnosis and appropriate treatment or intervention are vital for older people's physical, social and emotional well-being and for the well-being of those in their informal networks.

- *Old people are a burden on their families* – some older people are supported by their families. However, these relationships are often reciprocal, with older people making substantial contributions to the lives of their families, for example as grandparents. Many families derive emotional, social or financial rewards from giving support to older members.
- *People change when they get old – their personalities change, they aren't interested in things and they just sit around all day. They're just waiting to die* – there is evidence that many people continue to have the same interests, value the same things and exhibit the same traits as they become older. However, their social and financial circumstances and ageist social attitudes can lead to some older people becoming depressed. Nevertheless, many older people remain active and continue to make a valuable contribution to their families and society. Rather than 'waiting to die', for many older people later life is a time of continued life satisfaction and enjoyment.
- *'Even though I'm 85 and struggling to manage, I'm not going to ask for help. I know there's not enough money to go round and I think it should go to helping children. I've had my life'* – an older person is of the same individual worth as anyone else and has as much right to services. Getting the right help can improve people's quality of life, no matter how many or few years of life they have left. The law says that local authorities have to help older people who have certain needs and there are resources available to do this. It is important to use the provision that exists. If older people do not take it up, the assumption will be that it's not needed and less might be provided in the future.

ACTIVITY 1.6 REFLECTING ON VALUES AND VALUE CONSTRAINTS

There are many difficulties and constraints that are likely to be encountered in implementing the values and principles in practice. They include:

- Pressure to process work as quickly as possible, which risks failing to treat an older person as an individual in her/his own right and not according her/him value and status.
- A tendency to see older people as only service users, rather than first and foremost as citizens.
- Negative social and cultural attitudes towards ageing, held by other people and by older people themselves, may be hard to change.
- The extent to which older people can control their own lives can be constrained by the lack of resources to enable them to do so.
- Standardised processes of assessment may make it difficult to ensure that older people participate fully.
- There may be severe limitations on the choices available to older people and some older people may need support to enable them to exercise meaningful choice.
- Services and activities for older people tend to be specialist, making it difficult for them to integrate into services and activities that are not age-specific.
- What is needed to enable older people to live the life they want might far exceed what is available.

ACTIVITY 1.7 PUTTING YOURSELF IN THE PICTURE

This is a very personal activity that is likely to evoke a wide range of responses. Some of our thoughts are that if we see our own later lives as primarily a time of loss and vulnerability this may lead to a protective and risk-averse approach to practice. Fears about our own ageing may lead to strategies that distance us from engaging with older people's experiences, perhaps allying ourselves more closely with carers' perspectives. Fear of ageing may be particularly strong among women, with concerns that include future ill-health, dependency, loneliness, loss of dignity and changed physical appearance (Bernard and Harding Davies 2000). However, positive features of growing older may be anticipated positively, rather than dreaded, for example more time and opportunity to pursue interests and activities. It is salutary to consider what we think would be the important dimensions of a good quality of life for us and what sort of support and services might be needed to help us maintain this. One report, based on two seminars for practitioners working in health and social care, asked them what support they would want for their old age and how this matched with current provision (Easterbrook 1999). The practitioners' responses highlighted the need for services to do more to promote the dignity, choice and autonomy of older people. Key issues identified included: the links between poverty and ill-health; the need to reach an understanding of individuals' life histories in order to offer appropriate services; the need to regard older people as equal partners; the importance of respecting older people's own (rather than professionally determined) standards about care and support; the importance of enabling older people to use 'ordinary services'; and the need for clear responsibilities and well-coordinated care arrangements.

However you responded, the central point of the activity is that you need to be aware of the potential impact of your own thoughts and feelings about ageing on your work with older people. 'Putting ourselves in the picture' by continuing to reflect on these issues needs to be part of our practice.

ACTIVITY 1.8 USING THEORIES TO MAKE SENSE OF OLDER PEOPLE'S EXPERIENCES

Disengagement and activity theories of ageing could be supported by a range of evidence from the sources mentioned, including:

- Margaret Simey had a retirement that was characterised by considerable activity until her fall, when social processes of disengagement began to operate. Disengagement was forced upon Margaret, rather than a matter of her choice.
- Ageism and other dimensions of inequality, such as poverty and lack of access to culturally appropriate activities and services, can force older people to disengage.
- Older people can engage actively during older age, having positive experiences and clear views about what they want from their lives.
- Involvement in social relationships and hobbies outside the home can be important sources of activity.
- Older people can feel forced into activity as a way of distancing themselves from stereotypes of old age.

- Home can become an important refuge; a place to disengage.
- Health and physical ability can be crucial components in shaping patterns of activity or disengagement.

These examples suggest that both theories can be ways of understanding an older person's situation and experiences and that it is important to approach their use carefully in relation to an older person's individual circumstances, rather than as either/or explanations of the experiences of *all* older people.

ACTIVITY 1.9 BILL WATERS

You could have responded to this scenario in a number of different ways. One response might be:

Bill's mobility problems constrain his subjectivity and have led to isolation in his flat, which is a form of disengagement. Key events in his life have removed what were previously important parts of his identity: his relationship with Annie, ballroom dancing, gardening and being a postman. These aspects of Bill's life course give some understanding of why he might find his present circumstances difficult. He has limited scope for reconstructing his identity in ways that would replace the major changes his sense of self has undergone. Whilst maintaining a sense of integrity about not owing money to anyone and remaining independent, an aspect of his identity that seems to have been maintained, he seems to be close to despair at the loss of Annie. Other unresolved losses in his life may include the death of his son and feelings of loss associated with his sister's dementia. Erikson's emphasis on integrity and despair may be relevant here, though not as all-encompassing either/or responses to older age. The friends from the allotments might provide some sense of continuity with his previous life. His position in the labour market until he retired has shaped the resources available to him now and has limited his options. His occupancy of a first floor flat creates environmental obstacles to social activity and engagement and reinforces his isolation. It also disrupts another thread of continuity, his enjoyment of the open air.

These brief references to some of the ways in which theories might contribute to understanding Bill's situation illustrate the earlier point in Chapter 1 that there are no 'off the peg' practice implications that can be read off from theory. Instead, using theories, or certain aspects or combinations of them, could only serve to guide and inform your approach as a social worker, as you crafted your work with Bill in ways that were sensitive to the various facets of his life and your theoretical understandings of them.

ACTIVITY 2.1 THE IMPACT OF RESEARCH ON POLICIES AND SERVICES

It might have been expected that these two studies would have prompted major changes in policy and practice for older people, with a shift towards prioritising services in people's own homes, including finding ways of supporting family carers, who were, and are, mainly women.

The impact of the research might have been limited by financial factors. There might have been concern that a comprehensive system of support to people in their own homes might be much more expensive than limited provision of residential care. There might have been fears that such support at home might undermine families' willingness to care, placing additional demands on the state's resources. Dominant social and political objectives at the time are also relevant. It was assumed that families 'should' provide care for older relatives and that it was 'natural' for women to assume these responsibilities as part of their nurturing role in the family. The dominant view of residential care was likely to have regarded it as a benign and homely form of provision, appropriate for the care of older people who were viewed as passive, dependent and 'disengaged' (see Chapter 1).

Many care homes are now provided by the independent sector and physical standards have improved dramatically from Townsend's description. This has been helped by the introduction of national minimum care standards in care homes and requirements for the regulation and inspection of homes (see Chapter 4). However, there continue to be concerns about the quality of care within homes, including lack of appropriate social activity, insufficient time for staff to engage with residents outside of providing physical care, reported scandals of abuse and neglect and lack of dignity for older people in the way care is provided (see Chapter 7).

A study by Phillipson *et al.* (2001) revisited Bethnal Green, the area in which Townsend's study of family life was located (the Phillipson *et al.* study also included other areas where studies of family life were carried out in the 1940s and 1950s) to see how family and community life had changed. Patterns of family life were noted to be more diverse, influenced by a number of factors including social class, age and migration histories. Family networks were still important in the lives of older people, though they were now more restricted to immediate rather than extended family, and relationships between couples and with friends were found to have gained in significance.

ACTIVITY 2.2 REALISING GAINS FROM SPECIAL PROJECTS

You might have drawn on your reading and/or experience in a number of ways to respond to this activity. Overall we suspect that your conclusion will have been that current community care practice does not achieve the gains identified from the Kent community care project or only achieves them to a much more limited extent than in the project. For example, it is rare for current community care practice actively to seek out new needs. In the text that follows the activity in Chapter 2, we have provided pointers as to why the gains have tended not to be realised in current community care practice.

ACTIVITY 2.3 FRAGMENTING THE PROCESS OF ASSESSMENT AND CARE MANAGEMENT

From the local authority's point of view, functional specialisation may be seen as increasing the efficiency and cost-effectiveness of the service, improving the 'throughput' of work, and providing greater managerial control over the different parts of the care management process. The social worker/care manager might feel that s/he is only responsible for limited aspects of the intervention and might find it frustrating not to have the opportunity to work with older people throughout the whole social work process. Most social work models and approaches encompass the stages of assessment, intervention, review and evaluation, so restriction of the social worker's involvement to one or two stages can make it difficult for social workers to see the relevance of 'theory' or to perceive their role in the way it has been constructed in their professional education. The work can seem like 'managing care' rather than professional social work (see Chapter 5). This may have an impact on their morale and job satisfaction. The older person using the services might find the arrangements confusing and might not be able to work out who has overall responsibility for her/his support and whom s/he should approach if there is a problem. Research has shown that older people value highly the personal relationships developed with care staff. The fragmentation of the care management role is likely to disrupt the continuity necessary for developing a positive relationship between the social worker and older person. This has implications for the satisfaction of both parties (see studies by Postle 2002 and Ware et al. 2003).

ACTIVITY 2.4 REALISING THE VISION?

Some of the features of New Labour policy are:

- An acceptance of the 'mixed economy of care' introduced by the Conservatives but with more stress on standards and outcomes.
- Prevention of admission to hospital, and early discharge for those who are admitted.
- Changing the balance of service provision by a greater emphasis on prevention in order to reduce expenditure on high levels of need.
- Improving partnership working between different agencies and promoting multi-disciplinary work.

Some of the obstacles to realising New Labour policy goals are:

- The tight control over standards and outcomes can lead to local authorities 'performing to target'.
- Most policy initiatives are seen as being achievable through better use of existing resources rather than as needing additional funding.
- Greater emphasis on prevention may not lead to reduced expenditure on high level needs.
- There are technical and organisational problems that hinder partnership working, such as incompatibility of IT systems, different geographical boundaries and a history of difficulty in establishing successful collaborative mechanisms.

ACTIVITY 3.1 THE IMPACT OF THE QUALITY OF ASSESSMENT ON OUTCOMES

- Mr A. was met on a greater number of occasions.
- His expressed wishes about returning home have been taken seriously as the starting point for assessment.
- The kitchen assessment has been undertaken in his home environment with which he is familiar.
- There has been active engagement with Mr A.'s relatives.
- The discharge planning meeting was open to considering options instead of only contemplating one possible decision.
- The assessment takes account of Mr A.'s strengths and coping mechanisms, not just his difficulties.
- The way in which the support services are being provided and the workers are being introduced is being adapted to meet his specific needs.
- A key worker is designated to monitor the care plan.
- A review after a specified time has been agreed.

ACTIVITY 3.2 PERSON-HELD RECORDS

- It is important that older people give *informed* consent to information about them being shared with others. The processes and implications of person-held records may not have been fully explained to older people, in which case they would not have given informed consent.
- Some older people may not be able to 'manage' the records.
- To be meaningful to older people, person-held records will have to be prepared in such a way that older people themselves can access the information contained in the record. This means that facilities are needed to produce records in various formats, for example in different languages, in Braille, on audiotape, and using picture-based communication systems, depending on the needs of the older person concerned.
- The ability of workers to complete records in ways that are accessible and helpful to the older person is likely to vary.
- The older person may not be able to understand the content of the records, if it is written in professional jargon and/or produced in an inaccessible computerised format.
- Workers may not be aware of the existence of the records or they may be aware of them but fail to keep them up to date.
- The records may become lost in people's homes and professionals would not then be able to update them.
- Although the principles of putting the older person in control of their own records and sharing information openly with them are laudable, in practice professionals may record certain information in records held elsewhere that are not accessible to the older person.
- Practitioners may also be wary of sharing information with colleagues from other professions. Each profession could continue to maintain its own records with only basic details noted in the person-held record.

- It could be easy for other people entering the older person's home to access confidential information about them if the record is left in an easily visible place.

ACTIVITY 3.3 ASSESSMENT OBJECTIVES

- Identifying needs – questions about problematic aspects of older people's lives that fall within the remit of what the agency thinks is important. Often this will be about physical needs, for example: 'Are you able to get yourself washed and dressed?' 'Can you get to the toilet unaided?'
- Evaluating risks – questions about areas that pose threats to older people's safety or well-being. Often this will be about physical risks, for example: 'How would you get help in an emergency?', 'How many times have you fallen in the last few weeks?', 'How often do you have a cooked meal?'
- Promoting independence and well-being – questions that recognise older people's rights to participate in society as citizens. These questions would seek to find out about how older people would like their lives to be and the support they need to achieve this, for example: 'What things are most important in helping you to enjoy life?', 'What would help you to go out more?', 'Can we check whether you are getting all of the money/benefits that you are entitled to?'

There could have been a range of possible responses based on your material from Activity 1.1, depending on the sources used when that activity was completed. Whereas professionals may be concerned with narrow definitions of needs and risks, focusing largely on physical aspects, older people's concerns and priorities are likely to be much broader and encompass social and emotional dimensions of well-being. It is therefore likely that promoting independence and well-being is the approach to assessment that has emerged from reviewing your Activity 1.1 material as most likely to address the needs and concerns of older people.

ACTIVITY 3.4 ASSESSING TO PROMOTE CITIZENSHIP

Possible headings are in **bold** below and examples of prompts that might be used as an assessment framework follow them. The text within brackets (*in bold and italics*) shows where these issues could be addressed within the SAP domains.

Health (physical and mental) and impairments: health difficulties and assets; the impact of health problems or physical or sensory impairments on the older person's life; what the older person thinks might help to alleviate or offset difficulties; action needed to promote or maintain health or prevent deterioration. (*Clinical background, disease prevention, senses, mental health, personal care and physical well-being*)

Personal and social well-being: personal and social difficulties and strengths; the impact these have on the older person's life; what the older person thinks might help to alleviate or offset difficulties. (*Personal care, mental health, relationships*)

Housing and home: satisfaction with current housing; aspects of home and garden that are especially valued; views or concerns about future housing needs; difficulties or concerns about managing or maintaining the home or garden; specific risk factors within the home; any action directed at the home or locality that would improve the older person's access to the community. *(Immediate environment and resources)*

Community participation: involvement, or aspirations to be involved, in community activities, for example, through volunteering; barriers to community participation, for example, environmental obstacles or safety issues, such as fear of crime. *(Immediate environment and resources)*

Financial and other resources: income and possible entitlement to additional welfare benefits; need for financial or debt management advice; material resources that could address or alleviate difficulties and possible means of accessing these. *(Immediate environment and resources)*

Social, cultural, education, work and leisure needs and interests: current activities and those that the older person would like to begin, continue or resume; nature of the barriers preventing this and ways of addressing them; cultural, religious and spiritual needs and how these are/could be met; aspirations regarding future learning or leisure opportunities. *(Relationships)*

Access to services: for example, need for specific information or advice, interpreting services or advocacy. *(Immediate environment and resources)*

Needs and concerns of those in the informal network: this would include those involved in providing immediate support (with the older person's consent), but also anyone else that the older person felt that it was relevant to include. *(Relationships)*

The framework offered by the SAP domains and sub-domains does allow scope for issues such as social relationships, leisure, work and learning opportunities, housing and access to local services to be addressed within the assessment. However, the emphasis overall in the SAP is on health-related issues (Age Concern 2005b: 7), rather than wider citizenship and well-being concerns. There are a number of separate domains devoted to health-related issues in SAP, whereas significant issues concerning social and community participation are rolled together. This is likely to lead to less attention and priority being given to these areas in an assessment. Although 'user's perspective' constitutes a domain within the SAP, arguably this should be integrated throughout all domains of the assessment, rather than separated out in one domain. In a 'person-centred' assessment concerned with promoting the older person's well-being, we would expect to see the older person's perspective reflected throughout all areas of the assessment, with clear indications of points on which the older person's perspective differs from that of other parties to the assessment.

ACTIVITY 4.1 DRAWING UP A CARE PLAN

An outline care plan might look like this:

Needs and risks	Objectives	Services	Outcomes
To keep warm and avoid the risk of hypothermia	To make sure Ada's home is properly insulated to avoid heat loss. To have the central heating serviced to check it is working effectively. To ensure Ada is receiving all of the welfare benefits to which she is entitled.	Home improvement agency to carry out repairs. Access to approved tradesperson through Age Concern scheme. Visit from Welfare Rights Advice agency.	Ada is warm within her home and can afford to pay the heating bills.
To have a well-maintained property	To carry out essential repairs to the property. To give Ada information about local handyperson service run by Age Concern.	Home improvement agency to carry out property repairs. Handyperson scheme to deal with ongoing home maintenance problems as they arise.	Essential property repairs are carried out satisfactorily and any further home maintenance problems are dealt with to Ada's satisfaction.
To have adequate nutrition to avoid the risk of vitamin deficiency	To ensure that Ada has at least one proper meal a day.	A mobile meals service to provide a meal four times a week. Ada to attend local lunch club two days a week (transport provided). Befriender to visit and eat a meal with Ada once a week.	Ada has gained in weight and her physical health has improved.
To be safe within the home and avoid the risk of further falls.	To carry out a home safety assessment and address the hazards identified. Ada to have a full health check.	Occupational therapist to carry out a home assessment and fit rails, etc. GP to carry out full health check.	Hazards within the home are removed or managed (e.g. rugs removed, rails fitted). Ada has received any treatment necessary for physical health

Needs and risks	Objectives	Services	Outcomes
	To ensure that Ada can summon help if she falls.	Information to be given to Ada about pendant alarm to enable her to summon help in an emergency.	problems that contribute to the falls (e.g. anaemia/dizziness). Ada has no further falls or was able to summon help quickly in the event of a fall.
To improve mental well-being	To give Ada opportunities to talk about her feelings. Ada's mental health to be assessed within the health check.	Bereavement counselling. GP to check whether Ada needs treatment for depression.	Ada feels more content, better able to manage and her depressive symptoms have alleviated.
Social contact and activity to avoid the risks of isolation and loneliness	To enable Ada to get out more, enjoy the company of others and feel she has someone in whom she can confide.	Befriender to take Ada shopping once a week (prior to preparing and sharing a meal with her). Ada to attend local lunch club twice a week (transport provided). Ada given information about telephone counselling and support service run by Age Concern (linked to befriending service). Ada introduced by befriender to local 'Senior Action' group that meets fortnightly to make craft items to sell for charitable causes.	Ada's social contact has increased. She has people she can talk to. She feels as though she is involved in her local community and making a positive contribution to it.

The suggestions for interventions are only possible options. Ada could, of course, decide that she wishes to move to supported accommodation. (See page 98 for an example of weighing up different intervention options.) Clearly, too, the care plan formulated is dependent on the availability of appropriate services. In Ada's situation, this may be problematic, as she lives in an isolated rural area. If services are not available to meet the needs that have been identified in the assessment, this should be fed through to service planners and commissioners (see Chapter 3).

ACTIVITY 4.2 LAWFUL PRACTICE?

1   Mrs A. is someone for whom the local authority could potentially provide services, whether under the National Assistance Act (1948), the Health Services and Public Health Act (1968) or the Chronically Sick and Disabled Persons Act (1970). This means that there is a duty to assess Mrs A.'s need for services under the NHS and Community Care (1990) Section 47. Assessment of need should be carried out without reference to eligibility criteria, which relate to whether or not services should be provided, not whether or not needs are assessed. The local authority could well have breached its duty to carry out an assessment of need. However, it is not clear legally speaking what counts as an assessment. Depending on the nature of the telephone call and the level of expertise of the person asking the questions, the local authority could argue that this constituted its assessment of need and that the 'assessment' indicated that Mrs A.'s needs were not eligible for services to be provided. The local authority would need to show that it had taken account of guidance and case law in the way the assessment was carried out, for example, that needs were assessed holistically and that the views of the older person had been fully considered. If the telephone call amounted to no more than a superficial 'screening out' process, rather than an assessment, there could be a breach of the statutory duty to assess need.

2   Eligibility criteria have to be applied fairly and consistently to all individuals. The local authority is not at liberty to depart from its eligibility criteria in individual cases simply because of its financial resources, even if this is in the service user's favour. This would undermine the legal principle of 'fairness'.

3   Once need has been assessed as 'eligible', there is a statutory duty to meet it, regardless of the local authority's budget at the time. In not providing the service purely for financial reasons, the local authority is not fulfilling its duty to meet eligible need. This is different from Mr C. needing a specific service to meet his needs, this not being immediately available and his being placed on a waiting list for the particular service. Even here, however, the local authority would be expected to make the best possible alternative arrangements to meet the eligible need, pending the preferred option being available.

4   As established in the Gloucestershire case, each individual's needs have to be reassessed before services can be reduced or withdrawn. It is possible that Miss D.'s needs have increased since the original assessment and do now fall within the 'substantial' category. If her needs are reassessed as still in the 'moderate' category, her services can be withdrawn, though the reasons should be clearly explained to her and she should be given information on how to complain. Also, the local authority would have to consider the likely risks to her independence if the current

services were withdrawn and this, again, might indicate that her needs should be considered 'substantial'.

5   Local authorities have to be 'reasonable' in carrying out their functions and also be compliant with the Human Rights Act (1998). If they set their eligibility criteria too high, only providing services to those in very extreme need, they could be behaving unreasonably, in legal as well as moral terms, and be breaching human rights.

ACTIVITY 4.3 THE IMPLICATIONS OF DIRECT PAYMENTS

The points that would need to be covered in the visit (or subsequent visits) to Ada would include:

*   Finding out from Ada her preferences and requirements regarding services and what to her are the most important dimensions of a quality service. This would provide a starting point for advising Ada about the options available.
*   Explaining in detail and in clear terms exactly what a direct payment is. It would be helpful to have written information that could be left with Ada. The government has produced guidance on direct payments for service users (Department of Health 2004c) so a copy of this could be given to Ada.
*   Discussing with Ada the advantages and disadvantages of direct payments. Advantages would include the greater flexibility offered by direct payments, such as the freedom to choose who will provide the service, when this will be provided and the exact nature of the tasks to be undertaken. The disadvantages would include the responsibilities involved in managing a direct payment, such as keeping accounts, and the issues involved in becoming an employer.
*   Informing Ada about the sources of information and advice that are available locally to help people manage direct payments. Again, it would be useful to leave written information about local procedures and support systems.
*   In order to make an informed decision, Ada would need to know about all of the options available. For example, there may be other agencies that could be approached if Ada is not satisfied with the service provided by the current agency, without her necessarily needing to become a user of direct payments.
*   Ada may need help to consider the implications of employing someone from the village to help her. Employing someone who lives locally to provide help should mean that help is more accessible and reliable. It might also serve to link Ada more with her local community. However, there is unlikely to be back-up cover if the person is ill, on holiday or leaves suddenly. Ada would need to be clear about the local authority's responsibilities in these situations.
*   Ada might need help to think about what she would like to know about the person's experience and skills and to plan the questions that she would want to ask if she was considering appointing her/him to support her.
*   Ada would require clear information about the needs for which the direct payment is being made and the services it is meant to cover, since she will have to show that the direct payment is being used for the purposes for which it is intended.
*   Ada would need to know how much the direct payment would be, what this could be expected to purchase and how much she would have to contribute towards the

costs as a consequence of the charging policy. Some of this information may not
be immediately available.

- Ada would need to be clear about how she would have to account for the direct
payment to the council and what might happen if the direct payment were not used
for the services for which it was intended.
- It may be that, if Ada is depressed and already feeling overwhelmed, she does
not at the present time want to assume the additional responsibilities associated
with direct payments. However, she needs to know what to do and who to contact
if she changes her mind at any point.
- This would almost certainly be too much information for Ada to take in during
one visit. Ada would need the chance to digest the information and think about
it. She would benefit from the opportunity of a second visit or contact so that she
can ask further questions.
- Ada could be asked if she would like to be put in touch with a local organisation
that provides support for people receiving direct payments and, perhaps, with
people already receiving payments who could share their experiences with her.

ACTIVITY 4.4 IMPROVING STANDARDS

In relation to the seven areas of the minimum standards, the following list gives examples
of action that might be appropriate.

Staffing

- Review the adequacy of staffing levels and the appropriateness of the skills,
experience and qualifications levels of staff.
- Require all staff to participate in training on fundamental values and principles
underpinning the care provided in the home. This would focus on older people's
human rights and personhood, encompassing the need for respect and dignity in
all aspects of care (see Chapter 7).
- Provide specific staff training on handling and lifting residents. New equipment
may need to be purchased.
- Provide training on continence and review practice in this area.
- Review staff recruitment, training, supervision and appraisal processes and ensure
that these encourage promotion of the values and skills necessary for high quality
care.

Health and personal care

- Arrange visits to the home by relevant professionals to provide basic health
screening, for example, dental and chiropody checks, and personal care services,
such as hairdressing.
- Review each individual resident's care plan and ensure that individual needs are
documented and that action is taken on issues such as the need for new glasses or
dentures. Ensure that care plans are regularly reviewed.

- Nominate a key worker to assume responsibility for implementing and monitoring each individual resident's care plan.

Daily life and social activities

- Consult with residents about their ideas and priorities for how the home can be improved.
- Consult with residents about the menu and address issues regarding food supply and preparation with cook and kitchen team. Again this may involve a review of catering staff recruitment and training.

Environment

- Review policies and practices regarding cleaning of the home. Set clear standards and ensure that domestic staff are able to deliver these.
- Review supply of bed linen and laundry arrangements to ensure an adequate supply of clean bed linen.

Complaints and protection

- Set up a clear system for residents to raise complaints and issues within the home and make sure they are all fully informed about this.
- Make sure that residents and their families know how to make representation and complaints to the Commission for Social Care Inspection.
- Establish a clear policy regarding the unlocking of doors. Ensure that residents and their families and friends are informed about this. Record and manage any risks that the new policy presents.

Management and administration

- As a new manager, spend time getting to know every resident and every member of staff.
- Establish a residents' and friends'/relatives' committee to give the residents and their friends and families a say in how the home is run and provide a forum for their views to be communicated to staff.
- Set up regular staff meetings to review progress on achieving improvement in standards.

Choice

- It is likely that the current residents had little choice about coming to the home and many will feel they have little choice about moving elsewhere. Their satisfaction with their current living arrangements should be discussed at every review meeting.

- The aim would be to make the home a pleasant place that the residents would want to live in and a home that is attractive to potential new residents.

(For an account of a project that focused on these kind of issues in improving the standards of residential care, see Baldwin *et al.* 1993.)

ACTIVITY 4.5 A NEEDS-LED SERVICE?

Deciding whether to carry out an assessment

No. When local authorities are aware that someone may be in need of community care services, they have a duty to assess the person's need for services, regardless of their resources or whether the services in question are likely to be provided following the assessment.

Deciding who should be given help

Yes. Local authorities can take account of their resources in setting their eligibility criteria for service provision. It is these criteria that determine whether or not someone will receive services.

Deciding what services to provide

Yes. Local authorities can consider their resources and select the most economical way of providing a service, providing that it meets the eligible needs that have been identified in the assessment. In following this course of action, they would need to show that the service user's wishes, and those of any carers, had been taken into account.

Deciding after a period of time whether to continue providing services

Yes. Resources may be relevant to this decision if the local authority has changed its eligibility criteria in order to manage resource shortfalls. A person might no longer be eligible for a service even though their needs had not changed.

Deciding whether to accept responsibility for providing residential care

No. The local authority has a duty to provide residential accommodation where someone needs care and attention that is not otherwise available to them. This duty applies regardless of the local authority's finances. However, the finances of service users are relevant to determining whether the local authority has a duty to provide care. If their capital limit is above the current threshold, they are deemed to have care and attention available to them and the local authority would not have to provide accommodation – though it would still have a duty to assess need and help make the care arrangements, if necessary.

ACTIVITY 5.1 IDENTIFYING AND ADDRESSING BARRIERS TO CARRYING OUT AN ASSESSMENT AS AN 'EXCHANGE'

There are a number of factors that might present barriers to the assessment being a genuine exchange between you, Ranjana and other members of the family including:

- Your sense of being under pressure to contain costs and to get the assessment completed as soon as possible.
- Communication difficulties, if you are not a Punjabi speaker, because of Ranjana's limited knowledge of spoken English, compounded by the limited use you can make of non-verbal communication because of her visual impairment.
- Difficulties in engaging Ali and Meena fully in the assessment – Meena because she is depressed and Ali because of the stress and exhaustion he is experiencing.
- Ali's reluctance to discuss the situation openly with his mother.
- The GP may already have led Ali to believe that a place in a care home is the only option.
- Ranjana may be aware of the threat of 'going into a home' and may be resistant to you.
- Possible expectations and pressure from the GP that you will simply do what he has recommended.
- Your awareness of the limited services available may lead to a 'service-led' rather than 'needs-led' assessment.

(For a more general discussion of barriers to an exchange approach, see page 132).

You might be able to address some of these barriers by:

- arranging for an interpreter to be with you;
- stressing that you are 'starting from scratch' and that you want to understand how everyone is feeling;
- being clear with everyone involved (including the GP) that you will be exploring with them all of the options to help them deal with the situation and that a place in a care home is only one possible option;
- considering seeing Ranjana, Meena and Ali separately for part of the time;
- liaising with the hospital social worker to ensure that Meena's needs are considered;
- liaising with the children and families team and/or carer support services to explore support and relief for Ali;
- highlighting to your manager the complexity of the situation and the need for time to carry out a comprehensive assessment. If necessary economic arguments could be used: a superficial assessment might result in a care home admission

which could be a costly long-term commitment for the organisation. More time will allow less costly alternatives to be explored and, if appropriate, new services to be commissioned to support Ranjana at home;

- considering the need for an advocate who speaks Punjabi to help Ranjana represent her wishes.

ACTIVITY 5.2 ENGAGING IN POSITIVE COMMUNICATION

Examples of negative communications:

- *Disempowerment*: not allowing Jack to use his ability to communicate using his eyes or to appreciate jazz music.
- *Infantilisation*: dealing with Jack's physical needs but ignoring the fact that he is an adult with feelings, wishes and preferences.
- *Invalidation*: failing to acknowledge the subjective reality of Jack's experience and ignoring the significance of his personal biography.
- *Banishment*: excluding Jack psychologically by giving him no part in communications nor allowing him to make any mark on his environment.
- *Objectification*: treating Jack as if he were an object with no feelings.
- *Ignoring*: behaving as though Jack were not there.
- *Withholding*: refusing to give attention to Jack as a person (as opposed to Jack as a physical body).

Examples of positive communications:

- *Recognition*: acknowledging Jack as a person with important life experiences, interests and relationships and affirming his uniqueness.
- *Collaboration*: working with Jack on the shared task of presenting photos, using a process that involves the abilities he still has, instead of casting him in a passive role.
- *Timalation*: facilitating Jack's enjoyment of jazz music.
- *Validation*: devising approaches rooted in an understanding of Jack's situation and what this means for him.
- *Facilitation*: enabling Jack to take part in communications and reap enjoyment from music and family reminiscences.
- *Creation*: creating opportunities for Jack to become part of interactions as staff now have prompts around which to initiate communication.

ACTIVITY 5.3 USING NARRATIVES IN ASSESSMENT

Listening to an older person's narrative would help a social worker carrying out a community care assessment by: drawing out the impact of past life experiences on present circumstances; encouraging a rounded consideration of relationships and social networks; allowing an older person to be seen holistically in her or his social context; giving her or him the opportunity to express her or his hopes and fears; provide an understanding of and respect for her or his unique situation and characteristics and an appreciation of issues of diversity.

Community care assessments tend not to allow scope for individuals to tell their stories because they are frequently reduced to ticking boxes in order to provide crude data, as the basis for a managerial assessment geared to the allocation of resources. Time pressures can make social workers reluctant to explore areas that fall outside of the information required by these bureaucratic procedures.

You could increase the opportunities for older people to tell their stories by asking them to tell you about themselves, their lives and how they see their current situation and then listening carefully and respectfully. You may need to consider other ways that older people can communicate their stories, for example, by sharing activities that are important to them or looking at photographs. Giving opportunities for people to communicate their stories will require time and a suitable environment.

Listening to older people's narratives is likely to improve their experience of the assessment process and its outcomes because they are likely to feel respected and validated and to consider that their concerns have been recognised. Having space to tell their stories is likely to contribute to the development of a relationship of trust and to generate feelings of self-worth in the older person.

ACTIVITY 5.4 POSITIVE PRACTICE IN RECORDING

Negative phrases	Examples of more positive phrases
Mrs Brown is incontinent.	Mrs Brown is able to use the toilet herself but she needs regular reminding to go; or, Mrs Brown needs help to get on and off the toilet; or, Mrs Brown wears pads during the day and at night.
Mr Green is immobile.	Mr Green has full use of his arms and hands but he needs help to walk; or, Mr Green uses a wheelchair.
Ms Purple has early stage dementia.	Ms Purple has a very good memory for things that happened in the past but finds it difficult to remember recent events; or, Ms Purple feels that she can manage well at home but she becomes confused and gets lost easily when she goes out.
Mr Grey is unable to perform any personal care tasks for himself.	Mr Grey's mind is very active and he enjoys conversation but he needs help with tasks such as eating, washing, dressing and going to the toilet.
Mrs White is housebound and socially isolated.	Mrs White can move around slowly within the house but she needs help to go outside. She enjoys watching TV but misses having visitors and being able to go out.

ACTIVITY 6.1 EXPERIENCES OF PARTNERSHIP WORKING

As your response to this activity draws on your personal experience of partnership, it is difficult to provide pointers for it. Instead, when you have completed it, you may want to go back over the previous section in the chapter, 'Achieving effective partnerships', to assess the extent to which your experience accords with ideas presented there about effective partnership.

ACTIVITY 6.2 DISCHARGE PLANNING

The different expectations you encounter may result in tensions and conflicts. Hospital managers' expectations are likely to focus on your role in assisting them to meet performance targets by ensuring 'bed-space' is used 'efficiently' through achieving speedy discharge of patients. Ward staff may share some of the managers' expectations and, even if they do not, will be feeling pressured to comply with them. Accordingly, they are also likely to exert pressure for discharge as soon as possible but are more likely than managers to have a focus on whether proper arrangements are in place to support the older person's return home and to ensure continuing rehabilitation. Community support services will want to have sufficient notice to arrange services and to have clear and detailed information about the person's support needs. Your line manager/budget holder is likely to be concerned about the possible financial consequences, under the 'reimbursement policy', of any delay in discharge. Your manager's primary concern may, therefore, be with ensuring that the discharge happens within the required timescale, rather than that the arrangements made are appropriate. Your social work professional values stress considering the older person as an individual and undertaking a comprehensive assessment of what s/he needs to make discharge effective in her/his own terms. Social work colleagues may share those values but there may be a workplace culture of completing assessments and discharge planning speedily because of work pressures on the team and an emphasis on everybody showing that they are contributing to reducing those pressures in the interests of everyone else in the team. The older person may want to return home as quickly as possible or may be fearful about returning home, if s/he was feeling at risk before her or his admission to hospital. Either way, s/he is likely to want to feel that things are being properly thought through and that proper arrangements are in place before s/he is discharged. Carer(s)/family members are likely to be worried about the older person being discharged before s/he is ready and to be concerned that they will be asked to take on more of the caring because services are not available. They are likely to want the discharge to be carefully planned, allowing adequate time to ensure that appropriate support is in place for when the person is discharged.

ACTIVITY 6.3 THE ROLE OF TELECARE

Older people might feel more secure if they know such monitoring systems are in place. The availability of systems to respond to difficulties if they arise (such as alarm systems) may enable older people to live their lives more freely, without worrying so much about risks. They may feel more independent if they are managing with less direct 'care' from others. On the other hand, they may find telecare systems intrusive, both into their personal privacy and their home environment. They may see equipment in their homes as a marker of their 'need' or 'dependence' to be resisted.

Informal carers may feel reassured that there is now a way of 'keeping an eye on things' when no-one is with the older person and this may give them times when they feel freed up to do other things. However, both carers and older people may be concerned about the decrease in human contact that such systems encourage (see Beresford 2005).

Funders/commissioners of services might be attracted to telecare as a cost-effective option that is claimed to have beneficial outcomes for older people. Although there are initial outlay costs for telecare, the ongoing running costs are likely to be low compared with the staffing costs involved in direct care.

Provider agencies might be concerned that telecare will enable funders/commissioners to cut back on the contracts with them for the purchase of services involving direct contact with paid carers.

ACTIVITY 6.4 THE IMPACT OF CARERS' LEGISLATION

The local authorities were probably not publicising widely the possibility of having a carer's assessment or mentioning it routinely to those carers with whom they were in contact. Social workers may have been reluctant to encourage carers to have an assessment if they felt it was unlikely to result in additional services. Carers themselves may not have requested assessment, either because they did not perceive themselves as a 'carer', they were not aware of their entitlement to an assessment or they did not think the assessment would benefit them.

To increase the number of carers receiving an assessment, there could be wider publicity explaining who 'carers' are, what services are available to support them and how they can access these services. Social workers should routinely inform carers of their right to an assessment when they make contact with a carer for the first time and then at key points subsequently. They should record that a carer's assessment has been offered and note the outcome. A carer's assessment should be seen as a valuable process for helping carers to explore their needs and the different options for addressing them, rather than only of relevance if it leads to services provided by the authority (so there are similar arguments to those made concerning assessment under *Fair Access to Care Services* in Chapter 3).

Increasing the uptake of services by carers following assessments would require an increase in resources to make more services available locally and reduce waiting lists. The quality of existing services also needs to be improved so that carers are willing to receive them. If charges are a factor in carers not taking up services, charging policies need to be reviewed so that these costs do not prohibit carers from receiving the support they need. Making high quality service provision available and encouraging older people who are reluctant to receive services to sample them might minimise their resistance to accepting assistance from someone other than their usual informal carer(s). Social workers need to undertake sensitive assessments with both carers and the older people the carers are supporting in order to ensure that the needs of all parties are considered (see Chapter 7).

ACTIVITY 6.5 ENGAGING WITH CARERS' NEEDS

Sonia may need emotional support to enable her to cope with the demands that caring for Joe are making on her. This may include the need for counselling to explore her feelings about the loss of contact with her father in her earlier life, the death of her mother, the influence these factors have had on her hopes and expectations about her current relationship with her father and her feelings regarding his physical and verbal abuse of her. She may need counselling, either individually or with her partner, to consider the impact that caring for Joe is having on their relationship and to consider decisions about Joe and her partner in the light of what is important to her at this point in her life. Sonia may need practical support, for example help with laundry, if Joe is sometimes incontinent, and help to manage Joe's other personal care needs. She may need advice about further aids and adaptations that would make looking after Joe easier. She may need the chance for a break and the opportunity to spend time with her partner. She may need advice about welfare benefits that she may be able to claim. She may also need advice and information about the effects of stroke and long-term alcohol misuse and how to manage these. Just because Sonia is a trained nurse, it should not be assumed that she already has all of this information. Dealing with difficulties at a personal level is different from managing them professionally and neither Sonia herself, nor others, should expect that she is any more able to 'cope' than other people.

In terms of services that may be useful, Sonia could gain support from a local carers' centre, which could provide information and advice on a range of issues and the opportunity to join carer support groups. National carers' organisations could also be useful points of contact. Local support groups for relatives of people who have had a stroke or who misuse alcohol might also be helpful to her. Sonia might benefit from respite care, whether this takes the form of someone coming to sit with Joe during the day or Joe having respite care away from the home to give Sonia and her partner a break. Home care, a laundry service and mobile meals may also help Sonia in looking after Joe.

Joe's needs and wishes need to be considered by undertaking a separate assessment. Some services provided for Joe may have direct benefits for Sonia also. For example, Joe may be struggling to cope with his loss of independence following the stroke. Speech therapy (if he did not have this at the time) may help him communicate better and ease his frustration. Joe may (or may not) want help to deal with his alcohol problem. He may be depressed and the alcohol use may be linked with this. It is not clear what part Joe played in the decision to move in with Sonia. This may not be his preferred option but he may feel powerless to change the situation. All of these issues need to be explored fully with Joe. It may be useful for an advocate to be involved to get to know Joe well over a period of time, learn to understand his speech and help to represent his wishes.

ACTIVITY 7.1 PROMOTING INVOLVEMENT

From the brief details given about Fryderyk, it is not possible to say definitively how he lacks power or exercises it as we do not know enough about how he lives his life or about the dynamics of his relationship with Julia. For example, it cannot be assumed that

Fryderyk has been disempowered by Julia's hospitalisation. If, for example, Julia was abusive towards Fryderyk, it could be that he experiences her absence as a relief and an opportunity to exercise more power himself. The main point of this activity is to demonstrate how analysing individuals' lack of power or exercise of power can provide pointers for ways in which they can be assisted to exercise greater control in, or through, the social work process. For example, it may be that Fryderyk feels comfortable and in control within his home environment. He has been using a wheelchair for about 30 years and, although he now needs help to transfer to and from the wheelchair, he may feel in charge of most daily personal care and other routines, albeit with assistance. He becomes easily disorientated but may still feel a sense of control if the routines by which his life is ordered – for example, the day care, and respite service – are maintained. If this is established, it becomes important in this situation to try to retain those aspects of the situation that give him a sense of power and minimise those aspects that detract from this, such as instability and disruption. In Julia's absence, some disruption is inevitable but other changes could be kept to a minimum. Fryderyk is also likely to feel a lack of power if he does not understand where Julia is or what is happening. If, at times of stress, he loses some of his grasp of English, this would be a further loss of power.

As far as Fryderyk is concerned, the social worker may be the person who has the power to enable him to stay at home. The social worker, however, may feel a lack of power to act in a way that accords with Fryderyk's wishes and best interests. This may be because the services are not available or because the preferred service options are costly compared with alternative ways of addressing Fryderyk's needs. How the social worker responds to Fryderyk could be very significant in determining how much or how little power he feels in the situation. Fryderyk's involvement in the process of reassessing his needs and devising a new care plan should begin from where he is in relation to what's happening – what does it mean to and for him? Actions that might help to increase Fryderyk's sense of power include: making sure that he is given very clear information, repeated many times if necessary, about where Julia is and what has happened; involving someone who speaks Polish to enable Fryderyk to communicate in the language with which he is most at ease; involving someone who is familiar to him, perhaps to take him to see Julia to help him understand what has happened; trying to establish Fryderyk's needs and wishes by building a relationship with him (though recognising that support arrangements will need to be made quickly); explaining clearly to him what the different options are and their implications for him; and, when decisions have been made (hopefully with Fryderyk's involvement) making sure he understands what is going to happen. For the social worker, a sense of power may come from being clear about legal responsibilities, local policies and services and from using this knowledge to argue for whatever is thought to be the best option for Fryderyk.

ACTIVITY 7.2 DIFFERENT APPROACHES TO DEALING WITH RISK

In scenario 1, safety first predominates. The emphasis is on Mr A.'s physical health through the concentration on his dementia. His disabilities are stressed – he cannot manage in the kitchen, cannot make a cup of tea, would not be able to cope, etc. He is seen as in danger because he is disoriented and tries to leave the ward. The preoccupation is with getting control of him and his situation by doing what the assessor thinks is right in these circumstances. Certain risks are removed without full consideration being given either to how these could be managed or to new risks that may be presented by Mr A.'s admission to a care home.

In scenario 2 the emphasis is more on consideration of risk-taking in the interests of what will promote Mr A.'s well-being. He seems to be seen as having a right to live where he wishes and the assessor's views and actions are geared to maximising his choices and opportunities, notwithstanding his dementia. There is a strong commitment to identifying what he can do, for example he can find his way around his home and make tea. The care plan builds on his strengths and is oriented to managing risks in a manner that is least disruptive to his preferred way of living.

ACTIVITY 7.3 MANAGING RISKS

The purpose of this exercise is to illustrate how a comprehensive risk assessment can inform a plan to address the risks identified. To carry out the exercise, it is necessary to make certain assumptions about the values and preferences of Ann Lee and her daughter. In practice, Ann and her daughter would, of course, be involved as fully as possible in formulating the plan.

A care plan that would address the risks identified might include the following:

Dangers	Action
Hypothermia as a result of wandering when inadequately dressed	If/when Ann receives assistance to dress, ensure she wears warm undergarments and several layers in cold weather. Place large notices on and near the door reminding her to put on a coat.
Disorientation/getting lost when wandering	Give Ann a discreet identity note that she can wear (for example, as a necklace or bracelet), with her name, address and a contact number. Identify key people at strategic points along Ann's preferred route (for example, staff in shops, petrol station, etc.) and give them a contact number to call if they notice Ann appearing to be lost or distressed (this would require Ann's consent).
Food poisoning	Home carer or daughter to check old food is discarded and help Ann to buy food that does not need cooking. Some cooked meals to be provided by mobile meals or home carer/daughter helping Ann to cook. All food could be clearly labelled, telling Ann how it is to be prepared.
Daughter becoming depressed	Provide alternative support for Ann (ideally in her own home) so that her daughter can have complete breaks at regular intervals. Her daughter can also be offered various carer support services, such as counselling, relaxation and support groups. She may also want help to take up or continue work, leisure or social interests that give her satisfaction and a respite from caring.

All of the requirements set out in the *Code of Practice for Social Care Workers* (General Social Care Council 2002) and the values statements that form part of the *National Occupational Standards for Social Workers* (Training Organisation for the Personal Social Services 2002) would be important in working with Ann and her daughter, in particular: treating each person as a unique individual; helping Ann to express her wishes; respecting the views and wishes of both Ann and her daughter and treating them as experts on their own situations; ensuring that the care plan respects Ann's dignity and privacy as far as possible; working to promote Ann's independence; respecting Ann and her daughter's culture and values in planning and arranging support; maximising the involvement of Ann and her daughter in the care planning process; communicating openly and clearly in a way that is appropriate for Ann (and for her daughter); helping Ann to exercise her rights (for example, to leave her home when she wants to); helping Ann to take steps to manage risks; with Ann's consent (or that of her daughter acting on her behalf, if necessary), informing other agencies, as relevant, of the plans to address risks.

ACTIVITY 7.4 PLANNING AND PROVIDING 'GOOD CARE'

In terms of Brechin's model of quality of care (see Figure 7.2), it would be important to consider the relationships from the perspectives of Nora, Alan and Sylvia. The aim would be to remove or reduce the damaging aspects of the relationships and increase the rewarding aspects for each party. As with the previous activity, we do not have detailed information about the different individuals' needs and perspectives, so we have to make certain assumptions for the purpose of completing the activity. In practice, the individuals concerned would themselves play the main role in identifying the positive and negative dimensions of the relationships. The following are therefore only examples of the ways the relationships might be analysed:

Nora: The rewards from her relationship with Alan may be his company and attention, as this relieves her loneliness. The damaging aspect might be the continual fear that Alan will move to Spain.
Alan: He may derive satisfaction from caring for his mother, feeling that this repays her for the support she has given him earlier in life. The damaging aspect may be the demands she makes on his time, the guilt this causes him if he does not respond and the resentment it generates in Sylvia if he does.
Sylvia: The rewards from her relationship with Nora may come from Alan's appreciation and gratitude for the practical support that she gives Nora. The damaging aspect may be the way that Nora's demands on Alan's time interfere with the relationship between Sylvia and Alan and their plans for their retirement.

A plan (which would, of course, have to be carefully negotiated with each party) to increase rewards and reduce damaging aspects of the relationships might include: helping Nora to find other avenues for companionship to reduce her need for Alan's time; encouraging Alan and Sylvia to agree plans for their future and communicate these to Nora to alleviate her continual anxiety about this issue; working out with Nora, Sylvia and Alan an agreed schedule for when Alan will see Nora and other times that will be reserved for Alan and Sylvia to do things together and encouraging them all to adhere to this; working with Sylvia and Nora to seek to improve their relationship so that Alan can spend time with both of them together.

In terms of the six senses identified by Nolan *et al.* (2003), additional approaches that may be indicated include:

- increasing Nora's sense of security within her home and community environment, by, for example: arranging a visit from the crime prevention service; helping Nora to buy a personal alarm to take when she goes out; finding a befriender to take her out so she is not alone; and introducing her to her neighbours to reduce her fears and suspicions about them and, hopefully, help her to see them as possible sources of support if she needs help;
- helping Alan to consider what gives him a sense of purpose: it may be that since retirement from work, he is gaining a sense of purpose from his role in Nora's life. The work may involve helping Sylvia to understand that meeting Nora's needs is giving Alan a sense of purpose, or it may involve considering with Alan and Sylvia sources of help to examine their relationship;
- helping Sylvia to increase her sense of significance: this may involve helping Alan to find ways to spend more time with Sylvia and/or show her that she is important to him; or it could mean helping Sylvia to find personally rewarding ways to spend her time when Alan is busy supporting Nora.

These are only examples; you may well have come up with different ideas based on the information given. Also, you will see that various possibilities are presented here by way of example. Detailed discussion and exploration would be needed with Nora, Alan and Sylvia to work out a plan that enabled each of them to increase the level at which their 'six senses' are met.

NOTES

INTRODUCTION

1 In Chapter 2, and throughout the rest of the book, any recent policy and legislation to which we refer either applies to the whole of the UK or applies specifically to England. For reasons of space we have been unable to provide comprehensive accounts of the ways in which the individual countries of the UK have moved along different trajectories.

1 UNDERSTANDING LATER LIFE

1 Whilst Butler, and this book, are concerned with connecting ageism to old age, people of any age can be subject to ageism. Teenagers, for example, may be subject to negative social stereotypes and hostile attitudes simply as a consequence of their age.

4 PLANNING AND PROVIDING SERVICES

1 See Clements (2004: ch. 5) for a review of this legal judgment and the other judgments mentioned in this section.

6 WORKING IN PARTNERSHIP

1 Carer's Addition is an extra component, paid on top of Pension Credit, for pensioners on low income who are entitled to Carer's Allowance but are not paid it because their pension exceeds the Carer's Allowance ('the overlapping benefit rule'). Carer's Addition can in these circumstances be claimed instead (Carers UK 2005).

BIBLIOGRAPHY

Acheson, D. (1998) *Independent Inquiry into Inequalities in Health Report*, Chaired by Sir Donald Acheson, London: Stationery Office.

Adams, S. (2003) 'Healthy homes, healthier lives', *Housing, Care and Support* 6: 21–6.

—— (2006) *Small Things Matter: The Key Role of Handyperson Services*, Nottingham: Care and Repair England.

Age Concern (2003) *One in Four Single Women Pensioners Lives in Poverty*, London: Age Concern England/Fawcett Society.

—— (2005a) *Modernising the Regulation of Social Care: Age Concern's Response to 'Inspecting Better Lives'*, London: Age Concern England.

—— (2005b) *Human Rights: Policy Position Paper*, London: Age Concern England.

—— (2006a) *How Ageist is Britain?* London: Age Concern England.

—— (2006b) *Dignity, Security, Opportunity: A Decent Income for Current and Future Pensioners*, London: Age Concern England.

—— (2006c) *What Older People Want from Community Health and Social Care Services*, London: Age Concern England.

—— (2006d) *Housing Policy Position Paper*, London: Age Concern England.

Age Concern England, Alzheimer's Society, Help the Aged and Royal College of Nursing (2006) *Guide to Fully Funded NHS Care*, London: Royal College of Nursing. Online at www.ace.org.uk/AgeConcern/Documents/Guide_to_fully_funded_NHS_care.pdf (accessed 27 November 2006).

Age Positive (2005) *Age Discrimination Legislation*. Online at www.agepositive.gov.uk (accessed 3 January 2006).

Andrews, M. (1999) 'The seductiveness of agelessness', *Ageing and Society* 19: 301–18.

Appleton, N. (2002) *Planning for the Majority: The Needs and Aspirations of Older People in General Housing*, York: York Publishing Services.

Arber, S. and Evandrou, M. (1993) 'Mapping the territory: ageing, independence and the life course', in S. Arber and M. Evandrou (eds) *Ageing, Independence and the Life Course*, London: Jessica Kingsley Publishers.

Arber, S. and Ginn, J. (eds) (1995) *Connecting Gender and Ageing: A Sociological Approach*, Buckingham: Open University Press.

Arber, S., Davidson, K. and Ginn, J. (eds) (2003a) *Gender and Ageing: Changing Roles and Relationships*, Maidenhead: Open University Press.

—— (2003b) 'Changing approaches to gender and later life', in S. Arber, K. Davidson and J. Ginn (eds) *Gender and Ageing: Changing Roles and Relationships*, Maidenhead: Open University Press.

Association of Directors of Social Services (2003) *All Our Tomorrows: Inverting the Triangle of Care*, London: Association of Directors of Social Services/Local Government Association.

Atchley, R. (1989) 'A continuity theory of normal ageing', *The Gerontologist* 29: 183–90.

Audit Commission (1986) *Making a Reality of Community Care*, London: HMSO.

—— (1997) *The Coming of Age: Improving Care Services for Older People*, London: Audit Commission.

—— (2004) *Older People – Independence and Well-being: The Challenge for Public Services*, London: Audit Commission.

Baldock, J. and Hadlow, J. (2002) 'Self-talk versus needs-talk: an exploration of the priorities of housebound older people', *Quality in Ageing – Policy, Practice and Research* 3: 42–8.

Baldock, J. and Ungerson, C. (1994) *Becoming Consumers of Community Care: Households Within the Mixed Economy of Welfare*, York: Joseph Rowntree Foundation.

Baldwin, M. (2000) *Care Management and Community Care: Social Work Discretion and the Construction of Policy*, Aldershot: Ashgate.

Baldwin, N. and Walker, L. (2005) 'Assessment', in R. Adams, L. Dominelli and M. Payne (eds) *Social Work Futures: Crossing Boundaries, Transforming Practice*, Basingstoke: Palgrave Macmillan.

Baldwin, N., Harris, John, Littlechild, R. and Pearson, M. (1993) *Residents' Rights: Key Issues in the Power to Care in Homes for Older People*, Aldershot: Avebury.

Ballinger, C. and Payne, S. (2002) 'The construction of the risk of falling among and by older people', *Ageing and Society* 22: 305–24.

Banks, S. (2001, 2nd edn) *Ethics and Values in Social Work*, Basingstoke: Palgrave.

Barnes, M. and Bennett, G. (1998) 'Frail bodies, courageous voices: older people influencing community care', *Health and Social Care in the Community* 6: 102–11.

Barnes, M., Blom, A., Cox, K., Lessof, C. and Walker, A. (2006) *New Horizons: The Social Exclusion of Older People – Secondary Analysis of the English Longitudinal Study of Ageing*, London: National Centre for Social Research and University of Sheffield.

Bauman, Z. (2004, 2nd edn) *Work, Consumerism and the New Poor*, Maidenhead: Open University Press.

Beaumont, G., Kenealy, P., Murrell, R., Callander, G., Kingsley, B. and Golden, A. (2002) 'Psychological processes and perceived quality of life in the healthy elderly', *Proceedings of the British Psychological Society* 10: 54.

Beckett, C. and Maynard, A. (2005) *Values and Ethics in Social Work: An Introduction*, London: Sage.

Bengtson, V., Putney, N. and Johnson, M. (2005) 'The problem of theory in gerontology today', in M. Johnson (ed.) with V. Bengtson, P. Coleman and T. Kirkwood (eds) *The Cambridge Handbook of Age and Ageing*, Cambridge: Cambridge University Press.

Bennett, K., Smith, P. and Hughes, G. (2004) *Older Widow(er)s: Bereavement and Gender Effects on Lifestyle and Participation*, Economic and Social Research Council, Growing Older Programme, Findings 6. Online at www.shef.ac.uk/uni/projects/gop (accessed 19 June 2004).

Beresford, P. (2003) *It's Our Lives: A Short Theory of Knowledge, Distance and Experience*, London: Citizen Press.

—— (2005) 'Gadgets don't care', *Community Care* 18–24 August: 16.

Beresford, P. and Croft, S. (2001) 'Service users' knowledges and the social construction of social work', *Journal of Social Work* 1: 295–316.

Bernard, M. and Harding Davies, V. (2000) 'Our ageing selves: reflections on growing older', in M. Bernard, J. Phillips, L. Machin and V. Harding Davies (eds) *Women Ageing: Changing Identities, Challenging Myths*, London: Routledge.

Better Government for Older People (2000) *All Our Futures*, London: Cabinet Office.

Bigby, C. (2004) *Ageing with a Lifelong Disability: A Guide to Practice, Program and Policy Issues for Human Services Professionals*, London: Jessica Kingsley.

Biggs, S. (1997) 'Choosing not to be old: masks, bodies and identity management in later life', *Ageing and Society* 18: 553–70.

—— (1999) *The Mature Imagination: Dynamics of Identity in Middle Life and Beyond*, Buckingham: Open University Press.

Biggs, S., Phillipson, C., Money, A. and Leach, R. (2006) 'The age-shift: observations on social policy, ageism and the dynamics of the adult life course', *Journal of Social Work Practice* 20: 239–50.

Blakemore, K. and Boneham, M. (1994) *Age, Race and Ethnicity: A Comparative Approach*, Buckingham: Open University Press.

Bond, J. and Corner, L. (2004) *Quality of Life and Older People*, Maidenhead: Open University Press.

Bornat, J. (1998) 'Anthology: voices from the institutions', in M. Allott and M. Robb (eds) *Understanding Health and Social Care: An Introductory Reader*, London: Sage.

—— (1999) 'Introduction', in J. Bornat (ed.) *Biographical Interviews: The Link Between Research and Practice*, London: Centre for Policy on Ageing.

—— (2005) 'Listening to the past: reminiscence and oral history', in M. Johnson (ed.) with V. Bengtson, P. Coleman and T. Kirkwood (eds) *The Cambridge Handbook of Age and Ageing*, Cambridge: Cambridge University Press.

Bovens, M. and Zouridis, S. (2002) 'From street-level to system-level bureaucracies: how information and communication technology is transforming administrative discretion and constitutional control', *Public Administration Review* 62: 174–84.

Bowes, A. (2006) 'Mainstreaming equality: implications of the provision of support at home for majority and minority ethnic older people', *Social Policy and Administration* 40(7): 739–57.

Bowes, A. and Sim, D. (2006) 'Advocacy for black and minority ethnic communities: understandings and expectations', *British Journal of Social Work* 36: 1209–25.

Bowling, A., Grundy, E. and Farhquar, M. (1997) *Living Well into Old Age: Three Studies of Health and Well-being Among Older People in East London and Essex*, London: Age Concern England.

Bradshaw, J. (1972) 'The concept of social need', *New Society* 30 March: 640–3.

Brammer, A. (2003) *Social Work Law*, Harlow: Pearson Education.

Brandstädter, J. and Greve, W. (1994) 'The ageing self: stabilizing and protective processes', *Developmental Review* 14: 52–80.

Braye, S. (2000) 'Participation and involvement in social care: an overview', in H. Kemshall and R. Littlechild (eds) *User Involvement and Participation in Social Care: Research Informing Practice*, London: Jessica Kingsley.

Braye, S. and Preston-Shoot, M. (1995) *Empowering Practice in Social Care*, Buckingham: Open University Press.

Brayne, H. and Carr, H. (2003, 8th edn) *Law for Social Workers*, Oxford: Oxford University Press.

Brearley, C. (1982) *Risks and Social Work: Hazards and Helping*, London: Routledge and Kegan Paul.

Brechin, A. (1998) 'What makes for good care?' in A. Brechin, J. Walmsley, J. Katz and S. Peace (eds) *Care Matters: Concepts, Practice and Research in Health and Social Care*, London: Sage.

—— (2000)'Introducing critical practice', in A. Brechin, H. Brown, and M. Eby (eds) *Critical Practice in Health and Social Care*, London: Sage.

Buchanan, J. and Carnwell, R. (2005) 'Developing best practice in partnership', in R. Carnwell and J. Buchanan (eds) *Effective Practice in Health and Social Care: A Partnership Approach*, Maidenhead: Open University Press.

Bury, M. and Holme, A. (1991) *Life After Ninety*, London: Routledge.

Butler, R. (1987) 'Ageism', in *The Encyclopaedia of Aging*, New York: Springer.

Butt, J. and Moriarty, J. (2004) 'Social support and ethnicity in old age', in A. Walker and C. Hagan Hennessy (eds) *Growing Older: Quality of Life in Old Age*, Buckingham: Open University Press.

Butt, J. and O'Neil, A. (2004) *'Let's Move On': Black and Minority Ethnic Older People's Views on Research Findings*, York: Joseph Rowntree Foundation.

Butt, J., Bignall, T. and Stone, E. (eds) (2000) 'Directing support: report from a workshop on direct payments and black and minority ethnic disabled people', unpublished, cited in K. Chahal (2004) *Experiencing Ethnicity: Discrimination and Service Provision*, York: Joseph Rowntree Foundation. Online at www.jrf.org.uk/knowledge/findings/foundations/pdf/914.pdf (accessed 27 October 2006).

Bytheway, B. (1995) *Ageism*, Buckingham: Open University Press.

Bytheway, B. and Johnson, J. (1998) 'The social construction of "carers"', in A. Symonds and A. Kelly (eds) *The Social Construction of Community Care*, Basingstoke: Macmillan.

Caldock, K. (1996) 'Multi-disciplinary assessment and care management', in J. Phillips and B. Penhale (eds) *Reviewing Care Management for Older People*, London: Jessica Kingsley Publishers.

Caldock, K. and Nolan, M. (1994) 'Assessment and community care: are the reforms working?', *Generations Review* 4: 2–7.

Care and Repair England (2006) *Facts and Figures: Health and Well-being*, Nottingham: Care and Repair England. Online at www.careandrepair-england.org.uk/factshwb.htm (accessed 14 September 2006).

Carers UK (2002) *Without Us? Calculating the Value of Carers' Support*, London: Carers UK.

—— (2005) *Caring and Pensioner Poverty: A Report on Older Carers, Employment and Benefits*, London: Carers UK.

Carnwell, R. and Carson, A. (2005) 'Understanding partnerships and collaboration', in R. Carnwell and J. Buchanan (eds) *Effective Practice in Health and Social Care: A Partnership Approach*, Maidenhead: Open University Press.

Carson, D. (1988) 'Taking risks with patients: your assessment strategy', *Professional Nurse* April: 247–50.

Carson, G. (2006) 'Significant cost-shunting from NHS to social care revealed by survey', *Community Care* 27 July–2 August 2006: 12.

Challis, D. (1994) *Implementing Caring For People. Care Management: Factors Influencing its Development in the Implementation of Community Care*, London: HMSO.

Challis, D. and Davies, B. (1986) *Case Management in Community Care: An Evaluated Experiment in the Home Care of the Elderly*, Aldershot: Gower.

Challis, D., Darton, R., Johnson, L., Stone, M. and Traske, K. (1990) *Case Management in Health and Social Care: An Evaluation of an Alternative to Long-stay Hospital Care for Frail Elderly People, Discussion Paper 696*, University of Kent: Personal Social Services Research Unit.

Chesterman, J., Challis, D. and Davies, B. (1994) 'Budget-devolved care management in two routine programmes: have they improved outcomes?', in D. Challis, B. Davies and K. Traske (eds) *Community Care: New Agendas and Challenges from the UK and Overseas*, Aldershot: Ashgate.

Clark, H., Dyer, S., and Horwood, J. (1998) *'That Bit of Help': The High Value of Low Level Preventative Services for Older People*, Bristol: The Policy Press.

Clark, H., Gough, H. and Macfarlane, A. (2004) *It Pays Dividends: Direct Payments and Older People*, Bristol/York: The Policy Press/Joseph Rowntree Foundation.

Clarke, J. and Langan, M. (1998) 'Review', in M. Langan (ed.) *Welfare: Needs, Rights and Risks*, London: Routledge.

Clarke, J., Gewirtz, S., Hughes, G. and Humphrey J. (2000) 'Guarding the public interest? Auditing public services', in J. Clarke, S. Gewirtz and E. McLaughlin (eds) *New Managerialism, New Welfare?*, London: Sage.

Clements, L. (2004, 3rd edn) *Community Care and the Law*, London: Legal Action Group.

Coleman, N. and Harris, John (forthcoming) 'Calling Social Work', *British Journal of Social Work*, advance online access 11/12/06, http://bjsw.oxfordjournals.org/cgi/reprint/bcl371v1

Coleman, P., Ivani-Chalian, C. and Robinson, M. (1998) 'The story continues: persistence of life themes in old age', *Ageing and Society* 18: 389–419.

Coleman, P., McKiernan, F., Mills, M. and Speck, P. (2002) 'Spiritual belief and quality of life: the experience of older bereaved spouses', *Quality in Ageing: Policy, Practice and Research* 3: 20–6.

Coleman, R. (2000) 'Design for later life: beyond a problem orientation', in A. Warnes, L. Warren and M. Nolan (eds) *Care Services for Later Life: Transformations and Critiques*, London: Jessica Kingsley Publishers.

Commission for Social Care Inspection (2004a) *Direct Payments: What are the Barriers?*, London: Commission for Social Care Inspection.

—— (2004b) *When I Get Older: What People Want from Social Care Services and Inspections as they Get Older*, London: Commission for Social Care Inspection.

—— (2004c) *Leaving Hospital: The Price of Delays*, London: Commission for Social Care Inspection.

—— (2005a) *Inspecting for Better Lives: Delivering Change*, London: Commission for Social Care Inspection. Online at www.csci.org.uk/publications/national_reports/ibl_2.pdf (accessed 31 July 2006).

—— (2005b) *Leaving Hospital – Revisited: A Follow-up Study of a Group of Older People who were Discharged from Hospital in March 2004*, London: Commission for Social Care Inspection.

—— (2006a) *Time to Care: An Overview of Home Care Services for Older People in England*, London: Commission for Social Care Inspection.

—— (2006b) *Making Choices: Taking Risks*, London: Commission for Social Care Inspection.

Community Care (2003) 'News', 30 Oct–5 Nov: 15.

Connidis, I. (2003) 'Bringing outsiders in: gay and lesbian family ties over the life course', in S. Arber, K. Davidson and J. Ginn (eds) *Gender and Ageing: Changing Roles and Relationships*, Maidenhead: Open University Press.

Cornes, M. and Manthorpe, J. (2004) 'Making partnership work', *Working with Older People* 8: 19–24.

Corrigan, P. and Leonard, P. (1978) *Social Work Practice Under Capitalism: A Marxist Approach*, London: Macmillan.

Coulshed, V. and Orme, J. (1998, 3rd edn) *Social Work Practice: An Introduction*, Basingstoke: Macmillan.

Craig, C. (2004) 'Reaching out with the arts: meeting with the person with dementia', in A. Innes, C. Archibald and C. Murphy (eds) *Dementia and Social Inclusion: Marginalised Groups and Marginalised Areas of Dementia Research, Care and Practice*, London: Jessica Kingsley Publishers.

Crane, M., Warnes, A. and Fu, R. (2006) 'Developing homelessness prevention practice: combining research evidence and professional knowledge', *Health and Social Care in the Community* 14: 156–66.

Croucher, K. (2006) *Making the Case for Retirement Villages*, York: Joseph Rowntree Foundation.

Cumming, E. and Henry, W. (1961) *Growing Old: The Process of Disengagement*, New York: Basic Books.

D'Aboville, E. (1994) *Promoting User Involvement*, London: King's Fund.

Daichman, L. (2005) 'Elder abuse in developing nations', in M. Johnson (ed.) with V. Bengtson, P. Coleman and T. Kirkwood (eds) *The Cambridge Handbook of Age and Ageing*, Cambridge: Cambridge University Press.

Davies, B. and Knapp, M. (eds) (1988) 'The production of welfare approach: evidence and argument from the PSSRU', *British Journal of Social Work*, supplement to vol. 18.

Davies, B., Baines, B. and Chesterman, J. (1996) 'The effects of care management on efficiency in long-term care: a new evaluation model applied to British and American data', in J. Phillips and B. Penhale (eds) *Reviewing Care Management for Older People*, London: Jessica Kingsley Publishers.

Davies, B., Bebbington, A. and Charnley, H. (1990) *Resources, Needs and Outcomes in Community-Based Care: A Comparative Study of the Production of Welfare for Elderly People in Ten Local Authorities in England and Wales*, Aldershot: Ashgate.

Department for Work and Pensions (2005) *Opportunity Age: Meeting the Challenges of Ageing in the 21st Century*, London: Department for Work and Pensions.

—— (2006) *Security in Retirement: Towards a New Pensions System*, London: Department for Work and Pensions.

Department of Constitutional Affairs (2005) *Human Rights Act Guidance for Public Authorities: Contracting for Services*, London: Department of Constitutional Affairs.

—— (2006) *Mental Capacity Act Draft Code of Practice (for Consultation)*, London: Department of Constitutional Affairs.

Department of Health (1989) *Caring for People: Community Care in the Next Decade and Beyond*, London: HMSO.

—— (1990) *Community Care in the Next Decade and Beyond: Policy Guidance*, London: HMSO.

—— (1992) *Memorandum on the Financing of Community Care Arrangements after April 1992*, London: Department of Health.

—— (1993) *Approvals and Directions for Arrangements from 1 April 1993 made under Section 8 to the NHS Act 1977 and Sections 21 and 29 of the National Assistance Act 1948*, (LAC[93]10), London: Department of Health.

—— (1997a) *Better Management, Better Care: The Sixth Annual Report of the Chief Inspector*, London: Social Services Inspectorate/Department of Health.

—— (1997b) *Better Services for Vulnerable People*, EL(97)62, CI(97)24, Department of Health.

—— (1997c) *The New NHS: Modern, Dependable*, London: Department of Health.

—— (1998a) *Modernising Social Services: Promoting Independence, Improving Protection, Raising Standards*, London: Department of Health.

—— (1998b) *A Sharper Focus: Inspection of Social Services for Adults who are Visually Impaired or Blind*, London: Department of Health.

—— (1999a) *That's the Way the Money Goes: Inspection of Commissioning Arrangements for Community Care Services*, London: Department of Health.

—— (1999b) *Modern Social Services – A Commitment to Improve: The Eighth Annual Report of the Chief Inspector of Social Services 1998/99*, London: Social Services Inspectorate/Department of Health.

—— (1999c) *Caring about Carers: A National Strategy for Carers*, London: Department of Health.

—— (2000) *The Government's Response to the Royal Commission on Long Term Care*, London: Department of Health.

—— (2001a) *The National Service Framework for Older People*, London: Department of Health.

—— (2001b) *Fairer Charging Policies for Home Care and other Non-Residential Social Services: Guidance for Councils with Social Services Responsibilities*, LAC (2001)32, London: Department of Health.

—— (2001c) *NHS Funded Nursing Care: Practice Guide and Work Book*, London: Department of Health.

—— (2001d) *Continuing Care: NHS and Local Councils' Responsibilities*, (HSC2001/15; LAC(2001)18), London: Department of Health.

—— (2001e) *Intermediate Care*, HSC 2001/001, LAC (2001)1, London: Department of Health.

—— (2001f) *Carers and People with Parental Responsibility for Disabled Children: Practice Guidance*, London: Department of Health.

—— (2002a) *Focus on the Future: Key Messages from Focus Groups about the Future of Social Work Training*, London: Department of Health.

—— (2002b) *Fair Access to Care Services*, London: Department of Health.

—— (2002c) *The Single Assessment Process for Older People*, London: Department of Health.

—— (2002d) *The Single Assessment Process Summary: A Worked Example*, London: Department of Health.

—— (2002e) *Fairer Charging Policies for Home Care and other Non-residential Services: Practice Guidance*, London: Department of Health.

—— (2003a) *The Community Care, Services for Carers and Children's Services (Direct Payments) (England) Regulations 2003*, London: Department of Health.

—— (2003b) *Direct Payments Guidance: Community Care, Services for Carers and Children's Services (Direct Payments)*, London: Department of Health.

—— (2003c) *Fairer Charging Policies for Home Care and Other Non-residential Social Services: Practice Guidance*, London: Department of Health.

—— (2003d, 3rd edn) *Care Homes for Older People: National Minimum Standards and Care Homes Regulations 2001*, London: Department of Health.

—— (2003e) *Domiciliary Care: National Minimum Standards*, London: Department of Health.

—— (2004a) *The Community Care Assessment Directions 2004, LAC(2004)24*, London: Department of Health.

—— (2004b) *Guidance on the National Assistance Act 1948 (Choice of Accommodation Directions 1992 and National Assistance (Residential Accommodation) (Additional Payments and Assessment of Resources) (Amendment) (England) Regulations 2001, LAC (2004)20*, London: Department of Health.

—— (2004c) *A Guide to Receiving Direct Payments from your Local Council: A Route to Independent Living*, London: Department of Health.

—— (2005a) *Independence, Well-Being and Choice: Our Vision for the Future of Social Care for Adults in England and Wales*, Cm 6499, London: Department of Health.

—— (2005b) *Responses to the Consultation on Adult Social Care in England: Analysis of Feedback from the Green Paper 'Independence, Well-being and Choice'*, London: Department of Health.

—— (2005c) *Building Telecare in England*, London: Department of Health.

—— (2005d) *Carers and Disabled Children Act 2000 and Carers (Equal Opportunities) Act 2004: Combined Policy Guidance*, London: Department of Health.

—— (2006a) *A New Ambition for Old Age: Next Steps in Implementing the National Service Framework for Older People*, London: Department of Health.

—— (2006b) *Our Health, Our Care, Our Say: A New Direction for Community Services*, Cm 6737, London: Department of Health.

—— (2006c) *Making it Happen: Pilots, Early Implementers and Demonstration Sites – Health and Social Care Working in Partnership*, London: Department of Health.

—— (2006d) *Partnerships for Older People Projects Grant: Guidance Note for Applications for 2007/2008*, London: Department of Health.

—— (2006e) *The Mental Health Bill: Plans to Amend the Mental Health Act 1993. Briefing Sheets on Key Policy Areas where Changes are Proposed*, London: Department of Health.

—— (2006f) *The Caldicott Guardian Manual 2006*, London: Department of Health.

—— (2006g) *About Dignity in Care*, London: Department of Health. Online at http://www.dh.gov.uk/en/Policyandguidance/Healthandsocialcaretopics/Socialcare/Dignityincare/DH_4134922 (accessed 2 December 2006).

—— (2007) *Charges for Residential Accommodation – CRAG Amendment no. 26, LAC (2007) 4*, London: Department of Health.

Department of Health/Office of the Deputy Prime Minister (2000) *Quality and Choice in Older People's Housing*, London: Department of Health/Office of the Deputy Prime Minister.

Department of Health/Price Waterhouse (1991) *Implementing Community Care: Purchaser, Commissioner and Provider Roles*, London: HMSO.

Descombes, C. (2004) 'The smoke and mirrors of empowerment: a critique of user-professional partnership', in M. Robb, S. Barrett, C. Komaromy and A. Rogers (eds) *Communication, Relationships and Care: A Reader*, London: Routledge.

Dominelli, L. (2002) *Anti-Oppressive Social Work Theory and Practice*, Basingstoke: Macmillan.

Drakeford, M. (2006) 'Ownership, regulation and the public interest: the case of residential care for older people', *Critical Social Policy* 26: 932–44.

Dunning, A. (2005) *Information, Advice and Advocacy for Older People: Defining and Developing Services*, York: Joseph Rowntree Foundation.

Dwyer, S. (2005) 'Older people and permanent care: whose decision?', *British Journal of Social Work* 35: 1081–92.

Easterbrook, L. (1999) *When We are Very Old: Reflections on Treatment, Care and Support of Older People*, London: King's Fund.

—— (2002) *Healthier Homes, Healthier Lives*, Nottingham: Care and Repair England.

Ellis, K., Davis, A. and Rummery, K. (1999) 'Needs assessment, street-level bureaucracy and the new community care', *Social Policy and Administration* 33: 262–80.

Ely, M., Vinz, R., Downing, M. and Anzul, M. (1997) *On Writing Qualitative Research: Living by Words*, London: Falmer Press.

Erikson, E. (1977) *Childhood and Society*, London: Paladin.

Estes, C., Biggs, S. and Phillipson, C. (2003) *Social Theory, Social Policy and Ageing: A Critical Introduction*, Maidenhead: Open University Press.

Evans, T. and Harris, John (2004a) 'Citizenship, social inclusion and confidentiality' (with Tony Evans), *British Journal of Social Work* 34: 69–91.

—— (2004b) 'Street-level bureaucracy, social work and the (exaggerated) death of discretion', *British Journal of Social Work* 34: 871–95.

Featherstone, M. and Hepworth, M. (1989) 'Ageing and old age: reflections on the postmodern life course', in B. Bytheway, T. Keil, P. Allat and A. Bryman (eds) *Becoming and Being Old*, London: Sage.

Fernandez-Ballesteros, R., Zamarron, M. and Ruiz, M. (2001) 'The contribution of socio-demographic and psychosocial factors to life satisfaction', *Ageing and Society* 21: 25–43.

Finch, J. and Groves, D. (1980) 'Community care and the family: a case for equal opportunities?' *Journal of Social Policy* 9: 487–514.

Flynn, N. (1993, 2nd edn) *Public Sector Management*, Hemel Hempstead: Harvester Wheatsheaf.

Fook, J. (2002) *Social Work: Critical Theory and Practice*, London: Sage.

Froggett, L. (2002) *Love, Hate and Welfare: Psychosocial Approaches to Policy and Practice*, Bristol: The Policy Press.

Gabriel, Z. and Bowling, A. (2004) 'Quality of life in old age from the perspectives of older people', in A. Walker and C. Hagan Hennessy (eds) *Growing Older: Quality of Life in Old Age*, Maidenhead: Open University Press.

Gainsbury, S. (2006) 'NHS debts fuel bed-blocking surge', *Public Finance*, news analysis, 19 May. Online at www.publicfinance.co.uk (accessed 12 July 2006).

Gearing B. and Coleman, P. (1996) 'Biographical assessment in community care', in J. Birren, G. Kenyon, J. Ruth, J. Schroots and T. Svensson (eds) *Ageing and Biography: Explorations in Adult Development*, New York: Springer Publishing.

General Social Care Council (2002) *Code of Practice for Social Care Workers*, London: GSCC.

George, L. and Bearon, L. (1980) *Quality of Life in Older Persons: Meaning and Measurement*, New York: Human Science Press.

Gibson, F. (1993) 'The use of the past', in A. Chapman and M. Marshall (eds), *Dementia: New Skills for Social Workers*, London: Jessica Kingsley Publishers.

Gilleard, C. (1996) 'Consumption and identity in later life: toward a cultural gerontology', *Ageing and Society* 16: 489–98.

Glasby, J. (2004) 'Social services and the Single Assessment Process: early warning signs?', *Journal of Interprofessional Care* 18: 129–39.

Glasby, J. and Littlechild, R. (2002) *Social Work and Direct Payments*, Bristol: The Policy Press.

—— (2004) *The Health and Social Care Divide: The Experiences of Older People*, Bristol: The Policy Press.

Godfrey, M. (2001) 'Prevention: developing a framework for conceptualising and evaluating outcomes of preventive services for older people', *Health and Social Care in the Community* 9(2): 89–99.

Godfrey, M. and Callaghan, G. (2000) *Exploring Unmet Need: The Challenge of a User-centred Response*, York: Joseph Rowntree Foundation.

Godfrey, M. and Denby, T. (2004) *Depression and Older People: Towards Securing Well-being in Later Life*, Bristol: The Policy Press/Help the Aged.

Godfrey, M., Townsend, J. and Denby, T. (2004) *Building a Good Life for Older People in Local Communities: The Experience of Ageing in Time and Place*, York: Joseph Rowntree Foundation.

Gorman, H. (2003) 'Which skills do care managers need? A research project on skills, competency and continuing professional development', *Social Work Education* 22: 245–61.

Gough, O. (2001) 'The impact of the gender pay gap on post-retirement earnings', *Critical Social Policy* 21: 311–34.

Graham, H. (1983) 'Caring: a labour of love', in J. Finch and D. Groves (eds) *A Labour of Love: Women, Work and Caring*, London: Routledge and Kegan Paul.

Grant, L. (1999) *Remind Me Who I Am, Again*, London: Granta Books.

Grenier, A. (2004) 'Older women negotiating uncertainty in everyday life: contesting risk management systems', in L. Davies and P. Leonard (eds) *Social Work in a Corporate Era: Practices of Power and Resistance*, Aldershot: Ashgate.

—— (2006) 'The distinction between being and feeling frail: exploring emotional experiences in health and social care', *Journal of Social Work Practice* 20: 299–313.

Grewal, I., Nazroo, J., Bajekal, M., Blane, D. and Lewis, J. (2004) 'Influences on quality of life: a qualitative investigation of ethnic differences among older people in England', *Journal of Ethnic and Migration Studies* 30: 737–61.

Griffin, J. (1999) 'Abuse in a safe environment', in J. Pritchard (ed.) *Elder Abuse Work: Best Practice in Britain and Canada*, London: Jessica Kingsley.

Griffiths Report (1988) *Community Care: An Agenda for Action*, London: HMSO.

Gubrium, J. and Wallace, J. (1990) 'Who theorises age?', *Ageing and Society* 10: 131–49.

Gunaratnam, Y. (1997) 'Breaking the silence: black and ethnic minority carers and service provision', in J. Bornat, J. Johnson, C. Pereira, D. Pilgrim and F. Williams (eds) *Community Care: A Reader*, Basingstoke: Macmillan.

Hadley, R. and Clough, R. (1997) *Care in Chaos: Frustration and Challenge in Community Care*, London: Cassell.

Harris, John (1998) 'Scientific management, bureau-professionalism and new managerialism: the labour process of state social work', *British Journal of Social Work* 28, 839–62.

—— (1999) 'State social work and social citizenship', *British Journal of Social Work* 29: 915–37.

—— (2001) '"Better government for older people": citizens' participation in social policy at the local level', in P. Salustowicz (ed.) *Civil Society and Social Development*, Bern: Peter Lang.

—— (2002) 'Caring for citizenship', *British Journal of Social Work* 32: 267–81.

—— (2003) *The Social Work Business*, London: Routledge.

Harris, John and Hopkins, T. (1994) 'Beyond anti-ageism: reminiscence groups and the development of anti-discriminatory social work education and practice', in J. Bornat (ed.) *Reminiscence Reviewed: Perspectives, Evaluations, Achievements*, Buckingham: Open University Press.

Harris, Joy (2005) 'Speech and language therapy', in M. Marshall (ed.) *Perspectives on Rehabilitation and Dementia*, London: Jessica Kingsley Publishers.

Harrison, L. and Heywood, F. (2000) *Health Begins at Home: Planning at the Health–Housing Interface for Older People*, Bristol: The Policy Press.

Havighurst, R. and Albrecht, R. (1953) *Older People*, London: Longmans Green.

Hayden, C. and Boaz, A. (2000) *Making a Difference: Better Government for Older People Evaluation Report*, Coventry: University of Warwick, Local Government Centre.

Healthcare Commission/Commission for Social Care Inspection/Audit Commission (2006) *Living Well in Later Life: A Review of Progress Against the National Service Framework for Older People. Summary Report.* London: Commission for Healthcare Audit and Inspection.

Healy, K. (2005) *Social Work Theories in Context: Creating Frameworks for Practice*, Basingstoke: Palgrave Macmillan.

Heine, C. and Browning, C. (2004) 'The communication and psychosocial perceptions of older adults with sensory loss: a qualitative study', *Ageing and Society* 24: 113–30.

Heine, C., Erber, N., Osborn, R. and Browning, C. (2002) 'Communication perceptions of older adults with sensory loss and their communication partners: implications for intervention', *Disability and Rehabilitation* 24: 356–63.

Henderson, J. and Forbat, L. (2002) 'Relationship-based social policy: personal and policy constructions of "care"', *Critical Social Policy* 22: 669–87.

Henwood, M., Lewis, H. and Waddington, E. (1998) *Listening to Users of Domiciliary Care Services*, Leeds: University of Leeds, Nuffield Institute for Health.

Hepworth, M. (2000) *Stories of Ageing*, Buckingham: Open University Press.

Heron, C. (1998) *Working with Carers*, London: Jessica Kingsley Publishers.

Hey, V. (1999) 'Frail elderly people: difficult questions and awkward answers', in S. Hood, B. Mayall and S. Oliver (eds) *Critical Issues in Social Research: Power and Prejudice*, Buckingham: Open University Press.

Heywood, F., Oldman, C. and Means, R. (2002) *Housing and Home in Later Life*, Buckingham: Open University Press.

Hill, A. and Brettle, A. (2006) 'Counselling older people: what can we learn from research evidence?', *Journal of Social Work Practice* 20(3): 281–97.

Hirsch, D. (2005) *Facing the Cost of Long-Term Care: Towards a Sustainable Funding System*, York: Joseph Rowntree Foundation.

Hockey, J. and James, J. (1993) *Growing Up and Growing Old*, London: Sage.

—— (2003) *Social Identities Across the Life Course*, Basingstoke: Palgrave Macmillan.

Hornstein, Z., Encel, S., Gunderson, M. and Neumark, D. (2001) *Outlawing Age Discrimination: Foreign Lessons, UK Choices*, Bristol: The Policy Press.

Houston, S. (2001) 'Beyond social constructionism: critical realism and social work', *British Journal of Social Work* 31: 845–61.

Hudson, B., Exworthy, M. and Peckham, S. (1998) *The Integration of Localised and Collaborative Purchasing: A Review of the Literature and Framework for Analysis*, Leeds: University of Leeds/University of Southampton, Nuffield Institute for Health, cited in R. Carnwell and A. Carson (2005) 'Understanding partnerships and collaboration', in R. Carnwell and J. Buchanan (eds) *Effective Practice in Health and Social Care: A Partnership Approach*, Maidenhead: Open University Press.

Hudson, B., Hardy, B., Henwood, M. and Wistow, G. (1997) *Inter-agency Collaboration: Primary Health Care Sub-study*, Final Report, December, Leeds: University of Leeds, Nuffield Institute for Health.

Hughes, B. (1995) *Older People and Community Care: Critical Theory and Practice*, Buckingham: Open University Press.

Inter-Ministerial Group on Older People (1998) *Building a Better Britain for Older People*, London: HMSO.

Johnson, C. and Barer, B. (1997) *Life Beyond 85 Years: The Aura of Survivorship*, New York: Springer Publishing.

Johnson, J. (1998) 'The emergence of care as a policy', in A. Brechin, J. Walmsley, J. Katz and S. Peace (eds) *Care Matters: Concepts, Practice and Research in Health and Social Care*, London: Sage.

Johnson, K. (2005) 'A late picking: narratives of older people with learning disabilities', in G. Grant, P. Goward, M. Richardson and P. Ramcharan (eds) *Learning Disability: A Life Cycle Approach to Valuing People*, Maidenhead: Open University Press.

Jones, C. (1999) 'Social work: regulation and managerialism', in M. Hexworthy and S. Halford (eds) *Professionals and the New Managerialism in the Public Sector*, Buckingham: Open University Press.

—— (2001) 'Voices from the front line: state social workers and New Labour', *British Journal of Social Work* 31: 547–62.

Jones, J. (2006) 'Social work'. E-mail (17 December).

Jordan, B. and Jordan C. (2000) *Social Work and the Third Way: Tough Love as Social Policy*, London: Sage.

Joseph Rowntree Foundation (2004) *Older People Shaping Policy and Practice*, York: Joseph Rowntree Foundation.

—— (2006) *Introducing Smart Homes*, York: Joseph Rowntree Foundation. Online at www.jrf.org.uk/housingandcare/smarthomes (accessed 29 June 2006).

Joseph Rowntree Foundation Task Group (2004) *From Welfare to Well-being – Planning for an Ageing Society: Summary Conclusions of the Joseph Rowntree Foundation Task Group on Housing, Money and Care for Older People*, York: Joseph Rowntree Foundation.

Katz, S. (2000) 'Busy bodies: activity, aging and the management of everyday life', *Journal of Aging Studies* 14: 135–52.

Kellaher, L., Peace, S. and Holland, C. (2004) 'Environment, identity and old age: quality of life or a life of quality?', in A. Walker and C. Hagan Hennessy (eds) *Growing Older: Quality of Life in Old Age*, Maidenhead: Open University Press.

Kemshall, H. (2002) *Risk, Social Policy and Welfare*, Buckingham: Open University Press.

Kendig, H., Browning, C. and Young, A. (2000) 'Impacts of illness and disability on the well-being of older people', *Disability and Rehabilitation* 22: 15–22.

Killick, J. and Allan, K. (2001) *Communication and the Care of People with Dementia*, Buckingham: Open University Press.

King's Fund (2005) *The Business of Caring: King's Fund Inquiry into Care Services for Older People in London*, London: King's Fund.

Kingston, P., Bernard, M., Biggs, S. and Nettleton, H. (2001) 'Assessing the health impact of age-specific housing', *Health and Social Care in the Community* 9: 228–34.

Kitwood, T. (1997) *Dementia Reconsidered: The Person Comes First*, Buckingham: Open University Press.

Knapp, M. (1984) *The Economics of Social Care*, London: Macmillan.

Koprowska, J. (2005) *Communication and Interpersonal Skills in Social Work*, Exeter: Learning Matters.

Kuhn, T. (1970) *The Structure of Scientific Revolutions*, Chicago: University of Chicago Press.

Kymlicka, W. and Norman, W. (1995) 'Return of the citizen: a survey of recent work on citizenship theory', in R. Beiner (ed.) *Theorizing Citizenship*, Albany, New York: State University of New York Press.

Langan, J., Means, R. and Rolfe, S. (1996) *Maintaining Independence in Later Life: Older People Speaking*, Oxford: Anchor Trust.

Langley, J. (2001) 'Developing anti-oppressive empowering social work practice with older lesbian and gay men', *British Journal of Social Work* 31: 917–32.

Le Mesurier, N. (2003) *'So Much More Than Just Walking!' An Evaluation of a Pilot Programme of Social Rehabilitation Projects Provided by Age Concerns in Five Locations in England*, London/Birmingham: Age Concern England/Birmingham Social Science in Medicine Group, University of Birmingham.

Lewis, I. (2006) *Letter to Launch Dignity in Care Campaign, Gateway Ref. 7388*, London: Department of Health. Online at www.dh.go.uk/assetRoot/04/14/04/66/04140466.pdf (accessed 2 December 2006).

Lewis, J. (2000) 'Gender and welfare regimes', in G. Lewis, S. Gewirtz and J. Clarke (eds) *Rethinking Social Policy*, London: Sage.

Lewis, J. and Glennerster, H. (1996) *Implementing the New Community Care*, Buckingham: Open University Press.

Lipsky, M. (1980) *Street-level Bureaucracy: The Dilemmas of Individuals in Public Service*, New York: Russell Sage Foundation.

Lishman, J. (1994) *Communication in Social Work*, Basingstoke: Macmillan.

Littlechild, R. and Blakeney, J. (1996) 'Risk and older people', in H. Kemshall and J. Pritchard (eds) *Good Practice in Risk Assessment and Risk Management*, London: Jessica Kingsley Publishers.

Litwin, H. and Shiovitz-Ezra, S. (2006) 'The association between activity and well-being in later life: what really matters', *Ageing and Society* 26: 225–42.

Lloyd, L. (2006a) 'A caring profession? The ethics of care and social work with older people', *British Journal of Social Work* 36: 1171–85.

—— (2006b) 'Call us carers: limitations and risks in campaigning for recognition and exclusivity', *Critical Social Policy* 26: 945–60.

Lloyd, M. (2002) 'Care management', in R. Adams, L. Dominelli and M. Payne (eds) *Critical Practice in Social Work*, Basingstoke: Palgrave.

Local Government Association (2005) *Briefing on Independence, Well-being and Choice*, London: Local Government Association.

—— (2006) *Social Care Finance Survey June 2006: The Impact of NHS Trust Financial Deficits on English Local Authorities*, London: Local Government Association.

Local Government Association/Association of Directors of Social Services (2003) *All Our Tomorrows: Inverting the Triangle of Care*, London: Local Government Association/ Association of Directors of Social Services. Online at www.adss.org.uk/publications/other/allourtomorrows.pdf (accessed 2 April 2007).

Lymbery, M. (1998) 'Care management and professional autonomy: the impact of community care legislation on social work with older people', *British Journal of Social Work* 28: 863–78.

—— (2004) 'Managerialism and care management practice with older people', in M. Lymbery and S. Butler (eds) *Social Work Ideals and Practice Realities*, Basingstoke: Palgrave Macmillan.

—— (2005) *Social Work with Older People*, London: Sage.

—— (2006) 'United we stand? Partnership working in health and social care and the role of social work in services for older people', *British Journal of Social Work* 36: 1119–34.

Lyon, J. (2005) 'A systems approach to direct payments: a response to "Friend or foe? Towards a critical assessment of direct payments"', *Critical Social Policy* 25: 240–52.

McDonald, A. and Taylor, M. (2006) *Older People and the Law*, Bristol: The Policy Press.

McDonald, C. (2006) *Challenging Social Work: The Institutional Context of Practice*, Basingstoke: Palgrave Macmillan.

Macgregor, G. and Hill, M. (2003) *Missed Opportunities: The Impact of New Rights for Carers*, London: Carers UK. Online at www.carersuk.org.uk/Policyandpractice/Research/ Missed OppsFullReport.pdf (accessed 2 February 2006).

McLeod, E. and Bywaters, P. (2000) *Social Work, Health and Equality*, London: Routledge.

McLeod, E., Bywaters, P., Tanner, D. and Hirsch, M. (forthcoming) 'For the sake of their health: older service users' requirements for social care to facilitate access to social networks following hospital discharge', *British Journal of Social Work*, advance online access 3/11/06, http://bjsw.oxfordjournals.org/cgi/reprint/bcl341v1.

Maddox, G. (1970) 'Themes and issues in sociological theories of human aging', *Human Development* 13: 17–27.

Mandelstam, M. (2005, 3rd edn) *Community Care Practice and the Law*, London: Jessica Kingsley Publishers.

Manthorpe, J. and Iliffe, S. (2005) 'Timely responses to dementia: exploring the social work role', *Journal of Social Work* 5: 191–203.

Manthorpe, J., Iliffe, S. and Eden, A. (2004) 'Early recognition of and responses to dementia: health professionals' views of social services' role and performance', *British Journal of Social Work* 34: 335–48.

Marcoen, A. (2005) 'Religion, spirituality and older people', in M. Johnson with V. Bengtson, P. Coleman and T. Kirkwood (eds) *The Cambridge Handbook of Age and Ageing*, Cambridge: Cambridge University Press.

Margiotta, P., Raynes, N., Pagidas, D., Lawson, J. and Temple, B. (2003) *Are You Listening? Current Practice in Information, Advice and Advocacy Services for Older People*, York: Joseph Rowntree Foundation.

Margrain, T. and Boulton, M. (2005) 'Sensory impairment', in M. Johnson with V. Bengtson, P. Coleman and T. Kirkwood (eds) *The Cambridge Handbook of Age and Ageing*, Cambridge: Cambridge University Press.

Marsh, A., Gordon, D., Pantazis, C. and Heslop, P. (2000) *Home Sweet Home? The Impact of Poor Housing on Health*, Bristol: The Policy Press.

Marshall, M. (2005) 'Perspectives on rehabilitation and dementia', in M. Marshall (ed) *Perspectives on Rehabilitation and Dementia*, London: Jessica Kingsley Publishers.

Mayo, M. (1994) *Communities and Caring: The Mixed Economy of Welfare*, Basingstoke: Macmillan.

Means, R. and Smith, R. (1998) *From Poor Law to Community Care? The Development of Welfare Services for Elderly People*, Bristol: The Policy Press.

Means, R., Morbey, H. and Smith, R. (2002) *From Community Care to Market Care? The Development of Welfare Services for Older People*, Bristol: The Policy Press.

Means, R., Richards, S. and Smith, R. (2003, 3rd edn) *Community Care: Policy and Practice*, Basingstoke: Macmillan Press.

Merrell, J., Kinsella, F., Murphy, F., Philpin, S. and Ali, A. (2006) 'Accessibility and equity of health and social care services: exploring the views and experiences of Bangladeshi carers in South Wales, UK', *Health and Social Care in the Community* 14: 197–205.

Milner, J. and O'Byrne, P. (2002, 2nd edn) *Assessment in Social Work*, Basingstoke: Palgrave Macmillan.

Minichiello, V., Browne, J. and Kendig, H. (2000) 'Perceptions and consequences of ageism: views of older people', *Ageing and Society* 30: 253–78.

Moriarty, J. and Butt, J. (2004) 'Social support and ethnicity in old age', in A. Walker and C. Hagan Hennessy (eds) *Growing Older: Quality of Life in Old Age*, Maidenhead: Open University Press.

Morris, J. (1993) *Independent Lives: Community Care and Disabled People*, Basingstoke: Macmillan.

——(1997) '"Us" and "them"? Feminist research and community care', in J. Bornat, J. Johnson, C. Pereira, D. Pilgrim and F. Williams (eds) *Community Care: A Reader*, Basingstoke: Macmillan.

Morrison, A. (2001) 'Improving the quality of written assessments: a participative approach', in V. White and J. Harris (eds) *Developing Good Practice in Community Care: Partnership and Participation*, London: Jessica Kingsley Publishers.

Moss, B. (2005) *Religion and Spirituality*, Lyme Regis: Russell House.

Mountain, G. (2005) 'Rehabilitation for people with dementia: pointers for practice from the evidence base', in M. Marshall (ed.) *Perspectives on Rehabilitation and Dementia*, London: Jessica Kingsley Publishers.

Myers, K. and Crawford, J. (1993) 'Assessment and care management of people with dementia and their carers', in A. Chapman and M. Marshall (eds), *Dementia: New Skills for Social Workers*, London: Jessica Kingsley Publishers.

National Statistics (2006a) *Community Care Statistics: Home Care Services for Adults England*, London: NHS Health and Social Care Information Centre. Online at www.ic.nhs.uk/pubs/commcare2005homehelpadulteng/MAINREPORT.pdf/file (accessed 30 December 2006).

—— (2006b) *Community Care Statistics: Supported Residents (Adults) England*, London: NHS Health and Social Care Information Centre.

Nazroo, J., Bajekal, M., Blane, D. and Grewal, I. (2004) 'Ethnic inequalities', in A. Walker and C. Hagan Hennessy (eds) *Growing Older: Quality of Life in Old Age*, Maidenhead: Open University Press.

Nelson, T. (2005) 'Ageism: prejudice against our own feared future self', *Journal of Social Issues* 61: 207–21.

Nolan, M. (2000) 'Towards person-centred care for older people', in A. Warnes, L. Warren and M. Nolan (eds) *Care Services for Later Life: Transformations and Critiques*, London: Jessica Kingsley Publishers.

Nolan, M., Davies, S. and Grant, G. (2001) 'Integrating perspectives', in M. Nolan, S. Davies and G. Grant (eds) *Working with Older People and their Families*, Buckingham: Open University Press.

Nolan, M., Grant, G. and Keady, J. (1996) *Understanding Family Care*, Buckingham: Open University Press.

Nolan, M., Grant, G., Keady, J. and Lundh, U. (2003) 'New directions for partnerships: relationship-centred care', in M. Nolan, U. Lundh, G. Grant and J. Keady (eds) *Partnerships in Family Care*, Maidenhead: Open University Press.

Office for National Statistics (2004) *Focus on Older People*. Online at www.statistics.gov.uk (accessed 24 November 2006).

Office of Fair Trading (2005) *Care Homes for Older People in the UK: A Market Study*, London: Office of Fair Trading.

Office of the Deputy Prime Minister (2006) *A Sure Start to Later Life: Ending Inequalities for Older People*, London: Office of the Deputy Prime Minister.

Older People's Advocacy Alliance (2006) *About OPAAL*. Online at www.opaal.org.uk (accessed 2 December 2006).

Oldman, C. (2002) 'The importance of housing and home', in B. Bytheway, V. Bacigalupo, J. Bornat, J. Johnson and S. Spurr (eds) *Understanding Care, Welfare and Community: A Reader*, London: Routledge.

Orme, J. (2001) *Gender and Community Care: Social Work and Social Care Perspectives*, Basingstoke: Palgrave.

Parker, J. and Penhale, B. (2007) *Working with Vulnerable Adults*, London: Routledge.

Parkinson, P. and Pierpoint, D. (2000) *Preventive Approaches in Housing: An Exploration of Good Practice*, Kidlington: Anchor Trust.

Parrott, L. (2005) 'The political drivers of working in partnership', in R. Carnwell and J. Buchanan (eds) *Effective Practice in Health and Social Care: A Partnership Approach*, Maidenhead: Open University Press.

Parry-Jones, B. and Soulsby, J. (2001) 'Needs-led assessment: the challenges and the reality', *Health and Social Care in the Community* 9: 414–28.

Parsons, M. (2005) 'The contribution of social work to the rehabilitation of older people with dementia: values in practice', in M. Marshall (ed) *Perspectives on Rehabilitation and Dementia*, London: Jessica Kingsley Publishers.

Parton, N. (1996) 'Social work, risk and "the blaming system"', in N. Parton (ed.) *Social Theory, Social Change and Social Work*, London: Routledge.

Parton, N. and Marshall, W. (1998) 'Postmodernism and discourse approaches to social work', in R. Adams, L. Dominelli and M. Payne (eds) *Social Work: Themes, Issues and Critical Debates*, Basingstoke: Macmillan.

Patmore, C. and McNulty, A. (2005) *Making Home Care for Older People more Flexible and Person-centred: Factors Which Promote This*, University of York: Social Policy Research Unit.

Patsios, D. and Davey, A. (2005) 'Formal and informal community care for older adults', in M. Johnson with V. Bengtson, P. Coleman and T. Kirkwood (eds) *The Cambridge Handbook of Age and Ageing*, Cambridge: Cambridge University Press.

Pawson, R., Boaz, A., Grayson, L., Long, A. and Barnes, C. (2003) *Types and Quality of Knowledge in Social Care: Knowledge Review 03*, London: Social Care Institute for Excellence.

Payne, M. (2005, 3rd edn) *Modern Social Work Theory*, Basingstoke: Palgrave Macmillan.

Payne, M., Adams, R. and Dominelli, L. (2002) 'On being critical', in R. Adams, L. Dominelli and M. Payne (eds) *Critical Practice in Social Work*, Basingstoke: Palgrave.

Peace, S. (1998) 'Caring in place', in A. Brechin, J. Walmsley, J. Katz and S. Peace (eds) *Care Matters: Concepts, Practice and Research in Health and Social Care*, London: Sage.

Peace, S., Holland, C. and Kellaher, L. (2006) *Environment and Identity in Later Life*, Maidenhead: Open University Press.

Percival, J. (2002) 'Domestic spaces: uses and meanings in the daily lives of older people', *Ageing and Society* 22(6): 729–49.

Percival, J. and Hanson, J. (2005) '"I'm like a tree a million miles from the water's edge": social care and inclusion of older people with visual impairment', *British Journal of Social Work* 35: 189–205.

Petch, A. (1996) 'New concepts, old responses: assessment and care management pilot projects in Scotland', in J. Phillips and B. Penhale (eds) *Reviewing Care Management for Older People*, London: Jessica Kingsley.

—— (2003) *Intermediate Care: What do we Know about Older People's Experiences?* York: Joseph Rowntree Foundation.

Phillips, J., Bernard, M., Phillipson, C. and Ogg, J. (2002) 'Social support in later life: a study of three areas', *British Journal of Social Work* 30: 837–54.

Phillipson, C. (1982) *Capitalism and the Construction of Old Age*, London: Macmillan.

—— (1998) *Reconstructing Old Age: New Agendas in Social Theory and Practice*, London: Sage.

Phillipson, C., Bernard, M., Phillips, J. and Ogg, J. (2001) *The Family and Community Life of Older People: Social Networks and Social Support in Three Urban Areas*, London: Routledge.

Philpot, T. (2004) 'What price a caring future?' *Search* 41: 14–15.

Policy Research Institute on Ageing and Ethnicity (2004) *Minority Elderly Health and Social Care in Europe: Summary Findings of the Minority Elderly Care (MEC) Project*, Leeds: Policy Research Institute on Ageing and Ethnicity.

—— (2005) *Black and Minority Ethnic Elders in the UK: Health and Social Care Research Findings*, Leeds: Policy Research Institute on Ageing and Ethnicity.

Postle, K. (2001) 'The social work side is disappearing. I guess it started with us being called care managers', *Practice* 13: 13–26.

—— (2002) 'Working "between the idea and the reality": ambiguities and tensions in care managers' work', *British Journal of Social Work* 32: 335–51.

Postle, K., Wright, P. and Beresford, P. (2005) 'Older people's participation in political activity – making their voices heard: a potential support role for welfare professionals in countering ageism and social exclusion', *Practice* 17: 173–89.

Preston-Shoot, M. (2002) 'Evaluating self-determination', in B. Bytheway, V. Bacigalupo, J. Bornat, J. Johnson and S. Spurr (eds) *Understanding Care, Welfare and Community: A Reader*, London: Routledge.

Price, D. (2006) 'The poverty of older people in the UK', *Journal of Social Work Practice* 20: 251–66.

Price, D. and Ginn, J. (2003) 'Sharing the crust: gender, partnership status and inequalities in pension accumulation', in S. Arber, K. Davidson and J. Ginn (eds) *Gender and Ageing: Changing Roles and Relationships*, Maidenhead: Open University Press.

Priestley, M. (1999) *Disability Politics and Community Care*, London: Jessica Kingsley Publishers.

Priestley, M. and Rabiee, P. (2002) 'Same difference? Older people's organisations and disability issues', *Disability and Society* 17: 597–611.

Pritchard, J. (1997) 'Vulnerable people taking risks: older people and residential care', in H. Kemshall and J. Pritchard (eds) *Good Practice in Risk Assessment and Risk Management*, London: Jessica Kingsley Publishers.

Proctor, G. (2001) 'Listening to older women with dementia: relationships, voices and power', *Disability and Society* 16: 361–76.

Quilgars, D. (2000) *Low Intensity Support Services: A Systematic Review of Effectiveness*, Bristol: The Policy Press.

Qureshi, H. and Walker, A. (1989) *The Caring Relationship: Elderly People and their Families*, Basingstoke: Macmillan.

Ray, M. and Phillips, J. (2002) 'Older people', in R. Adams, L. Dominelli and M. Payne (eds) *Critical Practice in Social Work*, Basingstoke: Palgrave.

Read, K. (2005) 'Intermediate care: the new pathway to rehabilitation or widening the chasm?', in M. Marshall (ed.) *Perspectives on Rehabilitation and Dementia*, London: Jessica Kingsley Publishers.

Reed, J., Stanley, D. and Clarke, C. (2004) *Health, Well-being and Older People*, Bristol: The Policy Press.

Reid, W. and Epstein, L. (1972) *Task-centred Casework*, New York: Columbia University Press.

Richards, S. (1994) 'Making sense of needs assessment', *Research, Policy and Planning* 12: 5–9.

—— (2000) 'Bridging the divide: elders and the assessment process', *British Journal of Social Work* 30: 37–49.

Richardson, S. and Asthana, S. (2006) 'Inter-agency information sharing in health and social care services: the role of professional culture', *British Journal of Social Work* 36: 657–69.

Richardson, S. and Pearson, M. (1995) 'Dignity and aspirations denied: unmet health and social care needs in an inner-city area', *Health and Social Care in the Community* 3: 279–87.

Ritzer, G. (2000) *The McDonaldization of Society*, New Century Edition, Thousand Oaks: Pine Forge Press.

Roberts, E. (2000) *Age Discrimination in Health and Social Care*, London: King's Fund.

Roberts, E., Robinson, J. and Seymour, L. (2002) *Old Habits Die Hard: Tackling Age Discrimination in Health and Social Care*, London: King's Fund.

Roberts, K. and Chapman, T. (2001) *Realising Participation: Elderly People as Active Users of Health and Social Care*, Aldershot: Ashgate.

Rogers, C. (1951) *Client-Centred Therapy: Its Current Practice, Implications and Theory*, London: Constable.

Rowe, D. (1994) *Time on our Side: Growing in Wisdom, not Growing Old*, London: Harper-Collins.

Royal Commission on Long-Term Care (1999) *With Respect to Old Age: a Report by the Royal Commission on Long-Term Care*, Cm 4192-II/1, London: The Stationery Office.

Ruth, J. and Oberg, P. (1996) 'Ways of life: old age in a life history perspective', in J. Birren, G. Kenyon, J. Ruth, J. Schroots and T. Svensson (eds) *Ageing and Biography: Explorations in Adult Development*, New York: Springer Publishing.

Sadler, E. and Biggs, S. (2006) 'Exploring the links between spirituality and "successful ageing"', *Journal of Social Work Practice* 20: 267–80.

Schwehr, B. (2000) 'The legal regulation of the powers and duties of local authorities with regard to disabled people', in J. Cooper (ed.) *Law, Rights and Disability*, London: Jessica Kingsley Publishers.

Scourfield, P. (2006) '"What matters is what works"? How discourses of modernisation have both silenced and limited debate on domiciliary care for older people', *Critical Social Policy* 26: 5–30.

Secker, J., Hill, R., Villeneau, L. and Parkman, S. (2003) 'Promoting independence: but promoting what and how?', *Ageing and Society* 23: 375–91.

Seebohm Report (1968) *Report of the Committee on Local Authority and Allied Personal Social Services, Cmnd 3703*, London: HMSO.

Sheppard, M. (1990) *Mental Health: The Role of the Approved Social Worker*, Sheffield: University of Sheffield, Social Services Monographs.

Sidenvall, B., Nydahl, M. and Fjellstrom, C. (2001) 'Managing food shopping and cooking: the experiences of older Swedish women', *Ageing and Society* 21: 151–68.

Simey, M. (2002) 'I want something to do', *Community Care* 24–30 October: 20.

Smale, G. and Tuson, G. (1993) *Empowerment, Assessment, Care Management and the Skilled Worker*, London: HMSO.

Smale, G., Tuson, G. and Statham, D. (2000) *Social Work and Social Problems: Working Towards Social Inclusion and Social Change*, Basingstoke: Macmillan.

Smart, G. and Means, R. (1997) *Housing and Community Care: Exploring the Role of Home Improvement Agencies*, Oxford: Anchor Trust/Care and Repair England.

Social Care Institute for Excellence (2004) *Aiding Communication with People with Dementia: Research Briefing 03*, London: Social Care Institute for Excellence. Online at www.scie.org.uk/publications/practiceguides/bpg2/index.asp (accessed 3 September 2006).

—— (2005) *Implementing the Carers (Equal Opportunities) Act 2004: Practice Guide 05*, London: Social Care Institute for Excellence. Online at www.scie.org.uk/publications/practiceguides/carersguidance/index.asp (accessed 11 November 2006).

—— (2006a) *Assessing the Mental Health Needs of Older People: Practice Guide 02*, London: Social Care Institute for Excellence. Online at www.scie.org.uk/publications/practice guides/bpg2/index.asp (accessed 3 September 2006).

—— (2006b) *Using Qualitative Research in Systematic Reviews: Older People's Views of Hospital Discharge*, London: Social Care Institute for Excellence.

—— (2006c) *Dignity in Care: Dignity Challenge, Practice Guide 09*, London: Social Care Institute for Excellence. Online at www.scie.org.uk/publications/practiceguides/bpg2/index.asp (accessed 12 November 2006).

Social Policy on Ageing Information Network (2005) *What Price Care in Old Age? Three Years on from SPAIN's 'Underfunding of Social Care' Paper, what has Changed?*. Online at www.cpa.org.uk/cpa/cpa_what_price_care.pdf (accessed 3 June 2005).

Social Services Inspectorate/Department of Health (1991a) *Care Management and Assessment: Practitioners' Guide*, London: Department of Health.

—— (1991b) *Care Management and Assessment: Managers' Guide*, London: Department of Health.

Spiers, P. (2004) 'A question of care', *Care and Health* 6–12 April: 38.

Stalker, K. (ed.) (2003) *Reconceptualising Work with 'Carers': New Directions for Policy and Practice*, London: Jessica Kingsley Publishers.

Stanley, N. (1999) 'User–practitioner transactions in the new culture of community care', *British Journal of Social Work* 29: 417–35.

Stevenson, O. (1999) 'Old people at risk', in P. Parsloe (ed.) *Risk Assessment in Social Care and Social Work*, London: Jessica Kingsley Publishers.

Stuart-Hamilton, S. (2000, 3rd edn) *The Psychology of Ageing: An Introduction*, London: Jessica Kingsley Publishers.

Tanner, D. (1998) 'The jeopardy of risk', *Practice* 10: 15–28.

—— (2001) 'Sustaining the self in later life: implications for community-based support', *Ageing and Society* 21(3): 255–78.

—— (2005) 'Promoting the well-being of older people: messages for social workers', *Practice* 17: 191–205.

Taylor, B. and Donnelly, M. (2006) 'Professional perspectives on decision-making about the long-term care of older people', *British Journal of Social Work* 36: 807–26.

Tester, S., Hubbard, G., Downs, M., MacDonald, C. and Murphy, J. (2004) 'Frailty and institutional life', in A. Walker and C. Hagan Hennessy (eds) *Growing Older: Quality of Life in Old Age*, Maidenhead: Open University Press.

Thompson, N. (1995) *Theory and Practice in Health and Social Welfare*, Buckingham: Open University Press.

—— (2005, 2nd edn) *Understanding Social Work: Preparing for Practice*, Basingstoke: Palgrave Macmillan.

Thompson, P., Itzin, C. and Abendstern, M. (1990) *I Don't Feel Old: The Experience of Later Life*, Oxford: Oxford University Press.

Titterton, M. (2005) *Risk and Risk-taking in Health and Social Welfare*, London: Jessica Kingsley Publishers.

Townsend, P. (1957) *The Family Life of Old People*, London: Routledge and Kegan Paul; reproduced in C. Phillipson, M. Bernard, J. Phillips and J. Ogg (2001) *The Family and Community Life of Older People: Social Networks and Social Support in Three Urban Areas*, London: Routledge.

—— (1962) *The Last Refuge: A Survey of Residential Institutions and Homes for the Aged in England and Wales*, London: Routledge and Kegan Paul; reproduced in J. Bornat (1998) 'Anthology: voices from the institutions', in M. Allott and M. Robb (eds) *Understanding Health and Social Care: An Introductory Reader*, London: Sage.

—— (1981) 'The structured dependency of the elderly: a creation of social policy in the twentieth century', *Ageing and Society* 1: 5–28.

Tozer, R. and Thornton, P. (1995) *A Meeting of Minds: Older People as Research Advisers. Social Policy Report No 5*, York: University of York, Social Policy Research Unit.

Training Organisation for the Personal Social Services (2002) *National Occupational Standards for Social Work*. Online at http://www.topssengland.net/files/cd/England/Main.htm (accessed 27 December 2006).

Trevithick, P. (2005, 2nd edn) *Social Work Skills: A Practice Handbook*, Maidenhead: Open University Press.

Turner, B. (1994) *Citizenship: Critical Concepts, Volume 1*, London: Routledge.

Turner, M. and Beresford, P. (2005) *User Controlled Research: Its Meanings and Potential, Final Report*, Brunel University: The Centre for Citizen Participation, Brunel University and Shaping Our Lives.

Twigg, J. (1998) 'The medical/social boundary', in M. Allott and M. Robb (eds) *Understanding Health and Social Care: An Introductory Reader*, London: Sage.

—— (2000) 'The medical–social boundary and the location of personal care', in A. Warnes, L. Warren and M. Nolan (eds) *Care Services for Later Life: Transformations and Critiques*, London: Jessica Kingsley.

—— (2002) 'Carework and bodywork', in B. Bytheway, V. Bacigalupo, J. Bornat, J. Johnson and S. Spurr (eds) *Understanding Care, Welfare and Community: A Reader*, London: Routledge.

Twigg, J. and Atkin, K. (1994) *Carers Perceived: Policy and Practice in Informal Care*, Buckingham: Open University Press.

Twine, F. (1994) *Citizenship and Social Rights*, London: Sage.

Victor, C. (2005) *The Social Context of Ageing: A Textbook of Gerontology*, London: Routledge.

Walker, A. (1981) 'Towards a political economy of old age', *Ageing and Society* 1(1): 73–94.

—— (1993, 2nd edn) 'Poverty and inequality in old age', in J. Bond, P. Coleman and S. Peace (eds) *Ageing in Society*, London: Sage.

—— (1996) 'Intergenerational relations and the provision of welfare', in A. Walker (ed.) *The New Generational Contract: Intergenerational Relations, Old Age and Welfare*, London: University College London Press.

Walker, A. and Hagan Hennessy, C. (eds) (2004) *Growing Older: Quality of Life in Old Age*, Maidenhead: Open University Press.

Wanless, D. (2006) *Securing Good Care for Older People: Taking a Long-term View*, London: King's Fund.

Ware, T., Matasevic, T., Hardy, B., Knapp, M., Kendall, J. and Farder, J. (2003) 'Commissioning care services for older people in England and Wales: the view from care managers, users and carers', *Ageing and Society* 23: 411–28.

Weinberg, A., Williamson, J., Challis, D. and Hughes, J. (2003) 'What do care managers do? A study of working practice in older people's services', *British Journal of Social Work* 33: 901–19.

West Midlands Regional Single Assessment Process Group (2004) *The Single Assessment Process and Cross Boundary Working Good Practice Guide*. Online at www.dh.gov.uk/assetRoot/04/09/86/37 (accessed 20 March 2006).

Wetherly, P. (1996) 'Basic needs and social policies', *Critical Social Policy* 16(1): 45–65.

White, M. and Epston, D. (1990) *Narrative Means to Therapeutic Ends*, New York: Norton.

White, V. and Harris, John (1999) 'Social Europe, social citizenship and social work', *European Journal of Social Work* 2: 3–14.

—— (2007) 'Management', in M. Lymbery and K. Postle (eds) *Social Work: A Companion to Learning*, London: Sage.

Williams, F. (1996) 'Postmodernism, feminism and the question of difference', in N. Parton (ed.) *Social Theory, Social Change and Social Work*, London: Routledge.

Williams, J., Netten, A., Hardy, B., Matosevic, T. and Ware, P. (2002) *Care Home Closures: The Provider Perspective, PSSRU Discussion Paper No. 1753/2*, Canterbury: University of Kent, Personal Social Services Research Unit.

Wilson, G. (1995) 'Low expectations reinforced: experiences of health services in advanced old age', in G. Wilson (ed.) *Community Care: Asking the User*, London: Chapman Hall.

—— (2000) *Understanding Old Age: Critical and Global Perspectives*, London: Sage.

—— (2001) 'Conceptual frameworks and emancipatory research in social gerontology', *Ageing and Society* 21: 471–87.

Wistow, G. (2006) *Better Governance for Better Well-being: Summary Document of Improving Services, Improving Governance*, London: Local Government Association.

Wistow, G. and Lewis, H. (1997) *Preventative Services for Older People: Current Approaches and Future Opportunities*, Oxford: Anchor Trust.

Wistow, G., Knapp, M., Hardy, B., Forder, J., Kendall, J. and Manning, R. (1996) *Social Care Markets: Progress and Prospects*, Buckingham: Open University Press.

Woods, B. (2005) 'Dementia', in M. Johnson (ed.) with V. Bengtson, P. Coleman and T. Kirkwood (eds) *The Cambridge Handbook of Age and Ageing*, Cambridge: Cambridge University Press.

Wynne-Harley, D. (1991) *Living Dangerously: Risk taking, Safety and Older People*, London: Centre for Policy on Ageing.

Yeandle, S. and Buckner, L. (2005) *Older Carers in the UK*, London: Carers UK/Sheffield Hallam University.

Young, I. (1995) 'Polity and group difference: a critique of the ideal of universal citizenship', in R. Beiner (ed.) *Theorizing Citizenship*, Albany, New York: State University of New York Press.

Young, J. and Stevenson, J. (2006) 'Intermediate care in England: where next?', *Age and Ageing* 35: 339–41.

Zifcak, S. (1994) *New Managerialism: Administrative Reform in Whitehall and Canberra*, Buckingham: Open University Press.

INDEX

Page numbers in *italics* refer to figures and tables

eBooks – at www.eBookstore.tandf.co.uk

A library at your fingertips!

eBooks are electronic versions of printed books. You can store them on your PC/laptop or browse them online.

They have advantages for anyone needing rapid access to a wide variety of published, copyright information.

eBooks can help your research by enabling you to bookmark chapters, annotate text and use instant searches to find specific words or phrases. Several eBook files would fit on even a small laptop or PDA.

NEW: Save money by eSubscribing: cheap, online access to any eBook for as long as you need it.

Annual subscription packages

We now offer special low-cost bulk subscriptions to packages of eBooks in certain subject areas. These are available to libraries or to individuals.

For more information please contact webmaster.ebooks@tandf.co.uk

We're continually developing the eBook concept, so keep up to date by visiting the website.

www.eBookstore.tandf.co.uk